ForeworD

A sense of enormous excitement and satisfaction prevails as we celebrate the 50th Anniversary of the School of Public Health and dedicate the McGavran-Greenberg Hall and the Baity Laboratory. At this critical juncture of our history, we need to pause and reflect on our origin, mission, and achievements, which are well documented in this volume.

The expansion of the school facilities, the growth of the faculty and student bodies, the quality and dedication of the staff, the superb quality of the research, the technical assistance and continuing education offered to professionals in North Carolina, and the commitment of the faculty to teaching excellence are all clear achievements of which we are proud. Of equal importance, this book chronicles the many contributions of individual faculty and staff, living and dead, who have had a profound effect on what we are today. It is most gratifying to me that we have the opportunity to review their many accomplishments and to acknowledge our debt to them.

At the same time, it is appropriate that we recognize that there have been disagreements over the appropriate mission of the school, and that sincere men and women have held different, sometimes radically different, views of what our school should be. Some of these differences have been resolved; others are with us today. So must it be, lest we not be true to our heritage, or to the spirit of inquiry that is the primary purpose of an academic institution.

At this moment in the evolution of the school it is appropriate to reflect on the lessons of our history. While it is instructive, indeed necessary, for us to understand how we have become what we are, we must also recognize that not all of the accommodations to past realities are appropriate for the future. To be consistently ranked in the top echelon of schools of public health would indicate an institution of considerable strength and vigor. Organizations, however, cannot be complacent and ignore the changing realities of a dynamic society. Our tradition of departmental autonomy, for example, presented few obstacles to interdisciplinary efforts when the entire faculty could, and often did, meet around one conference table. While maintaining strong departments necessary to address societal problems in the next decades, we must discover ways to enhance cooperative efforts, which our current structure sometimes discourages. While continuing to support a strong research orientation in our faculty, we cannot minimize the fundamental importance of encouraging outstanding teaching and service programs. And while the School of Public Health can be justly proud of the leadership we have shown in recruiting women and minority faculty, staff, and students, we still have a long way to go. We cannot rest on past success but must vigorously pursue a goal of greater representation by women and minorities in all areas of the school.

Robert Korstad has shown us in this volume where we have been and something of how we came to be what we are. I am proud of our accomplishments, grateful for our differences, and confident that the School of Public Health will continue to make progress in teaching, research, and service programs. Let us not forget that this is a professional school dedicated to the maintenance of health and prevention of disease. Public service is not only a slogan for us; it is our mission. We may disagree on the mechanisms, on strategies, even on definitions of health and disease. Whatever the future brings us, let it be known that we will always care. If this book teaches us anything, it is that good people did care.

Michel A. Ibrahim, M.D.
Dean

Dreaming Of A Time

The School of Public Health

THE
UNIVERSITY OF NORTH CAROLINA
at
CHAPEL HILL

1939–1989

Sally –
Another SPHian –
Best wishes
Bob Korstad

Robert Rodgers Korstad

Photograph Credits

Bradford Bachrach: p. 95.

Betty Ficquett: p. 41 *(left).*

Hilton Goulson: p. 99.

Dorothy Mayes: p. 134.

North Carolina Collection, University of North Carolina at Chapel Hill: pp. 14, 15, 20, 23 *(bottom),* 27, 34, 62.

North Carolina Division of Archives and History: pp. 5, 18, 24, 25, 30, 38, 74.

Daniel Okun: pp. 80, 81, 131.

Rockefeller Archive Center: pp. 8, 11, 16, 19.

Eunice Tyler: 39, 41 *(right),* 42, 43, 45, 46, 48 *(top),* 60.

Bailey Webb: pp. 32, 35, 36.

The other photographs in the book are part of the School of Public Health Collection.

Acknowledgments

Compiling a history of the School of Public Health at the University of North Carolina at Chapel Hill in the short time we had available required supportive efforts from many people. Dean Michel Ibrahim's enthusiasm made the whole thing possible. The members of the 50th Anniversary Dedication committee—Harriet Barr, Pam Horne, Richard House, Robert Moorhead, and Linda Parker—read every word more times than they would have liked, but always had helpful suggestions. Harriet Barr shared her knowledge and love of the school and the many photographs she has collected over the years. Mike Martin, Frances Weaver, and Marshall Bullock of the University Archives led me through the extensive records of the school and provided me with much useful information on the university. The Dean's Office staff—Melinda Walden, Shirley Clements, Terri Davis, Gail Gibbs, Delores Gold, Rosa Laney, Jennie Maurer, Mary McCurdy, Barbara Seago, Sylvia White, and Betty Sue Yow—helped me over and around many bureaucratic hurdles and helped make my eighteen months at the school particularly enjoyable. Jean Allen, Donna Cooper, and Nancy Gant showed me the ropes at the Kron building. Gail Gibbs located school records in remote corners of Rosenau Hall and took care of many administrative details. Jennie Maurer transcribed the interviews and navigated the minefields of word processing programs. Her good cheer and dependability saw me through some anxious moments. Linda Waldrop provided good advice along the way, but her special concern in the final stages made this a better book. Bill Herzog, Bert Kaplan, Daniel Okun, and Sharon Schramm gave the manuscript the benefit of their rich knowledge of the school. Jacquelyn Dowd Hall and James Leloudis of the Department of History read many drafts and DREAMING OF A TIME benefitted from their considerable intellectual and editorial abilities. Winston Fitzpatrick copy-edited the manuscript with great care and patience. Debbie Atkinson proof-read the final copy with a watchful eye. Cranine Brinkhous's design captured the spirit of the school, and her remarkable equanimity kept us on course. Finally, Bob Moorhead's love of history and his commitment to the School of Public Health made this book a reality.

Robert Rodgers Korstad
Chapel Hill, January, 1990

Chapter 1

PREPARING THE WAY

On June 7, 1940, the Board of Trustees of the University of North Carolina officially created the School of Public Health at Chapel Hill. That act represented the culmination of a twenty-year attempt to build a permanent educational center for public health professionals. No single incident marked the beginning of the school. There were many false starts and small beginnings. But a sequence of events in the fall of 1935 crystallized those efforts and did more than anything else to give direction and character to the enterprise. Dr. Carl V. Reynolds, state health officer from 1934 to 1948, recalled:

> It was my habit to read the [Raleigh] *News and Observer* on rising in the morning, realizing that if there were news of importance, with its eagle eye for news, that paper would have it. It was that morning of all mornings, I saw an announcement of Dr. Milton J. Rosenau's retirement from Harvard School of Medicine. I envisioned, if we could secure the services of that nationally and internationally known man of many parts and the father of preventive medicine, who sought to give a healthier, happier and more abundant life to his fellow man, it would be the fulfillment of a fond dream come true. Realizing that an official invitation would have to come from the University of North Carolina, I hastened without notifying my office, to Chapel Hill for a conference with the dean of the medical school and my friend Dr. Charles S. Mangum. After [I made] my wishes known, Charles's reply was, "Carl, you can't get Rosenau to come here." My answer was a challenge, "Hell's Fire, shoot at the moon and you might hit it." The Dean surrendered and said, "Well, Carl if you feel that strongly about it, I will risk a three cent stamp on him."[1]

Dean Mangum promptly wrote to Rosenau, describing the university's plans to establish a public health training program and the importance of finding the right man to head the effort. "It occurred to me," he concluded, "that it might be possible that you could be interested in coming to this delightful climate and spend a while in Chapel Hill, in the foothills of the famous Piedmont section of North Carolina, so near Pinehurst, where we have flowers in bloom and play tennis and golf the year round."[2]

Unbeknownst to either Reynolds or Mangum, Rosenau had not retired voluntarily. Harvard required mandatory retirement at age sixty-five, but Rosenau had no desire to leave his life's work. (He later confided to a colleague, "You can't retire a man who's not tired.") Rosenau immediately expressed interest in the position and set in motion a series of exchanges that would lead to his appointment as director of the Division of Public Health in the School of Medicine.[3]

Milton J. Rosenau was at the time one of the premier figures in public health in the United States, and his presence gave the division instant national exposure. Born in Philadelphia in 1869, Rosenau received his M.D. from the University of Pennsylvania before doing postgraduate work in Germany. He joined the United States Public Health and Marine Hospital Service in 1890, directing the service's hygienic laboratory (the forerunner of the National Institutes of Health) from 1899 to 1909. In 1909 Rosenau took a newly established chair in preventive medicine at Harvard Medical School, the first of its kind in the United States, which he held until his retirement in 1935. There he helped establish and direct the first university-based public health training center, the Harvard-Massachusetts Institute of Technology School for Health Officers.

Rosenau's medical and research interests ranged widely. His work at the hygienic laboratory included standardization of diphtheria and tetanus antitoxins; controls for yellow fever, tuberculosis, smallpox, and rabies; and methods for pasteurizing milk. At Harvard he trained a new generation of doctors and health officials in the techniques of preventive medicine. His book, *Preventive Medicine and Hygiene*, published in 1913, became the standard text in the field and in revised form is still in use today.[4]

Rosenau no doubt deserved the appellation "Father of Preventive Medicine," but the modern public health movement can trace its roots back nearly two centuries to the industrial revolution in Great Britain. "The same process that created the market economy, the factory, and the modern urban environment," wrote historian George Rosen, "also brought into being the health problems that made necessary new means of disease prevention and health protection." Poverty, overcrowding, poor sanitation, and geographical mobility, which were the negative outcomes of urbanization and industrialization, created conditions favorable to the spread of diseases that threatened all segments of society.[5]

Until the end of the nineteenth century, two schools of thought concerning the cause and prevention of disease predominated. Contagionists located the cause of disease in infective agents that could be transferred by people, by intermediate carriers, or through the air. They advocated strict quarantine to protect the community at large. Adherents of a miasmatic theory contended that communicable diseases arose from effluvia produced by decaying organic matter. They fought for sanitary reform. Generally, some combination of these two theories defined public health policy, and the engineers, social reformers, and physicians who shared the leadership of the movement focused their efforts on cleaning up the environment, maintaining a clean water supply, and quarantining affected areas.[6]

Revolutionary changes in the scientific understanding of disease and its prevention took place in the late nineteenth century. A series of discoveries by European scientists established "that specific microscopic creatures rather than vague chemical miasmas produce[d] infectious diseases." As this germ theory gained wide acceptance, the individual, rather than the whole society, became the focus of public health. Bacteriology superseded engineering as the science of public health, and the medical doctor began to challenge the engineer as the spokesman for the movement.[7]

During the Progressive Era, American reformers used these discoveries to attack the health problems that multiplied as waves of immigrants filled the slums and sweatshops of northern cities. One wing of the public health movement focused on the inefficiency of unregulated economic activity that neglected the public and private needs of the less fortunate. This group advocated the expansion of scientific knowledge and the application of sound business practices to the delivery of health services. A smaller group of reformers highlighted the injustices of a competitive marketplace. They too believed scientific advancements held the answer to many health problems, but they also stressed the need for improvements in housing, working conditions, and access to medical services.

Prominent among those who stressed the larger social environment were Alice Hamilton and Charles-Edward A. Winslow. In 1920 Hamilton discovered that lead poisoning was killing thousands of American workers. Campaigning for the improvement of working conditions, she almost single-handedly founded the practice of industrial hygiene. Winslow, whose thinking would have an impact on some of the major figures in public health at Chapel Hill, advocated an expansive definition of public health as "the science and art of preventing disease, prolonging life, and promoting physical health and efficiency through organized community efforts."[8]

The trajectory of public health efforts in the South paralleled that in Europe and the northern United States; only the timing differed. The persistence of a rural, agricultural economy precluded a dramatic increase in public health problems in the antebellum South. North Carolina and other southern states had their share of illnesses, early deaths, and even occasional epidemics, but these struck the slave population disproportionately. They were seen, in any case, as natural occurrences, not something to be prevented by man. Sustained efforts to improve the health of the South's citizens began in the years after the Civil War. Smallpox and typhoid epidemics swept the region as Confederate soldiers returned home, and freed men and women gathered in towns. After the war, the creation of a free labor market, the rise of sharecropping, the expansion of the tobacco manufacturing and cotton textile industries, and the growth of Piedmont urban areas created even greater health problems.

In 1877 the North Carolina legislature established the State Board of Health to advise lawmakers on sanitary matters affecting the health of citizens. Initially, the board had little power and few resources; its primary objective was to educate North Carolinians about possible health risks. But over the years the efforts of its first two secretaries, Dr. Thomas F. Wood and Dr. Richard H. Lewis, and growing public awareness of health issues increased the board's influence. The board became involved in the control and prevention of contagious diseases, the improvement of sanitary conditions, the collection of vital statistics, and the organization of county health boards. The board's *Health Bulletin* was the first state publication in the country to issue monthly reports on public health.[9]

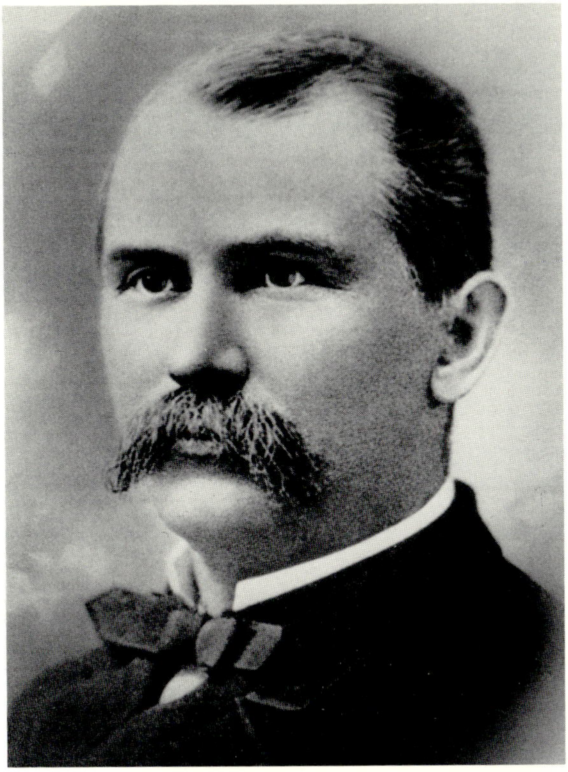

Dr. Thomas Fanning Wood, *Secretary of the State Board of Health*, 1877–92

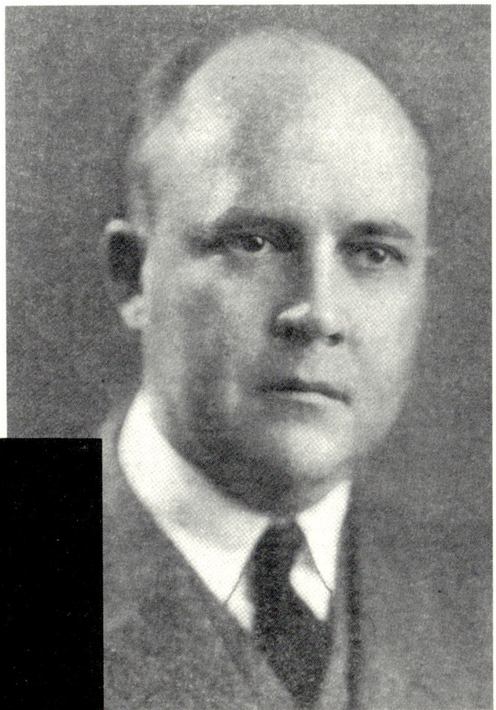

Dr. Watson Smith Rankin, *State Health Officer*, 1909–25

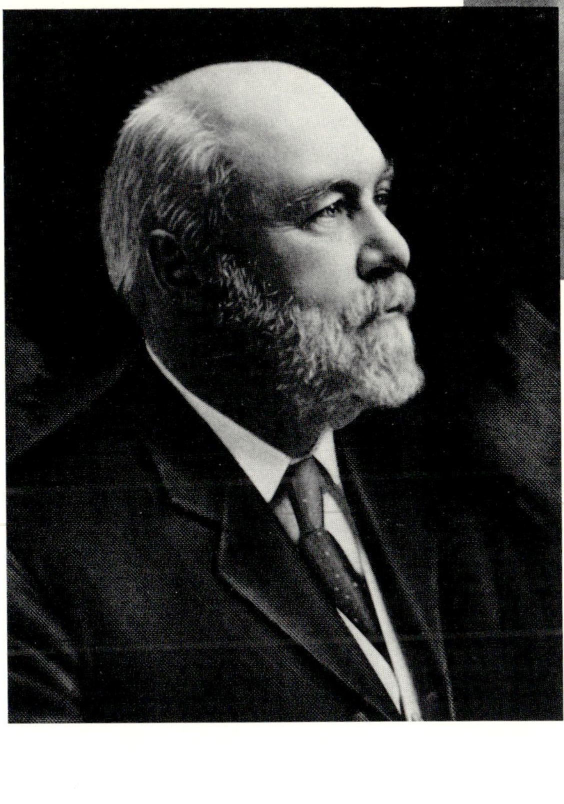

Dr. Richard Henry Lewis, *Secretary of the State Board of Health*, 1892–1909

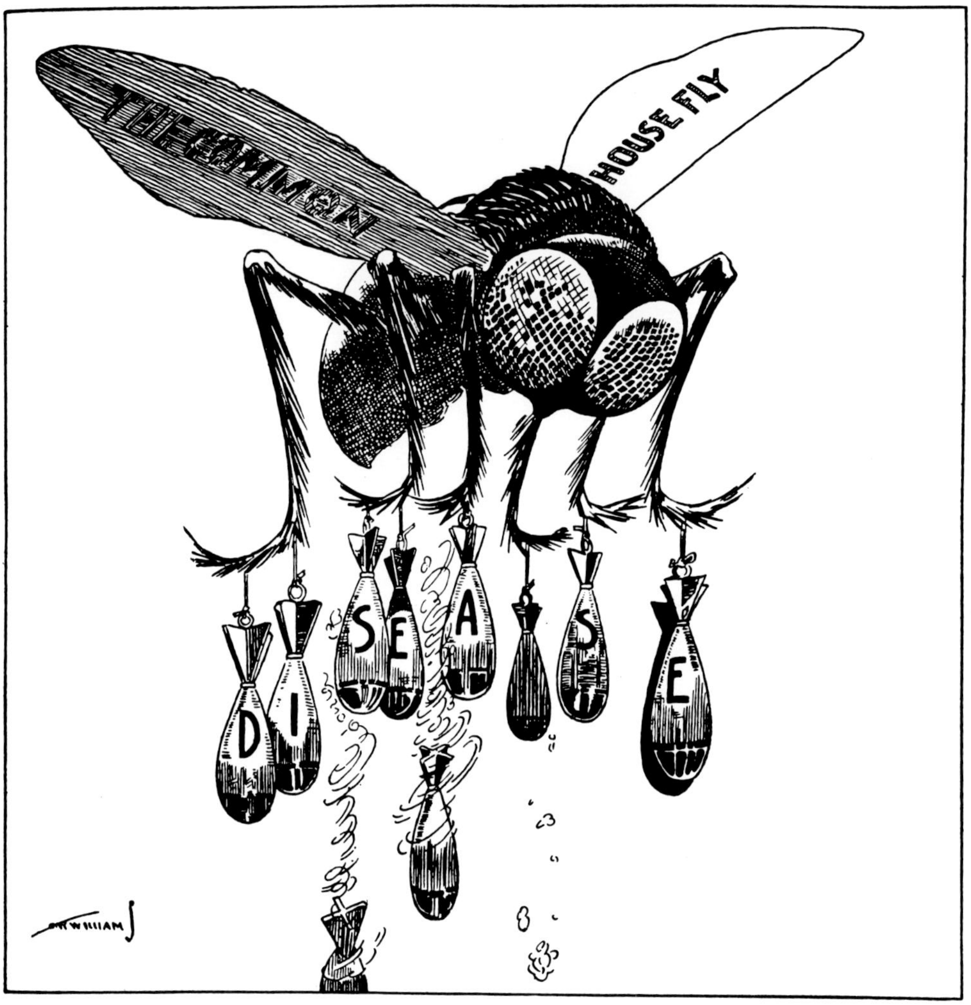

AN ENEMY TO MANKIND

It slays the tiny baby at mother's breast. Happy, joyous youth falls victim to poison it spreads. The strength of adult life is of no avail. The fly is no respecter of age, of sex, of color. It is the enemy of all. It must be fought and conquered.

An example of the graphics used in the *Health Bulletin* to educate North Carolinians about health issues.

The year 1909 marked a turning point in public health work in North Carolina. Dr. Lewis had served as president of the American Public Health Association, and he saw the need for an expansion and reorganization of public health forces in the state. He convinced law-makers to increase the State Board of Health's annual appropriation so that it could employ a full-time state health officer and maintain a tuberculosis sanatorium. The 1909 North Carolina General Assembly also gave the board greater authority over public water supplies.[10]

Dr. Watson Smith Rankin, dean of the Wake Forest medical school, replaced Lewis as secretary of the board and as the state's first full-time health officer. Rankin proved to be an unusually effective administrator, and during his tenure (1909–25) North Carolina was in the vanguard of the public health movement. Rankin oversaw phenomenal growth in public health activities in the state: the annual appropriation of the State Board of Health increased from $10,500 in 1909 to $340,000 in 1925. Like other Progressive Era reformers, Rankin argued that expenditures for public health were in the long run cost effective. But Rankin also maintained a relatively broad interpretation of public health that stressed education and immediate treatment, and he was not afraid at times to step on the toes of the medical profession. The State Board of Health gave the *Health Bulletin* a more popular design and expanded its circulation. Office staff produced movies and daily newspaper articles for statewide distribution, while doctors and dentists began examining children in the public schools, in many cases providing on-site treatment. This program of on-site treatment was viewed with alarm by some local doctors, who opposed the provision of any medical services by the state.[11]

Public health issues in North Carolina received a further boost when John D. Rockefeller gave $1 million to establish the Rockefeller Sanitary Commission for the Eradication of Hookworm Disease. Around the turn of the century, Dr. Charles W. Stiles, a zoologist connected with the United States Public Health Service, documented the prevalence of the disease among poor white farmers and mill workers in the South. Underestimating the effects of poverty caused by the Civil War, share-cropping, and industrial labor, he blamed the parasite for the "inferior physical development and mental powers" of the "cracker." Stiles had trouble convincing anyone of the seriousness of the problem, but by way of Walter Hines Page and the Country Life Commission—a national

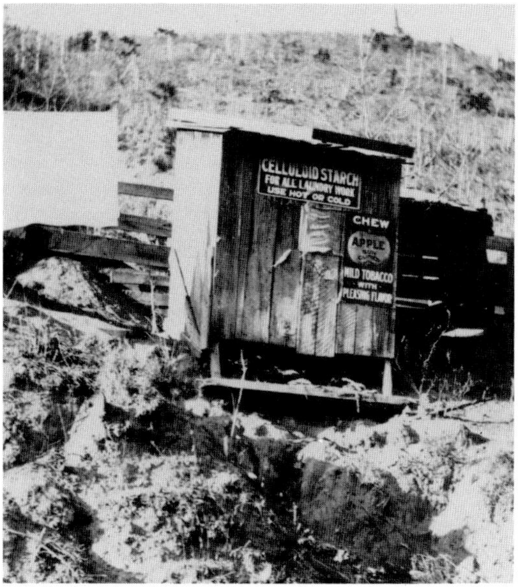

Improper privy construction was a major cause of hookworm infection in North Carolina.

campaign to uplift rural folk—he met Frederick Gates, who oversaw the Rockefeller philanthropies. Gates and the Rockefellers already had a strong interest in the regeneration of the southern economy through the General Educational Board. Improving the health and increasing the productivity of the region's workers fit squarely into their plans. Hookworm was also the perfect disease to highlight the benefits of public health and philanthropy. Diagnosis and cure were relatively simple and inexpensive, and the results were quick and dramatic.[12]

The Sanitary Commission identified North Carolina as one of eleven southern states where a significant number of people suffered from the disease. Because many North Carolinians distrusted the intentions of wealthy northerners like the Rockefellers, the Sanitary Commission worked through a Bureau for Hookworm Control established by the

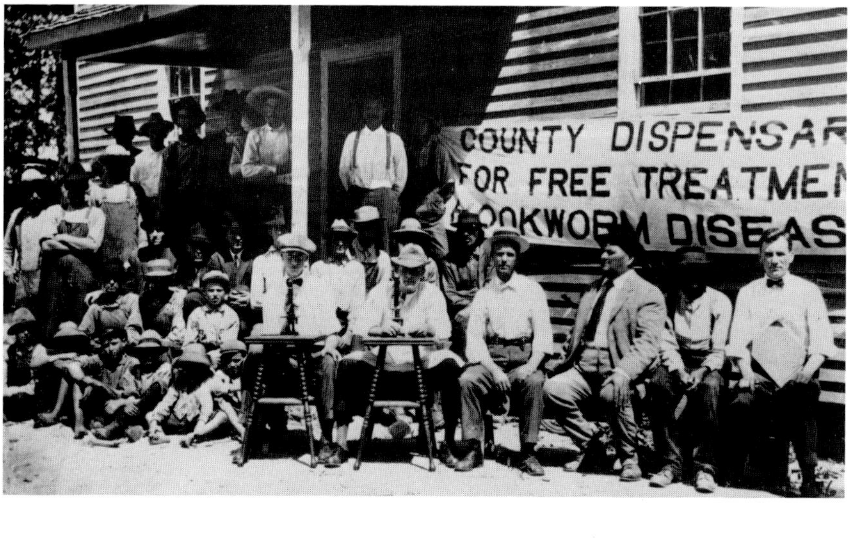

A hookworm dispensary in Lincoln County, North Carolina.

State Board of Health. The bureau identified the areas most heavily infected by the disease, then provided educational materials to schools and county health departments in the affected communities. In 1911 the campaign established dispensaries in which teams of doctors, microscopists, and record-keepers set up tents to educate and treat the local population.[13]

The campaign dramatically reduced the incidence of hookworm in the state, but perhaps more importantly it stimulated greater efforts in public health. Dr. Benjamin E. Washburn, a Rutherfordton physician who participated in the hookworm campaign, later observed that "[t]he cooperative work for the control of hookworm disease marked the beginning of active public health work in North Carolina and in the South." The campaign also served as an initiation for a number of North Carolina doctors like Washburn who went on to play important roles in the national and international public health movement.[14]

The hookworm campaign convinced Wickliffe Rose, director of the Sanitary Commission and its successor, the International Health Board, that the county was the most effective unit for public health work and the county health officer the most important administrator. But Rose remained equally certain that the movement could not rely on local physicians and volunteers; it needed trained, professional leaders. Efficiency-minded reformers such as Rose deplored interference by local political elites, who often viewed health officers as patronage appointments. In keeping with the general thrust of Progressive Era reform, public health advocates sought to develop a cadre of scientifically trained professionals who would be above partisan political squabbles.[15]

The Rockefeller Foundation's vast resources and experience in restructuring medical education put it in position to assume leadership in the training of these public health professionals. Under the leadership of Abraham Flexner, the Rockefeller Foundation's General Education Board had developed national standards for medical schools seeking philanthropic support. Schools had to be connected to a large university, research and educational programs had to be linked to clinical departments with access to laboratories and a university hospital, and teaching staffs had to be employed full time. Using Rockefeller funds, Flexner was able to develop a small group of elite medical schools that were clinically oriented. A similar strategy evolved in relation to schools of public health, and for twenty years, until the federal government took

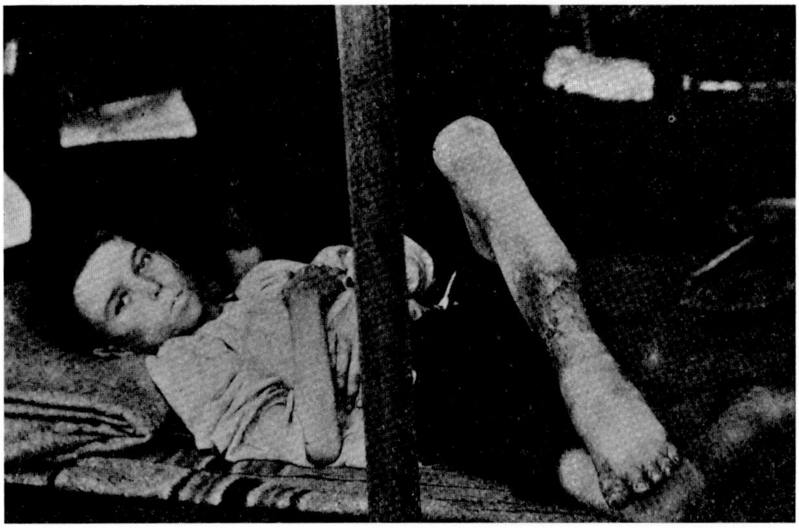

"Selma Ellis of Columbus county. Photograph made at county dispensary. Age 16, weight 62½ pounds; anemic ulcer on leg; ill 8 years. He was unable to go to school or work; in fact he was unable to sit or stand. Notice the change made in 7 weeks by a few cents worth of thymol."

Before and after photograph of hookworm carrier. Such formal portraits were often used to highlight the success of the hookworm treatment and reflected the reformers' hope that improved health would instill middle-class values in former victims.

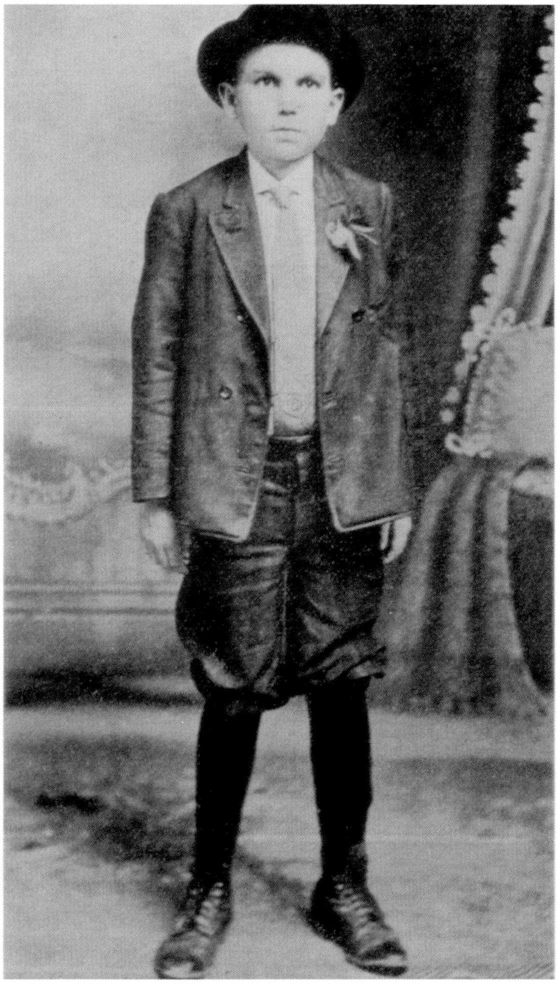

"Selma Ellis seven weeks later after taking the hookworm treatment. He was able to walk and run; weighed 79 pounds; and during the past winter he has been in school."

over in the 1930s, the foundation exercised enormous influence over public health instruction.[16]

In 1915 Wickliffe Rose drew up an initial plan calling for a national system of public health education, headed by a "central, scientific school" devoted to research and teaching and supplemented by state programs that were focused more on short courses and outreach and affiliated with a medical school and state health departments. In the end, however, the General Education Board announced its decision to fund a school at The Johns Hopkins University but made no mention of the practice-oriented state schools. As was the case with medical education, scientific research and clinical training remained foremost in the minds of foundation leaders.[17]

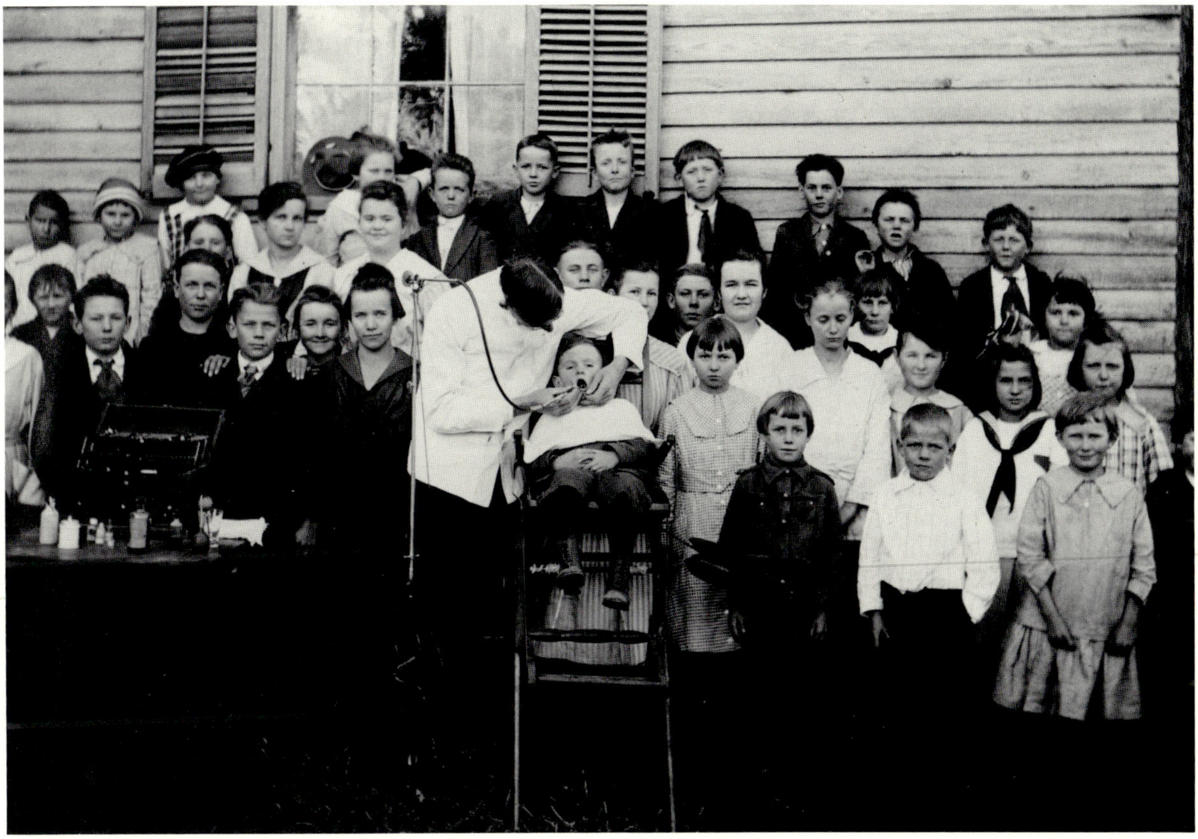

Outdoor dental health clinic at rural school in Wilson County, North Carolina.

Meanwhile, the push to find new markets and sources of raw materials had taken the industrialized nations into parts of the world where disease and unsanitary conditions prevented a full utilization of human and natural resources. Some means had to be found to train "foot soldiers" for the public health movement at home and abroad. The Rockefeller Foundation saw the South as another such underdeveloped region, and as it expanded its public health work overseas, it drew on its experience in the region. In 1913, for example, the foundation's International Health Board used the Sanitary Commission's work in North Carolina as a model for its hookworm campaign in the British West Indies. When the board decided to establish a training site that would serve as a model for local health departments, it also looked to North Carolina for a location, and to a North Carolinian for a director. Dr. Benjamin E. Washburn set up shop in Wilson County in 1916. State Health Officer Rankin was so impressed with the success of the training site that he asked Washburn to direct a new Bureau of County Health Work in the State Board of Health. The Rockefeller Foundation continued to pay Washburn's salary, and he moved quickly to set up county health departments modeled on the Wilson experiment.[18]

University of North Carolina officials, aware of the advances in public health work in the state, were eager to get involved. Health issues became the focus of much discussion on campus in the spring of 1919. The influenza epidemic of the previous winter and the surprisingly poor physical condition of recent army recruits prompted concern among politicians and educators. In response, the legislature allocated money for a campus health officer. Dr. William deB. MacNider of the University of North Carolina School of Medicine saw this as an opportunity to hire someone who, in addition to serving the university, might also cooperate with the Board of Health in providing training for public health workers. He put the idea to State Health Officer Rankin, who responded coolly, believing that the "scientific and theoretical training" given at the university would be impractical for public officials. MacNider eventually won the ear of Rankin's assistant, Benjamin Washburn, who convinced the board to submit to the university a tentative proposal for a training school. The board saw two related benefits from such a plan. First, university students who were exposed to "the rules of hygiene and sanitation" would become proponents of public health once back in their own communities. Second, the university could help train desperately needed health officers and public health nurses.[19]

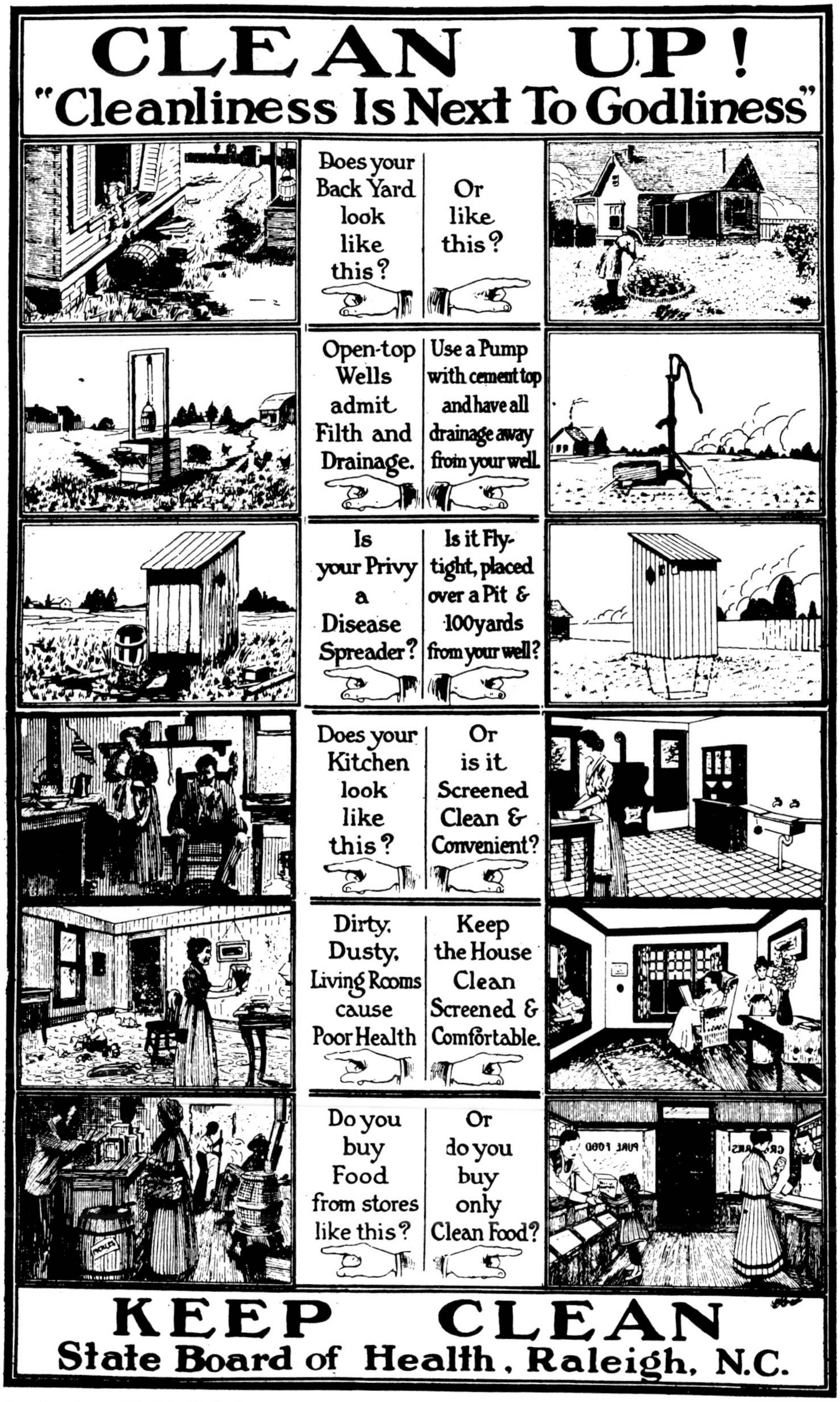
CLEAN UP!
"Cleanliness Is Next To Godliness"
Does your Back Yard look like this?
Or like this?
Open-top Wells admit Filth and Drainage.
Use a Pump with cement top and have all drainage away from your well.
Is your Privy a Disease Spreader?
Is it Fly-tight, placed over a Pit & 100 yards from your well?
Does your Kitchen look like this?
Or is it Screened Clean & Convenient?
Dirty. Dusty. Living Rooms cause Poor Health
Keep the House Clean Screened & Comfortable.
Do you buy Food from stores like this?
Or do you buy only Clean Food?
KEEP CLEAN
State Board of Health, Raleigh, N.C.

Graphic from *Health Bulletin*

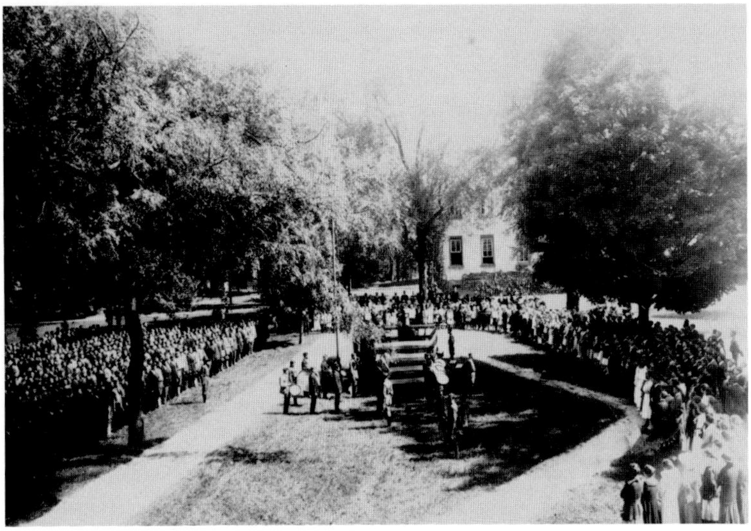

Students at the University of North Carolina being sworn into the Students Army Training Corps in 1918. The poor physical condition of student recruits prompted calls for health education on campus. Old East is in the background.

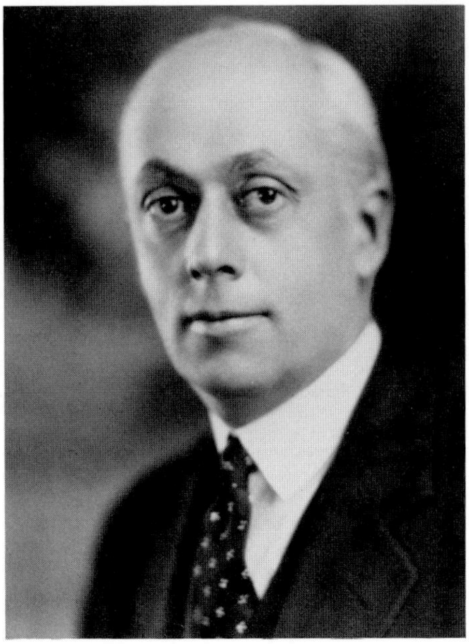

Harry Washburn Chase, *President of the University of North Carolina*, 1919–30

University President Harry Washburn Chase welcomed the board's proposal. He described his vision of the project in a letter to Dr. W. P. Jacocks, a leading candidate to head up the effort:

> It is not our ambition to develop here a school of public health, nor could we of course hope to compete with the work done at Harvard or The Hopkins, in case we desired to do so. We merely want to take a few practical steps toward making it a little easier for a medical graduate, who is interested in public health matters and who cannot spend the time to go to a school of public health, to get some training in the basic things he will need to meet.
>
> The supply of graduates of schools of public health is at present so limited that it seems clear that health positions in this section cannot for a number of years be filled from the ranks of such graduates. We therefore feel that if we work out a scheme whereby men could be given about three months' field work with the State Department of Health, and about three months' training, we will be meeting a need which is very real and very vital. Naturally such men would not have the grasp of their problems which graduates of the formal school of public health would have, but they would be in far better shape to handle their problems than they would be with no health training whatsoever. I believe that with the cooperation of our medical school and the engineering faculties, and the other departments which would be concerned, we could make the work very much worth while to such men as would come here.[20]

Unfortunately, these early plans for public health training faltered. The university lacked funds for the necessary equipment and capital improvements and had under consideration a competing plan by the United States Interdepartmental Hygiene Board to establish a Department of Hygiene. Rankin continued to voice doubts about the utility of university training, and there was dissent from professors who feared the training program might lower the standards of the university. Still, MacNider did not give up hope. "I would like to see," he wrote Chase, "and I believe it is our duty to establish a professorship of public health at the university."[21]

The 1920s proved a difficult time for the public health movement in North Carolina. Dr. Rankin continued to provide strong leadership during the early years of the decade, and the General Assembly, despite economic hard times after the end of World War I, steadily increased its appropriation to the State Board of Health. More and more counties established full-time health departments, and an ever greater number of people made use of their services. But the simple expansion of services could not cover up what Rankin and a number of other progressive

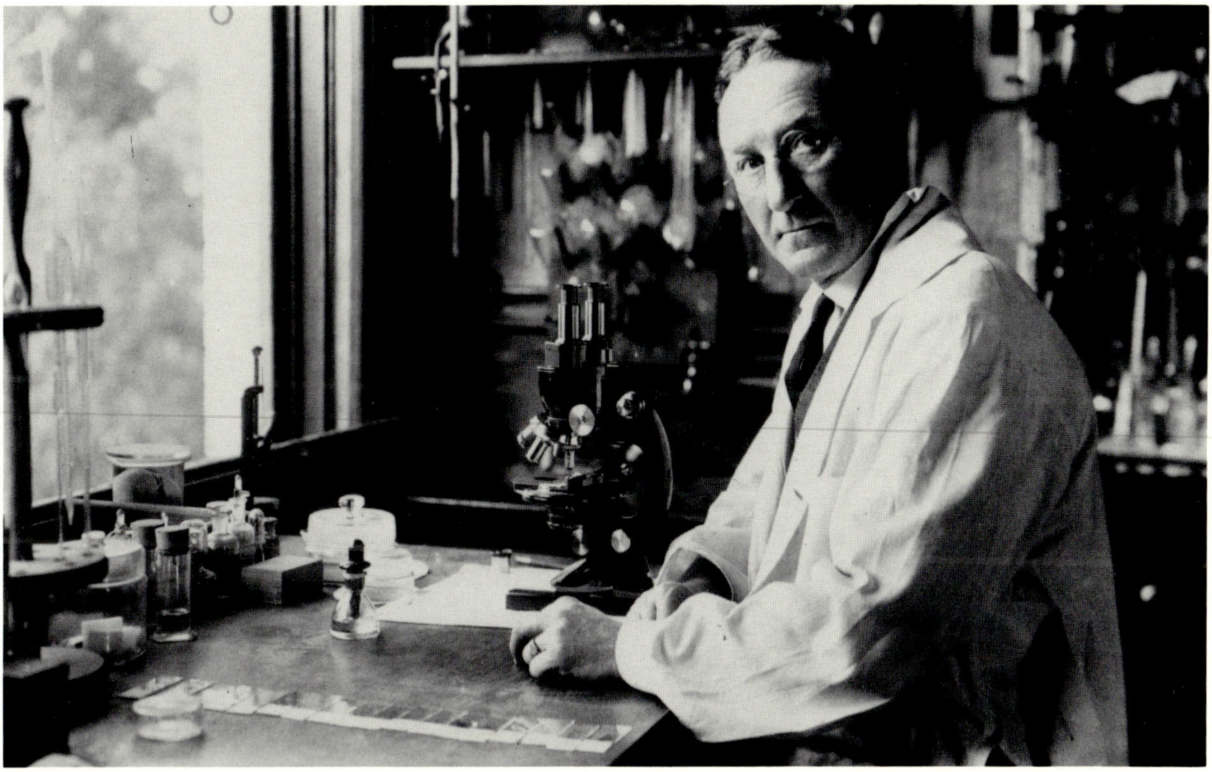

Dr. William deB. MacNider

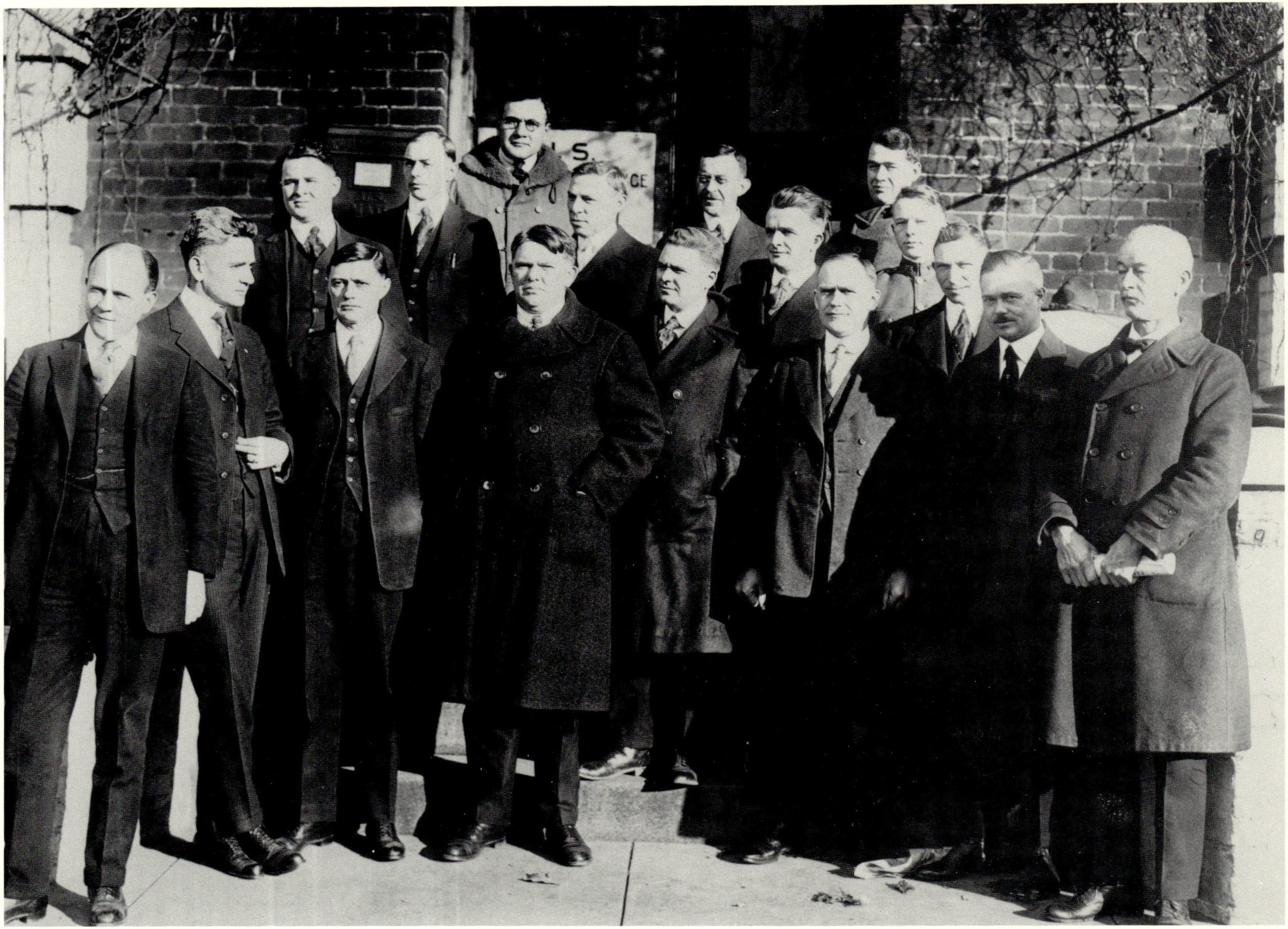

Conference of North Carolina Health Officers, December, 1919. Dr. Benjamin Washburn is fourth from left on front row.

public health leaders saw as some fundamental weaknesses of the movement: the continued political control of local health positions and the general inefficiency of most county health departments.[22]

Hoping to make the management of health services as "rational" as the laboratory dimension, Rankin introduced two schemes designed to improve the functioning of local health departments and local health officers. The first was a "piece-work" plan for allocating funds. For instance, instead of receiving general appropriations for vaccinations, counties submitted bills for the number they performed. Likewise, the State Board of Health began evaluating health officers on the basis of more precise, quantifiable criteria. Such policies had some impact on health services in the state, but most concerned observers continued to see the scientific training of public health professionals as the sine qua non of future progress.[23]

The resignation of Dr. Rankin in 1925 to become director of the Hospital and Orphan Division of the Duke Endowment seriously hampered public health activities in North Carolina. Although the State Board of Health continued to expand its operations until the early 1930s, much of the board's energy was taken up with personnel problems and intermittent conflicts with the State Medical Society. State Health Officer Charles O'H. Laughinghouse discussed starting a training station for health officers at the newly established Duke University Medical College, but the plan never materialized.[24]

The Great Depression unleashed forces that ultimately created a more favorable climate for a school of public health in Chapel Hill. President Frank Porter Graham's leadership put the university in the forefront of reform efforts in the South. Stringent purse tightening caused major changes in state government and brought new leadership to the State Board of Health. Finally, Franklin D. Roosevelt's New Deal provided funds for health and welfare programs.

The perceived need for greater efficiency in state government prompted Governor O. Max Gardner to ask the Brookings Institute in 1930 to "prepare for the consideration of the General Assembly a complete, modern, practical setup of government reorganization." The plan for public health called for the abolition of the State Board of Health and the relegation of the State Medical Society to an advisory position in public health matters. Authority would be centralized in an executive department headed by a commissioner appointed by the governor. The

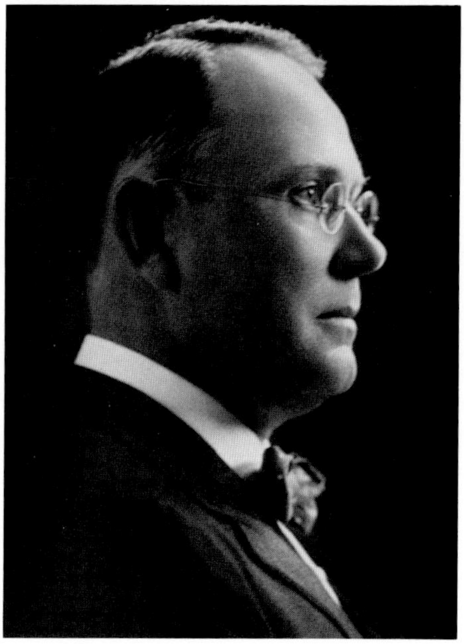

Dr. Charles O'H. Laughinghouse,
State Health Officer, 1926–1930

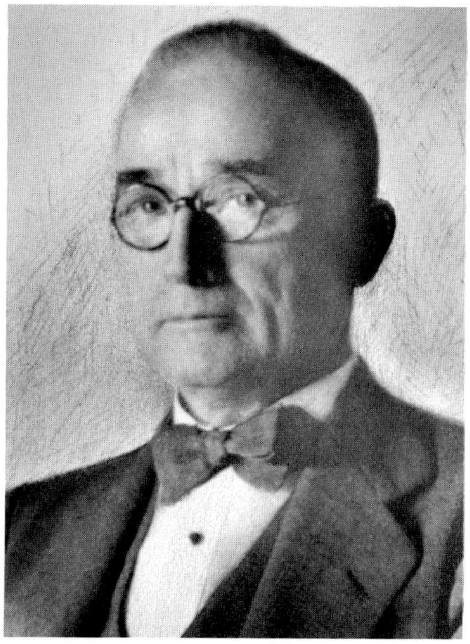

Dr. James M. Parrott,
State Health Officer, 1931–1934

state's medical profession successfully fought the proposed changes, but the legislature did force the resignation of the standing board and give the governor veto power over the selection of the state health officer.[25]

The new board selected Dr. James M. Parrott as state health officer. Parrott went to work quickly, reorganizing the divisions for more efficient functioning and withholding money from counties that appointed health officers who lacked training or experience in public health administration. The latter policy apparently forced Parrott to oppose the appointment of some long-time friends, but he persevered in his determination to improve the functioning of health officials throughout the state.[26]

Soon after taking office, Parrott approached Dr. John A. Ferrell, a North Carolinian who served as deputy-director of the Rockefeller Foundation's International Health Division, about a grant for a training base for county health officials. By requiring such training, he hoped to weed out "incompetent" doctors who might later be nominated by county boards of health. Ferrell could offer no encouragement. His response, in fact, pointed to what the Rockefeller Foundation saw as major deficiencies in the public health program in North Carolina. The first problem was the advanced age of many of the county health officers; the foundation did not encourage training for men over fifty, the average age of health officers in North Carolina. The second problem was the state's poverty and its dearth of public health professionals. The foundation would fund training bases only where the states contributed 50 percent of the costs and the instructors had "academic, medical and public

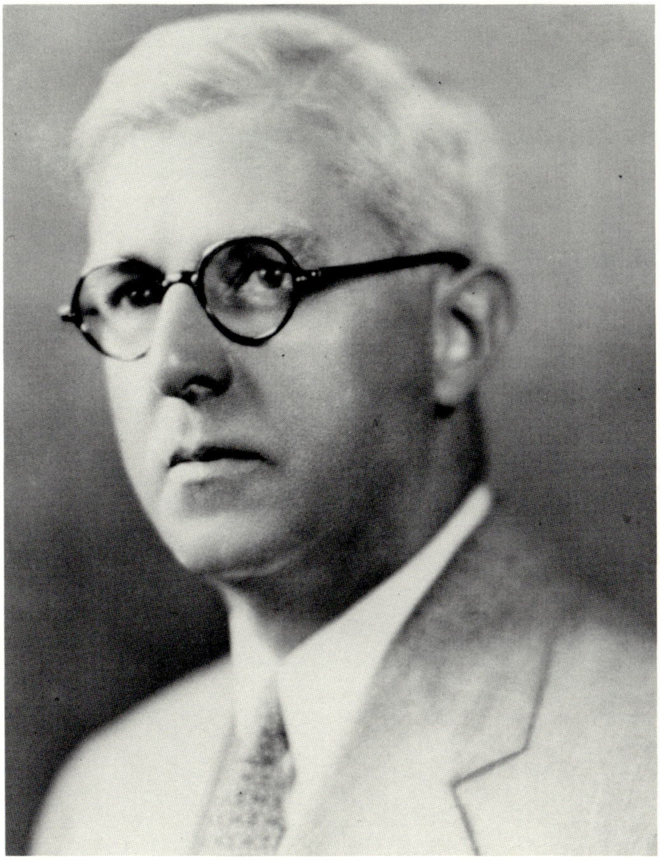

Dr. John A. Ferrell directed the State Board of Health's hookworm eradication program before joining the staff of the Rockefeller Foundation. He later returned to North Carolina as Executive Director of the Medical Care Commission.

health training" of the "first order." North Carolina obviously could not provide the money, and Ferrell questioned whether the state could find such instructors. "We had been hopeful," he wrote, "that each of the more important state health departments would arrange for their young and best prepared health officers to have courses in schools of public health, so that for administrative, epidemiological, or teaching assignments the needed personnel could be drawn from within the state." "North Carolina," he continued, "has not utilized the schools of public health as have other progressive states." Parrott reminded Ferrell that the state had produced many able public health men, such as W. S. Rankin, Benjamin Washburn, and Ferrell himself, only to have them snapped up by organizations like the Rockefeller Foundation and Duke Endowment.[27]

Parrott did not abandon his hopes for the training center. Together with officials of the university, the State Board of Health forged ahead with a plan for a school in Chapel Hill. Since Orange County did not have a full-time health officer, the director of the school would also serve in that capacity. A county nurse, sanitary officer, and health secretary would double as instructors. The director would offer a course in

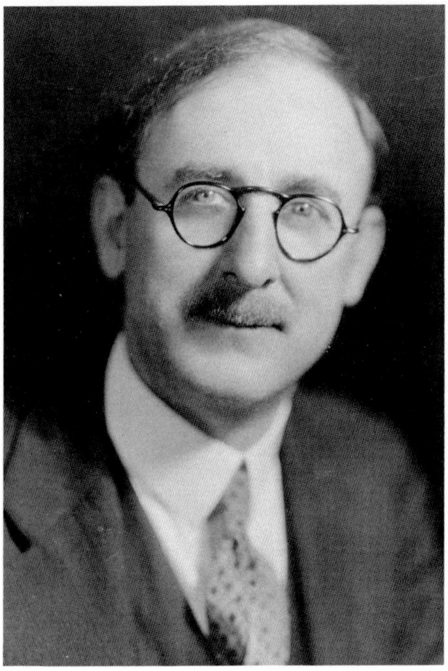

Howard Odum

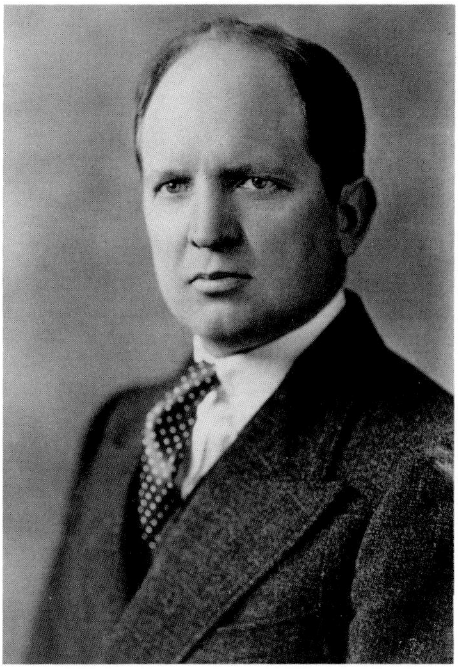

W. T. Couch

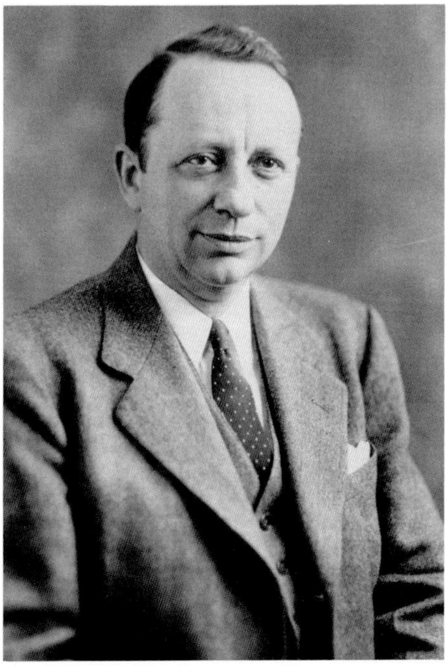

Albert Coates

"It is a strange thing, perhaps, that the University has grown in stature by getting down closer and closer to the earth and the people around it. . . . Its chief greatness now, it seems to me, lies in the fact that, in addition to the glory that was Greece, the grandeur that was Rome, the immensity of the cosmos, and the infiniteness of the atom, it has looked around at the human qualities of the State and the South. Red-necked farmers have become as important in its classrooms as Roman Senators once seemed to be, and for all I know, may be now. In the University, where students once paid a black man named Benny Booth a dime to let them split a plank over his skull, there is an increasing concern for what goes on in other black skulls and in an inescapably black and white Southern world. The new School of Public Health (headed by the world's leading sanitarian who is both a Yankee and a Jew) is an aspect of the University's public concern." (Jonathan Daniels, *TarHeels: A Portrait of North Carolina*) preventive medicine at the Medical School in hopes of attracting some physicians to the public health field. Frank Graham offered strong support for the effort. Dr. H. G. Baity, dean of the School of Engineering and a member of the State Board of Health, served as a liaison between the board and the university. Baity told board members, "We of the university [consider] none of our functions more vital or of greater value to the state than the adequate training of personnel who are engaged in conserving the health of our people, making life fuller, longer, and North Carolina a more wholesome place in which to live."[28]

Dr. Parrott's efforts greatly impressed Ferrell. "In my judgment," Ferrell wrote to a member of his staff, "conditions in North Carolina now merit liberal cooperation from our organization." Nevertheless, the Rockefeller Foundation could find no funds for the proposed training school. The Depression prohibited philanthropic contributions on the scale of those in the 1910s and 1920s, but the Rockefeller Foundation did provide scholarships for two State Board of Health officials and loaned a member of its own staff to the State Board of Health.[29]

By the early 1930s the university had become a center for reform-minded southerners. Frank Graham stood as a symbol of the school's liberality, but others like Howard Odum of the Institute for Research in Social Science and W. T. Couch of the University of North Carolina Press were also committed to addressing the region's economic and social problems.[30]

A more cautious group of university-based reformers concentrated on the waste and inefficiency caused by antiquated bureaucratic structures and poorly trained government employees. In the early 1930s, Albert Coates, a law professor at the university, established the Institute of Government, which offered short courses and provided technical advice for elected and appointed officials. "The need for training in our governmental personnel is painfully apparent," Coates told a gathering of government officials in 1932. "[T]he hope of popular government is not so much wrapped up in theories of government, centralized or localized, as in the effective and efficient handling of governmental affairs by effective and efficient governmental officers."[31]

In 1932 the university also established a School of Public Administration to provide more formal training for public officials. An important feature of the new curriculum was a program in public health administration designed for physicians who were already engaged in public health work or wished to enter the field. The faculty would be drawn from various schools on the Chapel Hill campus and from the State Board of Health in Raleigh. Unfortunately, when the school offered a "Short Course in Public Health Administration" in the fall of 1933, only three students registered, and the course had to be canceled. The shortage of state funds prevented some interested persons from applying, but the program also needed to build a constituency among health workers if it was to succeed.[32]

Meanwhile, efforts to devise some workable scheme for public health work continued. M. V. Ziegler of the Public Health Service prodded the Medical School, the School of Engineering, and the State Board of Health to cooperate in offering two twelve-week short courses during the 1934–35 academic year. The eleven students divided their time between classroom instruction in sanitary engineering, vital statistics, and epidemiology and "practical work" at State Board of Health facilities in Raleigh and at county health departments. The program failed to attract enough qualified in-state students to justify continuing the courses the next summer, but Medical School Dean Charles Mangum appealed to the Public Health Service to provide funding that would allow the university to accept students from other states. The Public Health Service responded favorably, and Mangum prepared a plan for the State Board of Health to submit to Washington.[33]

This time the plan took, thanks in large measure to heightened interest in public health at the federal level. Even as Mangum was drawing up his plan, Congress had under consideration the most far-reaching piece of social legislation in the nation's history, the Social Security Act. The act contained key provisions relating to public health. An advisory committee appointed by President Franklin Roosevelt in 1934 to study long-term economic problems recognized that "illness is one of the major causes of economic insecurity which threaten people of small means in good times as in bad." A logical way to deal with such suffering, the committee concluded, was to take steps to prevent sickness. The committee recommended grants to states for local health programs, funds for training public health workers, and additional personnel for the Public Health Service.[34]

Although allocations for public health paled in comparison to the cost of social security, they helped sway influential southern congressmen who were otherwise critical of the bill. Title VI earmarked much of the money for states where poverty had limited public health work, and

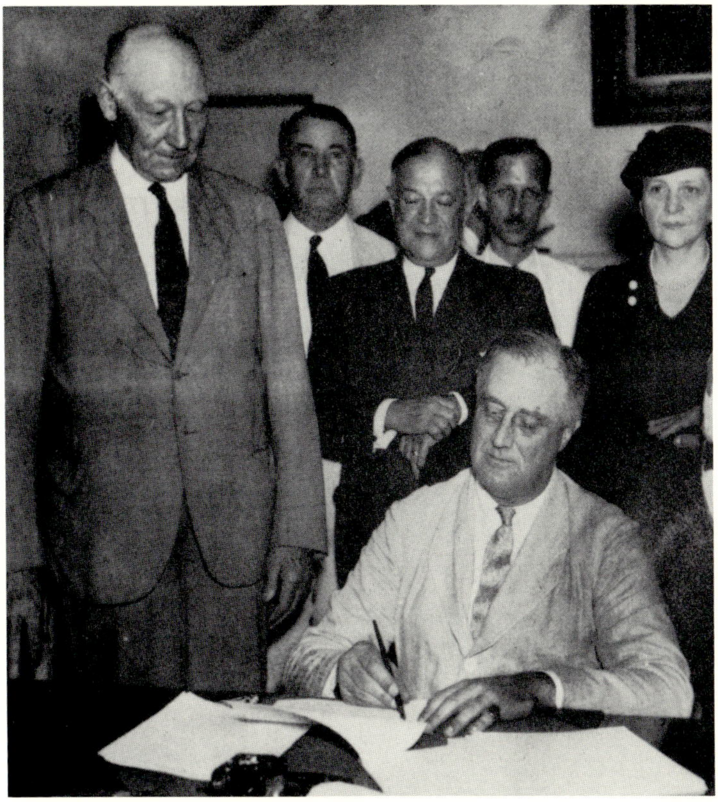

President Franklin D. Roosevelt signing the Social Security Act.

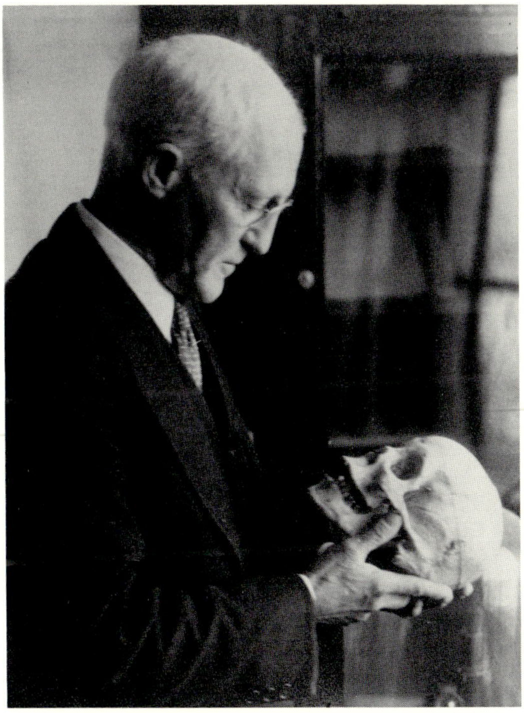

Dr. Charles Mangum

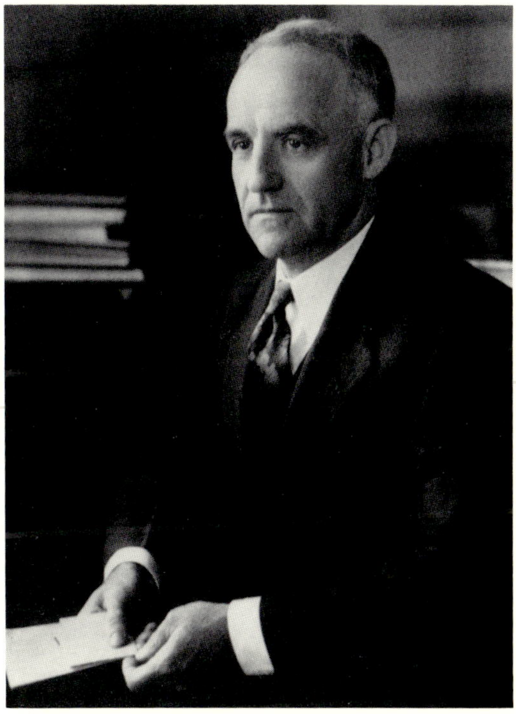

Frank Porter Graham

southern public health officials appeared before Congress to support the legislation. Conservatives also saw public health programs as a way to counter growing support for national health insurance. The House and Senate passed the bill in the summer of 1935, and President Roosevelt signed it on August 14.[35]

Anxious to take advantage of the availability of federal funding, Dean Mangum stepped up his search for someone to head the university's proposed public health program. State Health Officer Carl Reynolds's notice of Dr. Milton J. Rosenau's resignation that September came in the midst of this search. Once Rosenau expressed interest in coming to Chapel Hill, Dean Mangum invited him to meet with representatives of the university, the State Board of Health, and the Public Health Service. On December 13, 1935, the parties agreed to establish a Division of Public Health in the Medical School that would serve as a regional training center for public health workers in interstate Sanitary District Number 2, made up of Delaware, Florida, Georgia, Maryland, North Carolina, South Carolina, Virginia, and West Virginia. Rosenau accepted the position as director, and the university agreed to begin admitting students the following January.[36]

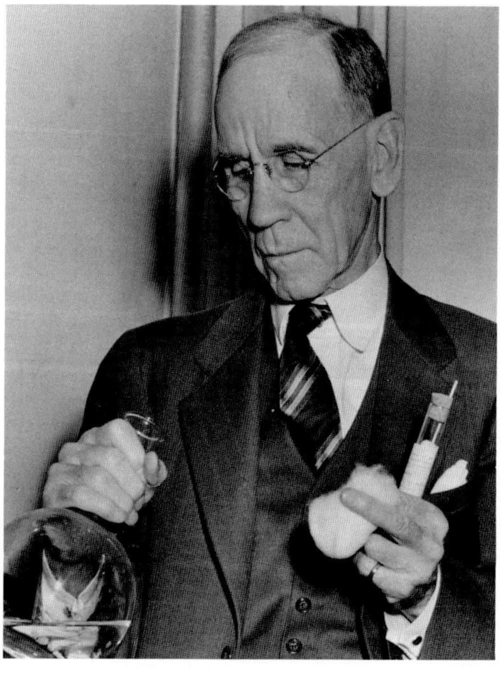

Dr. Carl Reynolds,
State Health Officer, 1934–1947

Chapter 2

THE EARLY YEARS

State and university officials greeted Dr. Rosenau's arrival in 1936 with great fanfare. "Your eminence, your training and experience, and your personality and spirit cause us to welcome you with sincere enthusiasm," wrote Frank Graham. Newspapers throughout North Carolina carried word of the new undertaking. State Health Officer Carl V. Reynolds called Rosenau "the foremost teacher of public health matters in the world" and the establishment of the school "one of the most

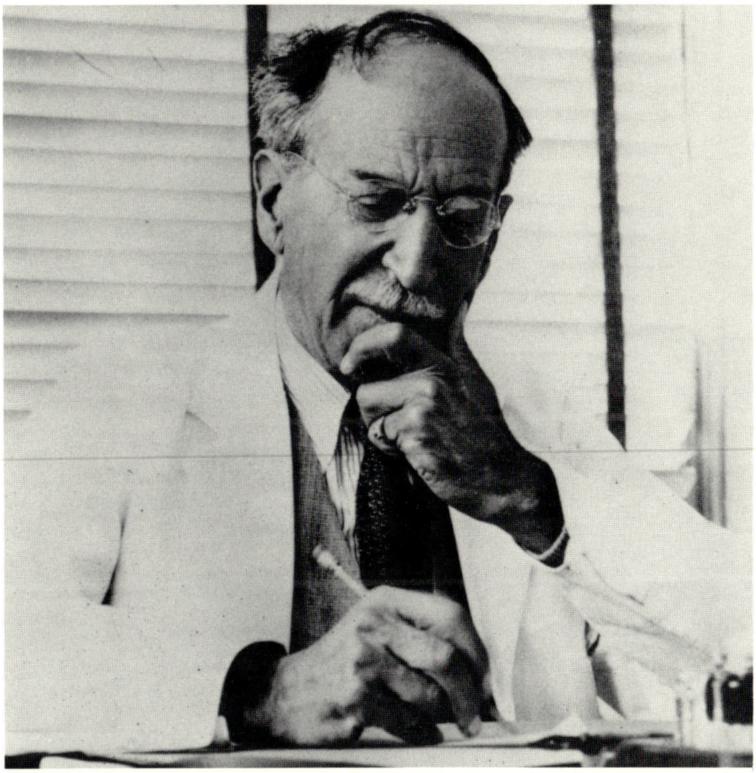

Dr. Milton J. Rosenau

important events in this state for the last 25 years." Members of the Buncombe County Medical Society welcomed the "increased influence and prestige and power" that would accrue to the university and the state with Rosenau's arrival.[1]

Rosenau met his admirers at a gathering of public health officials and medical educators on the Chapel Hill campus. Frank Graham's introduction praised Rosenau for his dedication to the cause of public health and for his willingness at the end of a life filled with honors and high position to lead the foundling program at Chapel Hill. Then Dr. Rosenau took the floor. "The epidemiologist is a disease detective," he told his audience. "[We] hunt and determine the causes of diseases and then track down the mode of transmission." To underscore the tragedy of epidemics, Rosenau described a plague in Stratford-on-Avon during Shakespeare's childhood. The great dramatist survived, but how many similar geniuses had been lost, he wondered. "We find monuments erected to heroes who have won wars, but we have none commemorating anyone who prevented a war. The same is true with epidemics. But preventive medicine is coming into its own."[2]

State and local health associations inundated Rosenau with requests to address their groups. They looked to him for inspiration for their own troops and for influence with local political officials. Rosenau ventured out when he could, but setting up the Division of Public Health required most of his time. Four health officer trainees registered for courses during the winter quarter, but they were only the beginning. Students supported by funds from the Social Security Act began arriving in the spring. By March 28, fifty-one health officers, sanitary engineers, sanitarians, and sanitary officers had registered. All the members of Interstate Sanitary District Number 2, with the exception of Maryland, sent representatives. Rosenau taught epidemiology and the medical faculty helped out, but the staff of the State Board of Health handled much of the instruction and classroom work. Without their efforts, the school could not have opened.[3]

Rosenau's most pressing tasks that first spring involved raising money and building a faculty. Unlike The Johns Hopkins and Harvard, which received substantial endowments as well as operating costs from the Rockefeller Foundation, the division at Chapel Hill relied on a small appropriation from the university, funds from the Public Health Service, and the tuition of students. Rosenau knew about Chapel Hill's limited resources when he took the job, but he had no intention of sitting still. He aspired to build a program to compete with Harvard and The Hopkins.[4]

Rosenau used his personal influence in Washington to secure an additional allocation from the Public Health Service for two full-time professors. "This is to relieve the strain on the State Board of Health and to make a nucleus of a small, well-knit, full-time faculty to carry on the bulk of the teaching," he wrote Dean Mangum. Dr. Robert E. Fox joined the faculty as professor of public health administration. As director of county health work for the State Board of Health, Fox had been involved in the initiation of public health training at the university. He taught on a full-time basis for six months of the year and worked for the board during the remaining time. This arrangement continued the close cooperation between the state and the university and allowed the division to grow gradually.[5]

Dr. Herman Glenn Baity, a professor of sanitary engineering, a former dean of the School of Engineering at Chapel Hill, and at the time director of the Public Works Administration (PWA) in North

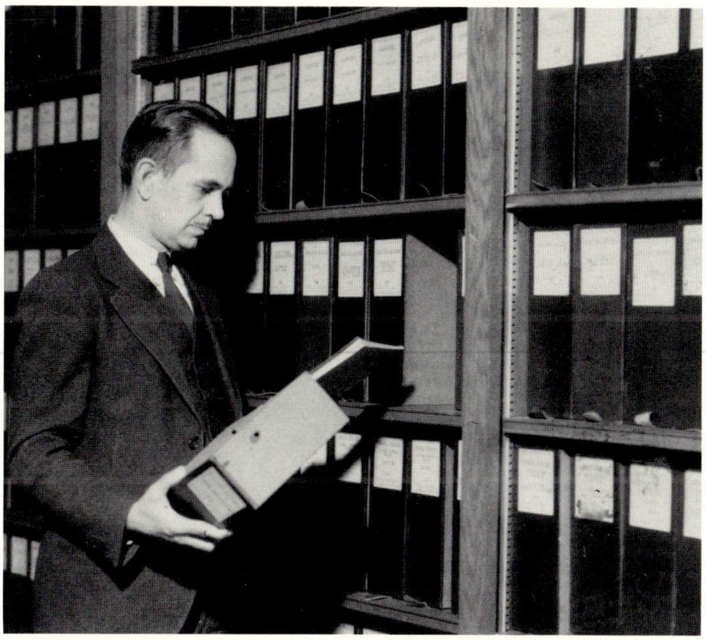

Dr. Herman G. Baity

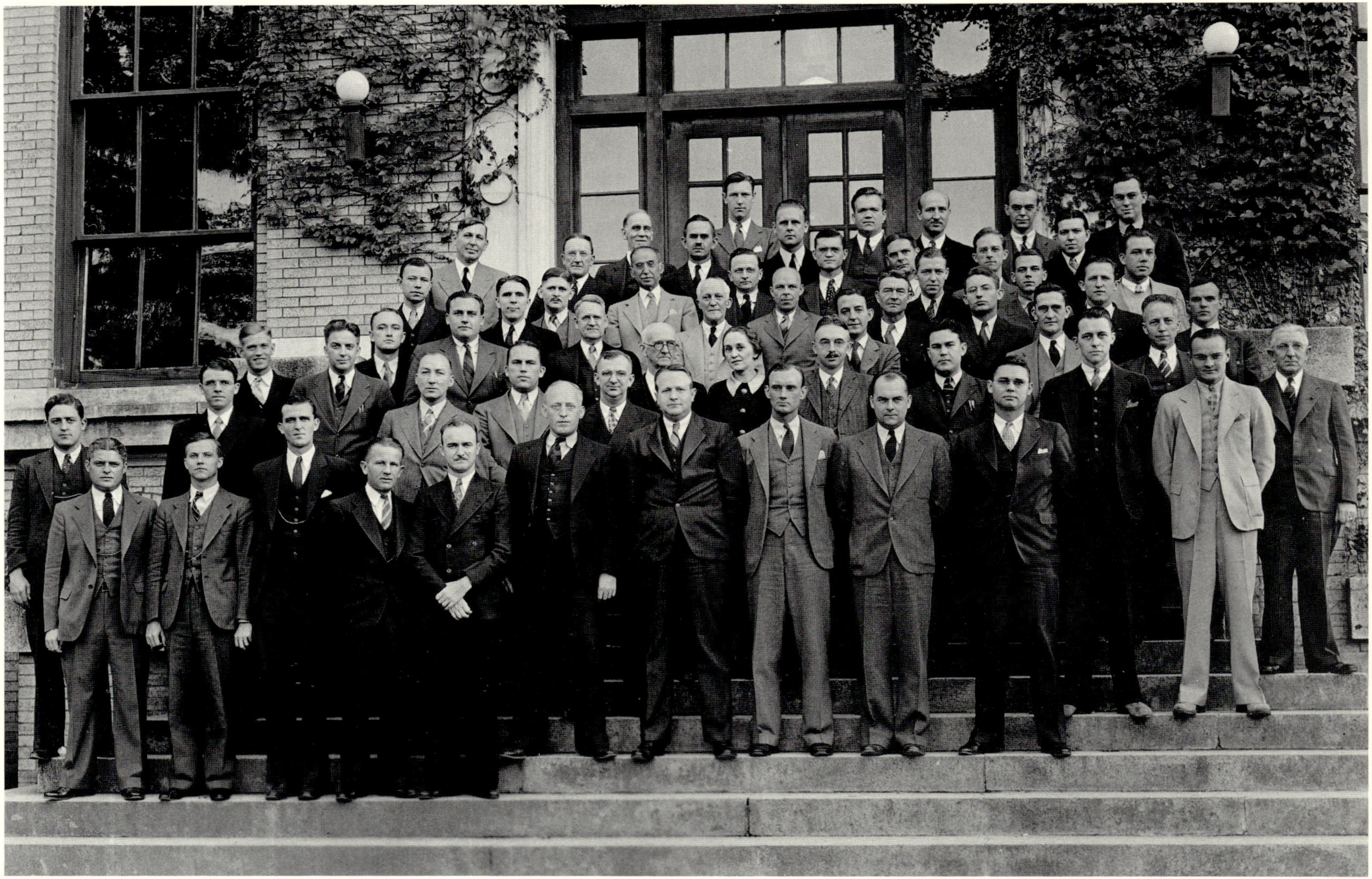

Fall Class (1936), Division of Public Health

Carolina, also came on board in the summer of 1936. Baity's appointment was anything but routine. The year before, the Board of Trustees, at the urging of Frank Graham, moved the School of Engineering at Chapel Hill to North Carolina State College in Raleigh as part of the 1933 consolidation of the schools in Greensboro, Chapel Hill, and Raleigh. Economics motivated Graham's decision, but the move also represented an effort to build up the Raleigh campus and make consolidation more equitable. Many Chapel Hill alumni and some faculty members voiced strong opposition to the proposal, Baity among them. As a concession, Graham placed engineering faculty who did not want to move to Raleigh in other departments at Chapel Hill. Baity moved the program in sanitary engineering into the Division of Public Health, where he retained some of his assistants, his laboratory, and the right to grant advanced degrees.[6]

Baity brought many qualities to his position as professor of sanitary engineering. He was a native North Carolinian, a graduate of the university (B.A. in liberal arts in 1917 and B.S. in engineering in 1922), a member of the State Board of Health, a nationally known sanitary engineer, and a Public Works administrator with strong connections in Washington. Among his many distinctions, Baity had been the first person to earn a doctorate in sanitary engineering (Harvard, 1928).[7]

When classes began in the fall of 1936, forty-six students enrolled in the Division of Public Health. Among them was A. Worth Petty, a recent graduate in sanitary engineering at North Carolina State College employed by the State Board of Health. The program "looked like a bonanza," he remembered, "because they were going to pay my salary and pick up all my travel, and a public health scholarship paid for the fees, tuition, and books. They broke us up into groups. If you didn't have a degree you were a sanitary officer. If you had a degree other than medicine or engineering you were a sanitarian. If you had a degree in engineering, of course, you were an engineer and a degree in medicine [made you] a health officer."[8]

Students took courses in public health administration, epidemiology, vital statistics, principles of sanitation, and child hygiene. "The big course was epidemiology with Dr. Rosenau," Petty recalled. "This big book he had written, thicker than the Sears & Roebuck catalog, was the whole story on everything to do with communicable diseases." Rosenau did not limit his instructional materials to the lectern, black-

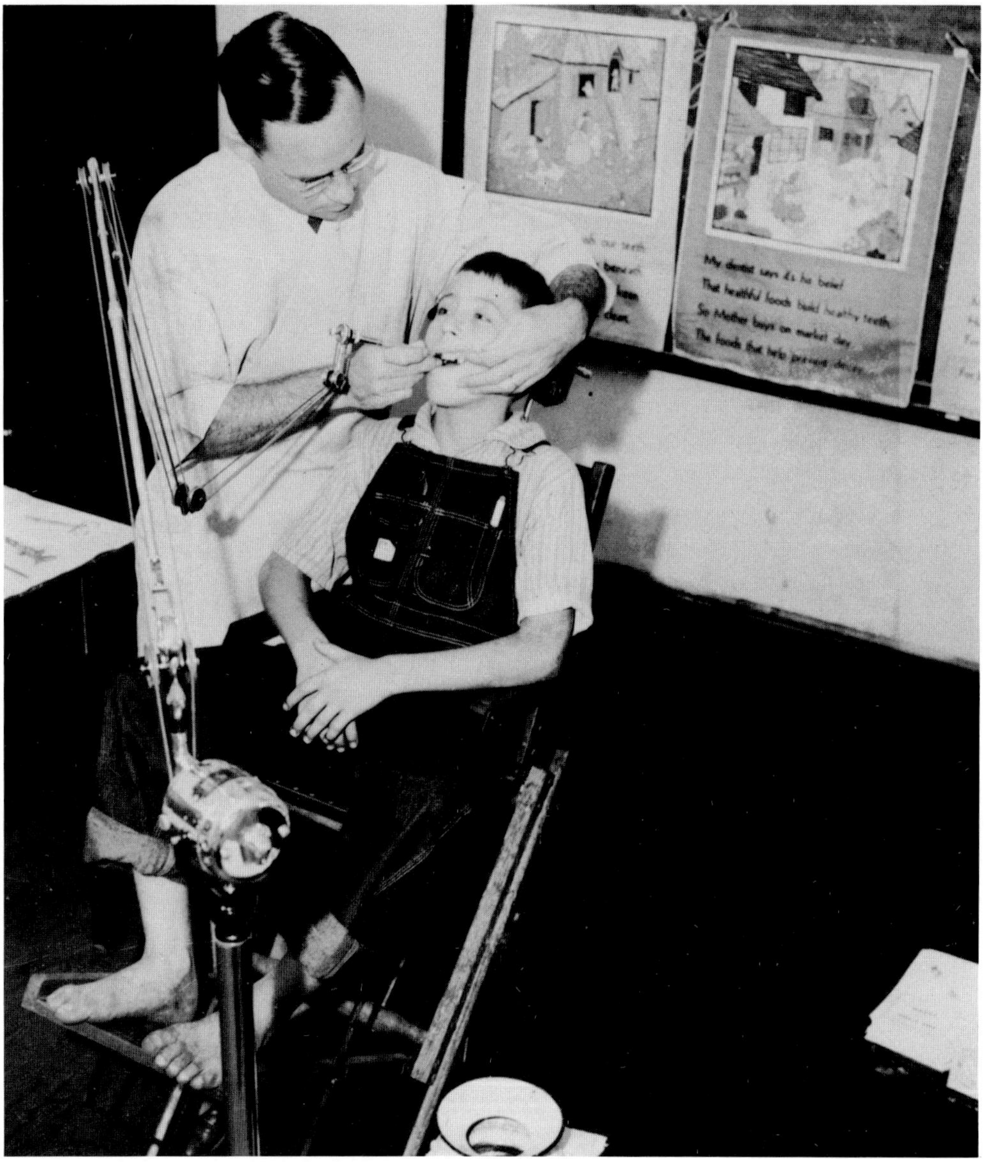

Among the early successes of the division was a summer short course in public health dentistry in 1936. The State Board of Health had initiated an oral hygiene program in public schools in 1918, and over the years the program had enjoyed great success. In 1937, the board had seventeen dentists on the staff, who spent their time in the public schools of North Carolina teaching oral hygiene, examining the mouths of school children, giving treatment to those who could not afford to consult a private dentist, and referring others to their family dentist. Unfortunately, the lack of funds prevented the continuation of the summer short course after a few years.

board, and textbook. The students staged a mock courtroom trial to demonstrate their knowledge of the social dimensions of disease control. Dr. Rosenau presided, dressed up in his black robe and wig. "It was a remarkable course," Petty recalled. "We thoroughly enjoyed it."[9]

Despite Rosenau's occasional clowning, the program proved quite rigorous. "Dr. Baity told us that the course they had at Harvard, a nine-month course with a thesis, was a master of public health; without a thesis it was a certificate of public health," one student remembered. "Basically [Chapel Hill] tried to jam nine months of class work without a thesis into three months. We went to school all day, five and a half days a week." The faculty realized the program was too intensive and discussed the possibility of starting a nine-month course. Baity and Rosenau favored the plan, but State Health Officer Carl Reynolds protested, saying it would be too difficult for health departments to send people for that length of time.[10]

Dr. Rosenau initially found office space in Caldwell Hall, home of the Medical School, but the influx of faculty and students into public health quickly depleted available space. Medical School Dean Charles Mangum persuaded President Graham to ask the state legislature for funds for a new building. The legislature appropriated $226,000 in 1937, but that fell far short of the amount needed. Graham then asked a committee to prepare a proposal for the Public Works Administration (PWA). Funds had dried up for PWA projects, but Graham thought that the federal government's "interest in medical science and public health" might persuade the agency.[11]

The committee's proposal to the PWA highlighted the South's acute health needs. Among these were the nation's highest infant and maternal death rates, as well as "shameful morbidity and mortality rates due to nutritional deficiencies." The proposal also pointed to the university's many efforts to eradicate these problems: the Institute for Research in Social Sciences, a division of social work and public welfare, and a division of public health. The lack of a proper building to house the Medical School and Division of Public Health, the proposal concluded, handicapped the functioning and expansion of both programs.[12]

Members of the university community used their considerable influence in Washington to speed along the review process and ultimately win approval for the proposal. H. G. Baity first wrote to Raymond Rosenberger, a friend on the PWA staff and a Chapel Hill alumnus,

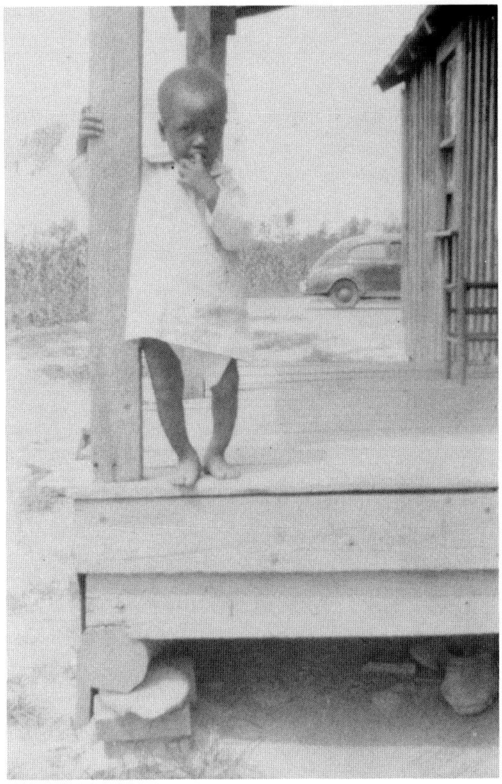

A child suffering from rickets, one of the many nutritional diseases afflicting southerners in the 1930s and 1940s.

asking him to "assume the personal responsibility of steering this application through the proper examining channels." Once the PWA staff passed on the application, the "next battle [was] to secure an allotment of funds." Baity wrote to Dr. Rosenau suggesting he contact friends in the Public Health Service, such as Surgeon General Thomas Parran. "Since the greatest social appeal can be made in the name of public health," Baity said, "such expression would have the greatest weight with the allocating agency." These efforts apparently paid off, for Parran wrote a strong letter on behalf of the application and it won approval.[13]

Rosenau achieved much in his first two years at Chapel Hill. The university remained a strong moral, if not financial, supporter of the program. Under Title VI of the Social Security Act, the Public Health Service continued to provide a substantial portion of the division's money. The students seemed enthusiastic about their classes. But public health remained a poor cousin to its academic neighbors, and the North Carolina program paled in comparison to its counterparts at Harvard and The Johns Hopkins. Short courses for public health practitioners were valuable endeavors, but until the division could begin granting advanced degrees, its scope remained limited and the enterprise lacked a secure future. Rosenau sought to remedy that situation by asking the administration to allow the division to confer baccalaureate, master's, and doctoral degrees in addition to certificates. The Graduate School

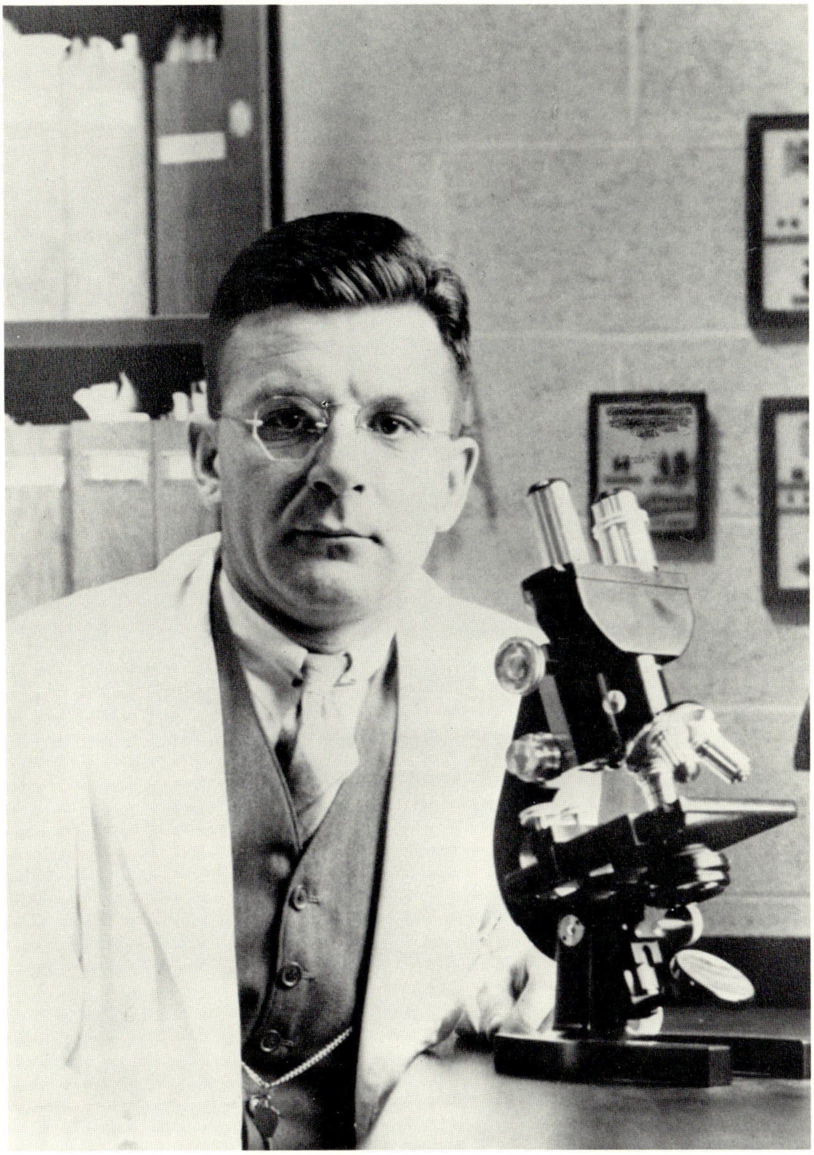

Dr. Harold Brown joined the faculty in 1937 and served as dean of the school from 1941–43.

"[It] looks as though we are developing into a real School of Public Health. That's the dream and I believe before long [it] will be a fait accompli."

M. J. Rosenau

approved the move, and the university administration acknowledged that approval as the first step in creating an independent School of Public Health.[14]

Continued support from the General Assembly and President Graham allowed Rosenau to expand his staff. Dr. Harold Brown joined the faculty in September, 1937, with probably the most impressive academic credentials of anyone in the field of public health. John Larsh, who came later to Chapel Hill to work with Brown, explained. "He had more degrees than anyone I ever knew. He had a bachelor's and a master's and took his doctorate in science at Hopkins just as I did. He went from Hopkins to Vanderbilt, teaching parasitology [while] he got his M.D. Later he went to Harvard and got a Doctor of Public Health. He was about thirty-five years old before he got his first job, down here." Harold Gotaas joined the Department of Sanitary Engineering that same year, and a year later John William Roy Norton came on board as professor of public health administration. With the addition of these men, Rosenau felt more hopeful about the future of the enter-

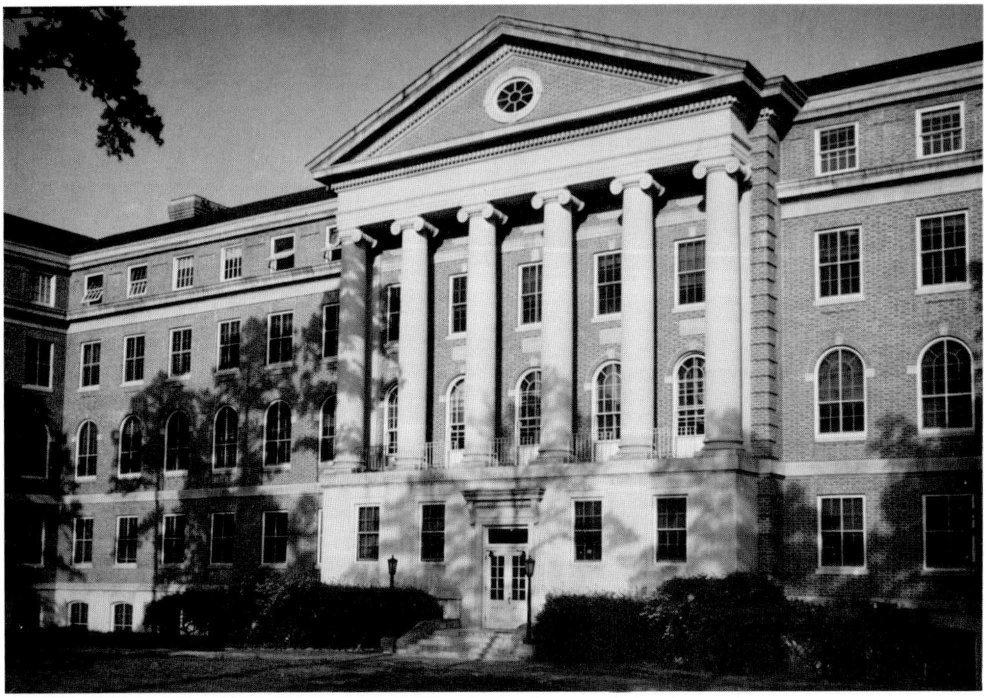

The Medical and Public Health Building (later named MacNider Hall)

prise in Chapel Hill. "[I]t looks as though we are developing into a real School of Public Health. That's the dream and I believe before long [it] will be a fait accompli."[15]

The 1939–40 academic year marked a watershed for public health at Chapel Hill. "We are testing fate on a higher level," Rosenau observed. First, the division moved into the new Medical and Public Health Building (now MacNider Hall). The "fine new building with shiny streamlined equipment" greatly impressed Dr. William A. McIntosh of the Rockefeller Foundation. "A model of architectural design," he noted. "Everyone who went through the building seemed to be impressed with the fact that much had been realized for the moderate cost involved both as to

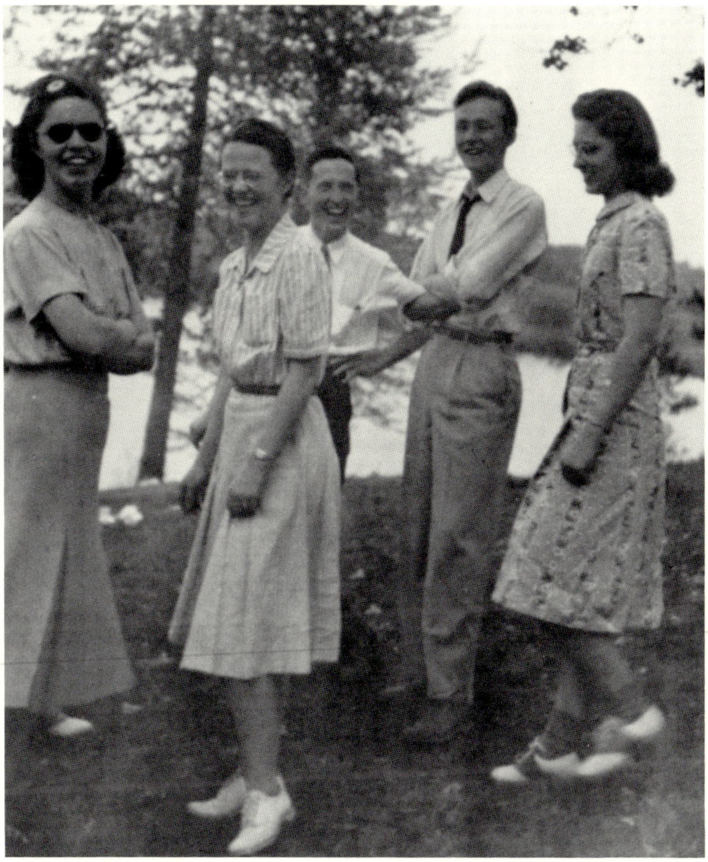

Center, Bailey Webb, Gene Cornatzer, and Bill Taylor, students in biochemistry. For many years public health had a strong presence in the Medical School. Harold Brown and later John Larsh taught parasitology to students at UNC and Duke.

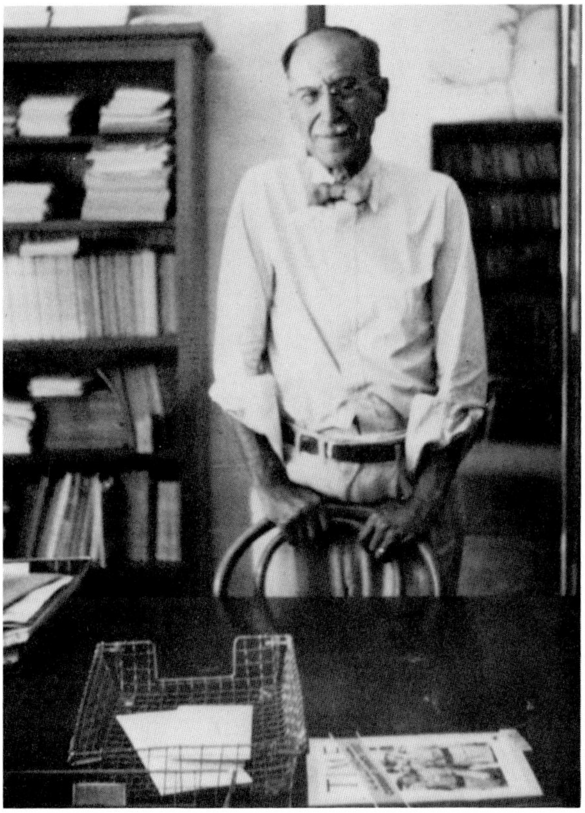

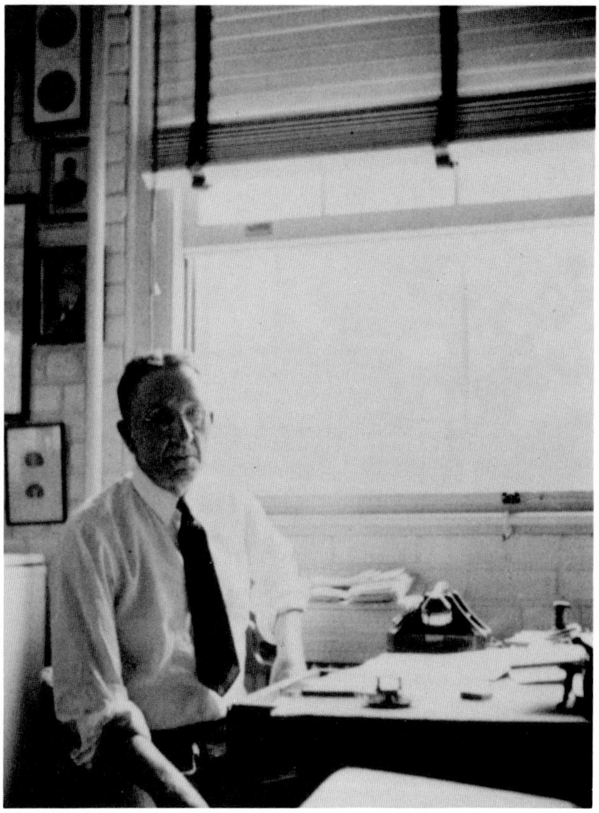

Disagreements between Dr. Rosenau *(left)* and Dr. MacNider *(right)* contributed to the creation of an independent School of Public Health.

the structure itself and its equipment." The division also offered the last short course that fall—"the last of the kindergarten stage," Rosenau remarked. Having been accepted into the graduate school, the division redesigned its curriculum and admitted fourteen graduate students.[16]

Emil Chanlett entered the master's program in sanitary engineering that year. He divided his time between chemistry and engineering courses on campus (some of the former engineering professors still taught in the math department) and public health courses in the new building. In those days the distance between the two parts of campus seemed imposing. The Medical and Public Health Building "stood out there by itself," Chanlett remembered, "almost like a monument. It was considered to be far away from the rest of the campus." Classroom and laboratory work consumed most of the students' time, but Chanlett and Buster Horton, along with two graduate students in parasitology, Bill Taylor and Thomas Brooks, managed to play handball every day and get over to Kenan Stadium for Saturday football games.[17]

A number of factors contributed to the decision to upgrade the Division of Public Health to a school in 1940, but most important was the public health profession's desire for independence. The General Education Board report that led to the founding of The Johns Hopkins School of Hygiene and Public Health in 1916 contained a strong recommendation that public health programs remain independent from medical schools, with their own faculties and budgets. The independent program at The Hopkins became the standard for other programs. During Rosenau's years at Harvard, medicine and public health were closely associated, with the Medical School being the more dominant power. The small size of the initial endeavor at Chapel Hill prevented the formation of a school on the model of The Hopkins, but Rosenau's strong personality and Dean Mangum's commitment to the program made for a healthy relationship. As the division grew, however, problems emerged. The new dean of the Medical School, William deB. MacNider, became impatient with what he saw as a conflict between the relative autonomy of the Division of Public Health and his responsibilities as dean. Rosenau and MacNider maintained a formal cordiality, but privately they did not see eye to eye on matters relating to the division. Finally, in the spring of 1940, the public health faculty petitioned President Graham for a change in the status of the Division of Public Health to the School of Public Health. Graham and the Board of Trustees approved the petition on June 7, 1940.[18]

The school also launched its first major research project at that time. Venereal disease had always been a major concern of public health officials. But society's unwillingness to separate medical issues from moral concerns prevented significant progress in eradicating the disease. The campaign against VD received a major boost in 1936 with President Roosevelt's appointment of Thomas Parran, Jr., as surgeon general. As former chief of the Public Health Service's Venereal Disease Division and most recently New York state health commissioner, Parran advocated public discussion of VD. The publication of Parran's *Shadow on the Land*, his identification of VD as the nation's number one health problem, the passage of the National Venereal Disease Control Act—all these helped change public attitudes and generate a commitment to bringing the problem under control.[19]

In this climate of increased national concern, the Z. Smith Reynolds Foundation announced in December, 1937, that income from its $7 million endowment would go to the North Carolina State Board of Health

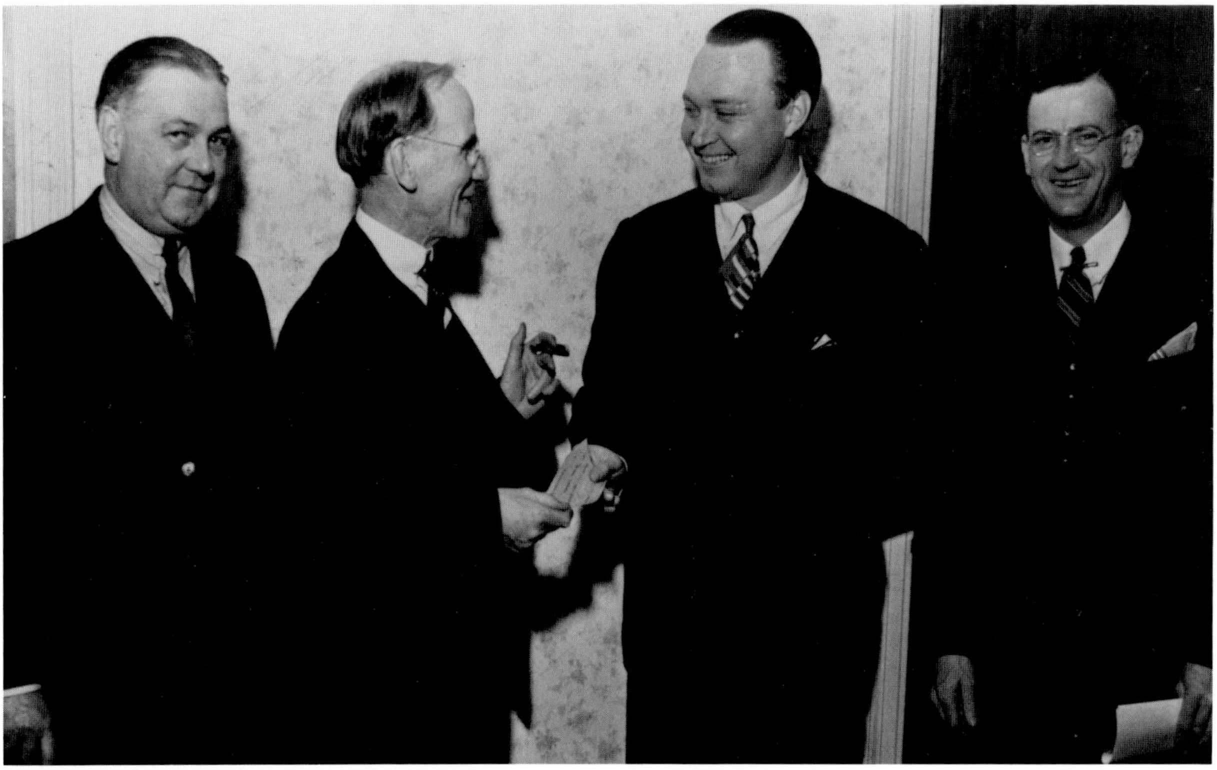

Dr. Carl Reynolds accepting from Richard Reynolds a check that established a major venereal disease control program in North Carolina.

to develop a VD control program. Z. Smith Reynolds, the youngest son of Winston-Salem tobacco manufacturer R. J. Reynolds, had died mysteriously in 1933, and his siblings established the foundation as a memorial. Mary Reynolds Babcock, Smith's sister, had strong ties to the American Social Hygiene Association, and she apparently directed the foundation's interest toward VD. The $100,000 the foundation allocated in the first year provided the stimulus for a campaign by the State Board of Health that lasted through 1946.[20]

The school's involvement in the campaign began a few years later when the State Board of Health allocated $17,500 for a professor of syphilogy and a staff to conduct research on venereal diseases. The school conducted a national search and selected Dr. William A. Fleming for the professorship. With a B.A. and M.D. from Vanderbilt University, where his father was a well-known southern historian, Fleming had gone on to The Johns Hopkins to study and conduct research on syphilis.[21]

Shortly after Fleming came on board, the Rockefeller Foundation contributed additional funds for a major epidemiological study of VD. The school selected Dr. John Wright, an M.D. from Vanderbilt University and a recent M.P.H. from The Johns Hopkins, to head the project. Initially the study targeted the Orange-Person-Chatham County Health District, but Wright soon realized the need to include a more urban area and added the Durham City-County Health Department. The project's goals included establishing the prevalence of syphilis in the area, gathering data to determine incident rates and trends, identifying the contacts of infected people, and developing programs to treat the afflicted. Wright and his staff used a number of innovative techniques. They collected data from a variety of sources and entered it on McBee keysort cards for analysis, the first application of computer technology at the school. Film strips provided an alternative method of instruction for patients, and recordings of nurse-patient interviews helped train public health nurses.[22]

These efforts to control and eradicate VD increased the demand for public health nurses and soon led to the establishment of the Department of Public Health Nursing. Nurses played a key role in the delivery of health care to the public, but from the beginning they had been excluded from schools of public health. Nurses in North Carolina expressed great interest in public health training when the division opened in 1936, and the North Carolina State Nurses' Association asked the university to develop a program in public health nursing. Rosenau

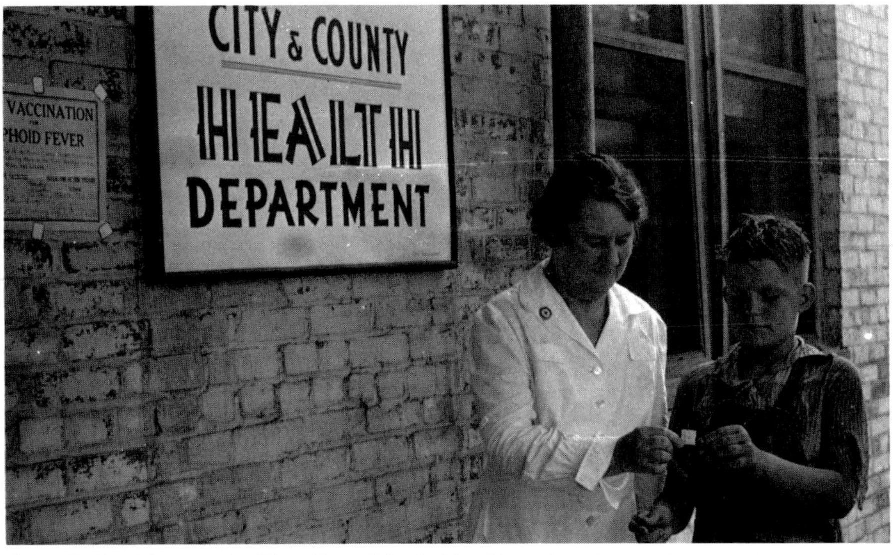

A public health nurse in New Bern, North Carolina, gives instructions on ways to eradicate rats.

recognized the need for such a program but said he lacked the personnel and resources to make it possible. By 1940 the addition of new faculty and the support of the State Board of Health changed all that.[23]

In that year State Health Officer Carl Reynolds requested an outline for a course in public health nursing. The School of Public Health submitted a plan that drew on existing faculty and called for the addition of two professors. Reynolds sent the proposal to the Public Health Service and the Children's Bureau, a branch of the U. S. Department of Labor that served as an advocate for the needs of children and mothers. Both agencies responded favorably. "We believe that training for public health nursing should be an integral part of a School of Public Health and with our setup we have an opportunity to establish this useful enterprise on a plane that will be without peer anywhere," wrote Rosenau. "There is at present a dearth of trained nurses for public health service, and a career in this field opens a new frontier for which there will be a growing and continuing demand."[24]

Among the people suggested to head a Department of Public Health Nursing was Ruth Hay, then on the faculty of the University of California at Berkeley. Writing to Dr. Rosenau, she expressed great interest in the possibilities at Chapel Hill. "The inclusion of training of all public health personnel in one school," she wrote, "is a plan that I have considered for some time as an ideal set-up." Rosenau offered her the job. Ruth Hay brought many years of experience as a teacher and a practicing public health nurse to the job at Chapel Hill. A native of Ohio, she received her B.A. from Ohio Wesleyan University and her M.S. from Western Reserve. Since 1931 she had taught public health nursing at Vanderbilt, Western Reserve, and at Berkeley. She recommended a colleague from Berkeley, Margaret Blee, to fill the other position in the department.[25]

In 1942 the presence of a well-qualified educator provided the stimulus for a second new program. In the fall of 1941, Dr. Lucy S. Morgan, a health educator with the Public Health Service, joined the staff of the State Board of Health as part of a "lend-lease program." The daughter of Harcourt A. Morgan, a former president of the University of Tennessee and at the time chairman of the Board of Directors of the Tennessee Valley Authority, Lucy Morgan possessed a keen awareness of the health problems of the South and a great deal of experience in addressing them. Before receiving her Ph.D. in public health from Yale

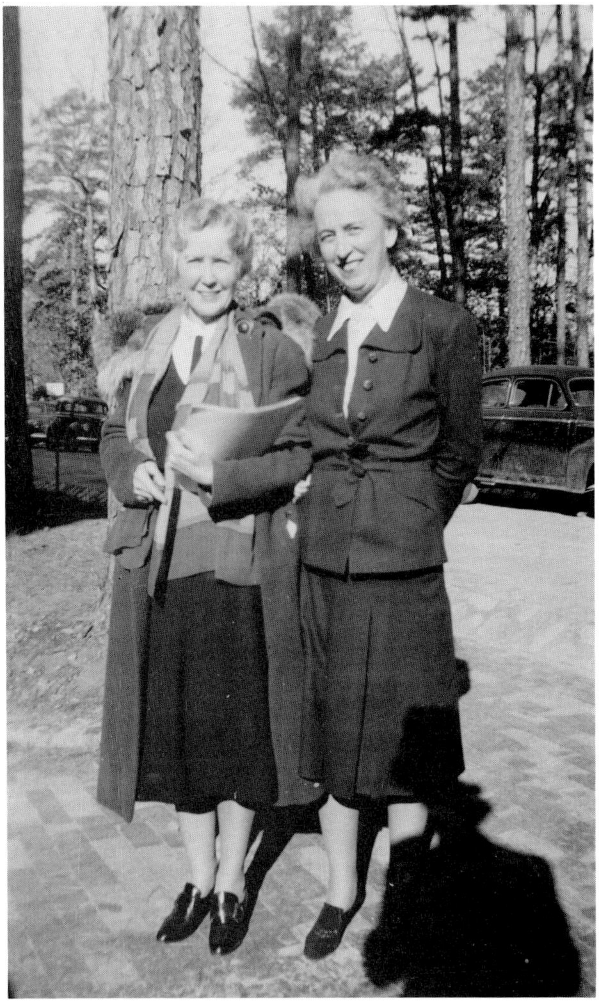

Ruth Hay and Margaret Blee shortly after they began teaching at Chapel Hill.

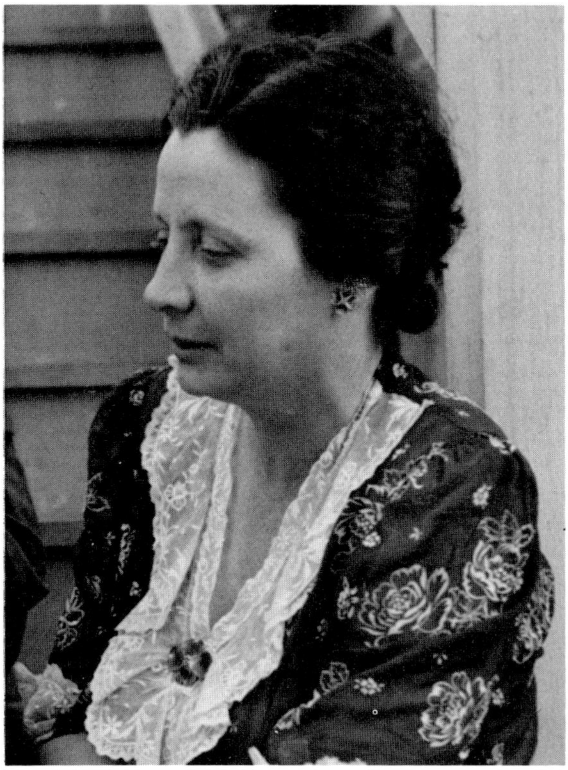

Dr. Lucy Shields Morgan

in 1938, Morgan taught school and worked as a health educator in Tennessee. After graduating, she developed a community health education program for the city of Hartford, Connecticut.[26]

Morgan joined the Public Health Service in 1941, which immediately "loaned" her to the North Carolina State Board of Health. State Health Officer Carl Reynolds assigned Dr. Morgan to the Cumberland County Health Department in Fayetteville with specific instructions to counter the increase of prostitution around Ft. Bragg. Wartime created numerous health problems for towns near military bases. There were housing shortages, a constant coming and going of civilians and soldiers, and an upsurge in venereal disease. Dr. Morgan applied imaginative community-organizing techniques to public and private health problems. By working through local black and white women's groups and relating the educational program to the war effort, she helped rally the com-

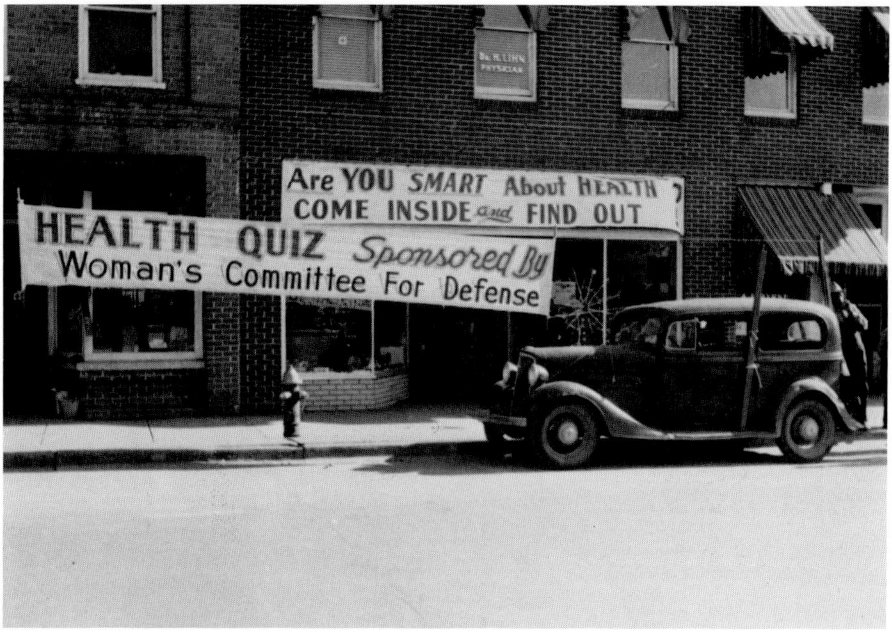
Are YOU SMART About HEALTH ?
COME INSIDE and FIND OUT
HEALTH QUIZ Sponsored By
Woman's Committee For Defense

Campaigns designed by health educators in North Carolina on loan from the Public Health Service.

munity around issues such as nutrition, venereal disease, sanitation, and tuberculosis.[27]

Soon more Public Health Service educators arrived in North Carolina, and similar programs developed in other cities. The success of these health educators spurred Dr. Reynolds to ask the School of Public Health to train some North Carolinians. The State Board of Health offered fellowships to three young women, and in the fall of 1942 they enrolled at Chapel Hill. At the same time, Dr. Rosenau requested the services of Dr. Morgan to develop a curriculum in health education and assist with the instruction of students. "We have already made a modest start in Public Health Education," Harold Brown wrote in requesting a faculty appointment for Lucy Morgan, "but this can be greatly augmented and made outstanding by a person of Dr. Morgan's ability and experience."[28]

Lucy Morgan produced a whirlwind of activity wherever she went. Thanks to twenty scholarships from the W. K. Kellogg Foundation, the first class of public health educators had twenty-five students in the spring of 1943. Morgan immediately put the students to work, with courses ranging from malariology to public speaking. Like nursing, health education had a somewhat experimental curriculum for the first few years. For instance, Dr. Morgan initially planned field training for the summer months, only to discover that vacations and the weather prevented quality interaction between the students and local practitioners. The next year the students took their training in the spring and spent the summer taking courses in Chapel Hill. Dr. Morgan did not limit the students' education to classroom instruction and field training. She

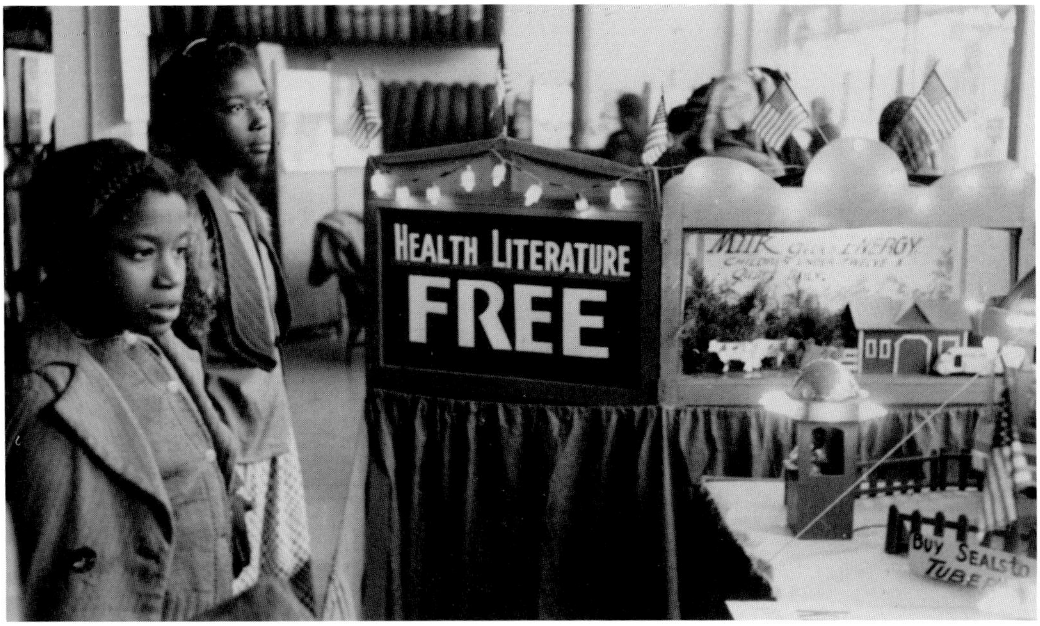

instituted a speakers series that brought in some of the most respected people in the field of public health.[29]

The addition of departments of public health nursing and education had not been part of Dr. Rosenau's original plan for the school. Like the men who guided the schools at The Johns Hopkins and Harvard, he envisioned a more scientific orientation for the program at Chapel Hill. But like so much that happened over the next fifty years at the school, demand for the service and the availability of resources brought about unintended change. The two new departments set a pattern for the future in another way as well: like most of the practice-oriented disciplines that would eventually be included in the curriculum, public health nursing and public health education were dominated by women. Dr. Margery Lord had broken the gender barrier as a student in 1940, and the presence of Ruth Hay, Margaret Blee, Lucy Morgan, and in 1945 Eunice Tyler made the school a unique enclave of female academics on the Chapel Hill campus.

Relationships with faculty at the university proved difficult for the pioneer women. "They thought next to nothing of women, " Lucy Morgan remembered, "and when we first got here, we weren't allowed to join the faculty club [even though] the only thing they did was go to the Carolina Inn for lunch and maybe they told jokes they thought we couldn't hear." In discussions with early civil rights groups Morgan used to pull out her Men's Faculty Club card—after they let women join—as proof that she belonged to "the most discriminated group in the world—women." "Even at Chapel Hill," she would add, "that great liberal institution." The situation at the school, however, proved quite

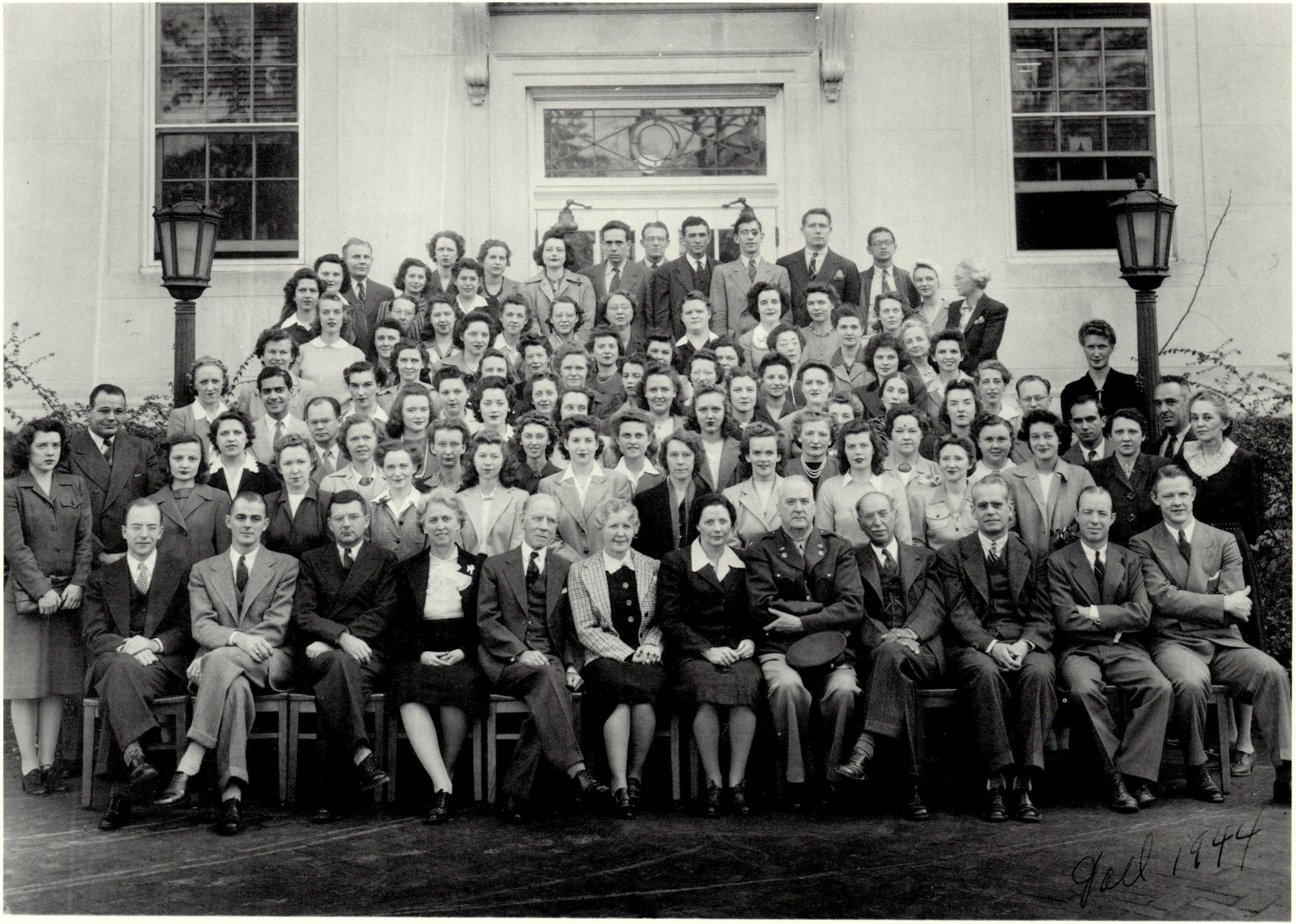

The faculty and student body in the fall of 1944. Women students in public health education and public health nursing helped keep the school afloat during World War II.

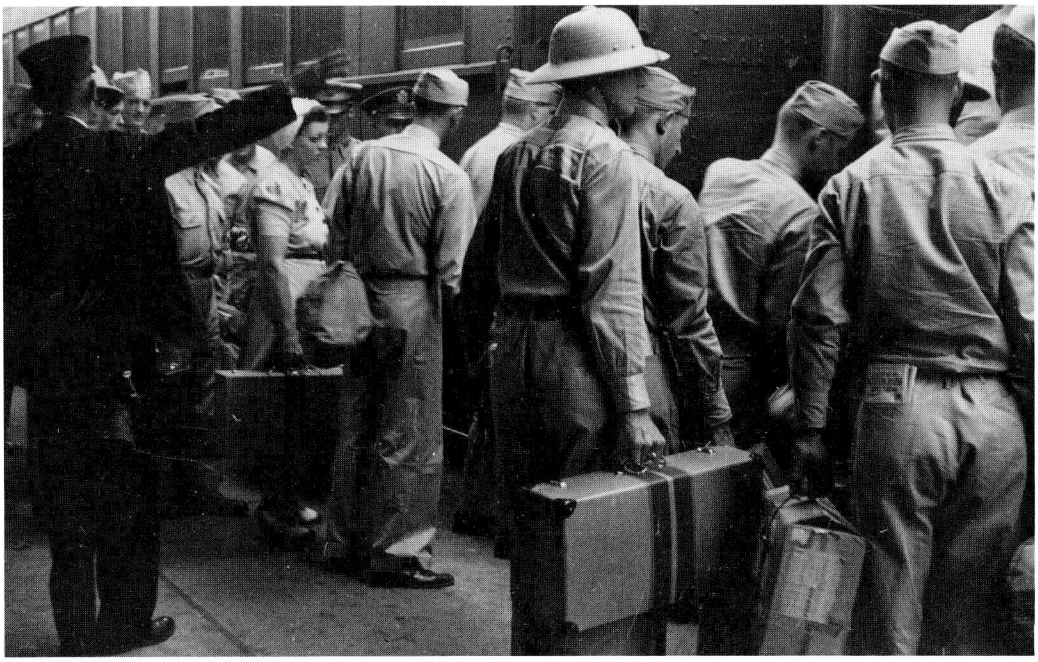

Troop departures in Fayetteville in 1942.

different. “There was no question with Rosenau [and later McGavran] about women,” Morgan remembered. “We would gather in Dr. Rosenau’s office and we would just talk over whatever it was. [Women] were treated exactly alike, your opinions were asked. We had a democratic institution.”[30]

Despite the success of nursing and health education, World War II imposed severe hardships on the school. The armed forces and the Public Health Service needed men and women with public health experience, so fewer people applied to the graduate programs. In addition, certain members of the faculty felt they could contribute most to the war effort by working outside the university. H. G. Baity spent part of the war in Brazil working for the Institute of Inter-American Affairs (the predecessor of the Agency for International Development), Harold Gotaas joined the same organization in Washington in 1942, and Roy Norton left for the army.

Determined not to let the school founder, Rosenau began looking for students to fill the classes. He was aided in this effort by Dr. Harold Brown, who was appointed dean of the school in 1941. The armed forces provided one obvious source of students, and the School of Public Health instituted short-term training for military men and women. The university also authorized the school to allow undergraduates with certain prerequisites to take their fourth year at the school and receive a B.S. in Public Health. Upon entering the armed forces, these graduates could be assigned to public health work. Short courses for public health nurses, dentists, sanitarians, and health educators filled out the schedule.[31]

During the war, the School of Public Health also began receiving students from outside the United States. The International Health Division of the Rockefeller Foundation, the Commonwealth Fund, and the Pan American Sanitary Bureau each made scholarships available, primarily for students in sanitary engineering. Luis Mantilla from Lima, Peru, and Tarik Bilginer from Istanbul, Turkey, were the first students on Rockefeller fellowships to attend.

Over the next two decades, hundreds of foreign students would take classes and receive degrees from the school. Virtually all of the faculty during that time would serve as consultants to health agencies in developing countries. Dr. Harold Gotaas, former faculty member at the school and later president of the Institute of Inter-American Affairs, offered an explanation for this development, which put the public health movement at the forefront of American expansion in the postwar world:

> The activities of the Inter-American Cooperative health program directed toward the control and reduction of infectious diseases and toward the elevation of health standards in the hemisphere serve in the interest of economic and efficient development of resources. With this development will come purchasing power and a higher standard of living which are necessary bases for the extension of trade and the support of commerce.
>
> Cooperative public health had already proven an efficient means for cementing friendship, understanding, and cooperation in the hemisphere. It is believed that public health will continue to develop as an instrument of neighborly friendship and for the demonstration and preservation of the democratic way of life.[32]

The comings and goings of faculty and students became commonplace during the war. Samuel Hopper and Brewster Snow taught sanitary engineering for a period. Dr. John Larsh joined the faculty in 1943. But the most unsettling departure was that of Dr. Harold Brown, who resigned as dean to go to Columbia University. Rosenau had groomed Brown as his replacement, and with Brown's promotion to the deanship everything seemed to be in place. But the New York school offered more money and better research facilities. Rosenau reclaimed the title of dean, but the search began almost immediately for a replacement.

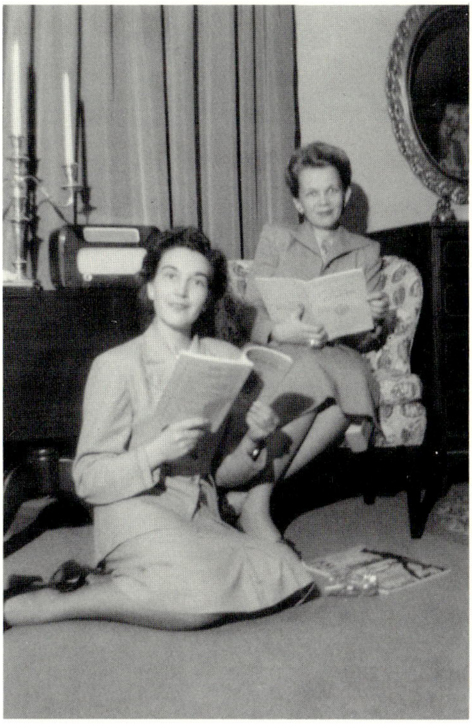

Elizabeth L. McMahan (*left*) and A. Helen Martikainen (*right*) at a journal club meeting. McMahan was a student and later a faculty member of the Department of Public Health Education. Martikainen was director of Health Education for the State Board of Health before becoming the first chief of health education for WHO.

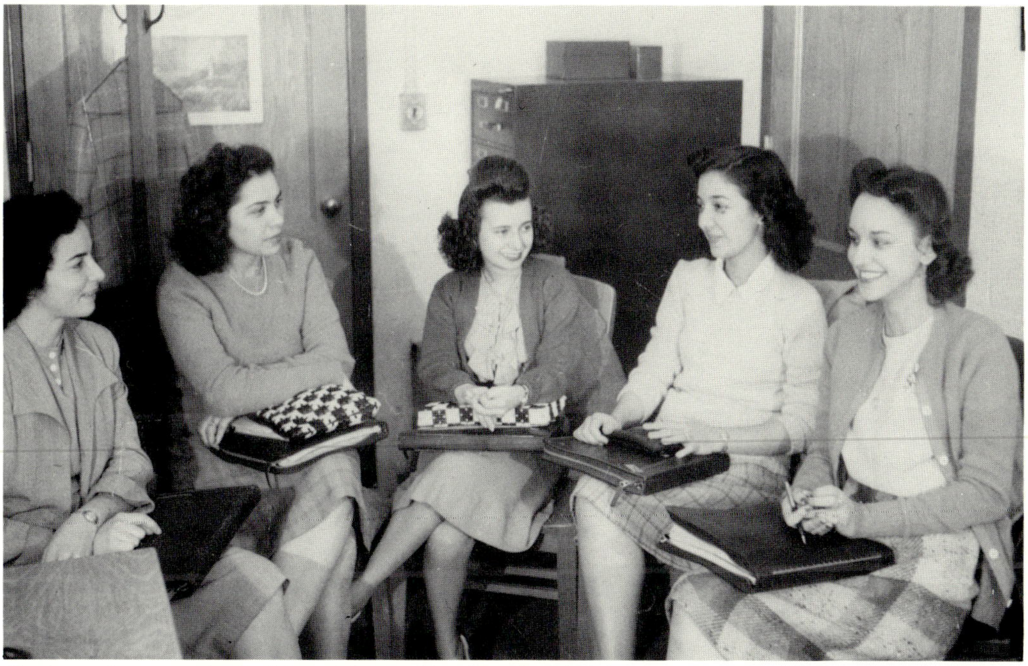

Students from outside the United States, like these health educators from Puerto Rico, became commonplace at the school during the 1940s.

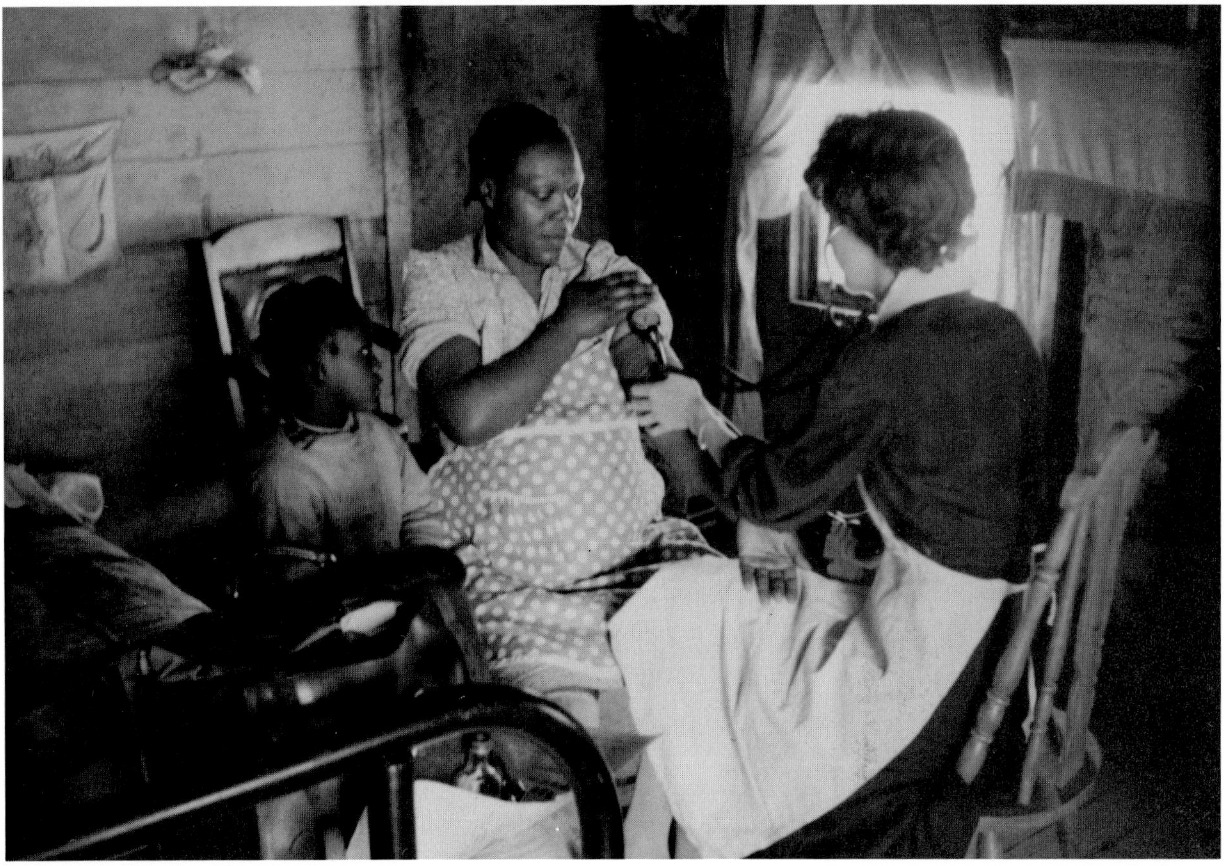

A public health nurse visits the home of a family in South Carolina in the 1940s. Training these front-line practitioners was an important part of the School of Public Health's mission in the 1940s.

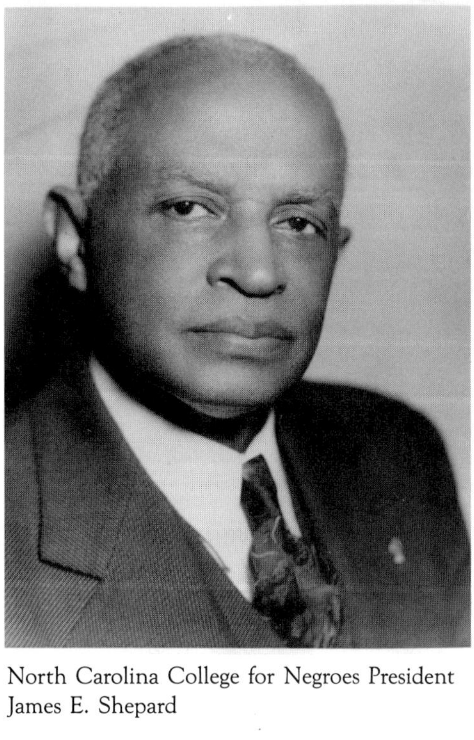

North Carolina College for Negroes President James E. Shepard

Chapter 3

DOCTORS OF THE BODY POLITIC

The prospect of peace buoyed the spirits at the school during the spring and summer of 1945, and the staff began looking expectantly toward the future. Dr. Rosenau expressed that enthusiasm upon his return for the fall semester. "I am just back after a bully vacation," he wrote a friend, "and I am in a hot spot trying to hold down the lid. Our school is booming and prospects are glamorous."[1]

The world had changed dramatically during the previous four years. Fascist movements in Germany, Japan, and Italy had been defeated; the Soviet Union had become a world power; and the nineteenth-century colonial empire had come apart. The United States had emerged from the war virtually unscathed, determined to play a leading role in world affairs. The United Nations had been created, along with agencies such as UNESCO, UNICEF, and WHO.

On the home front, the federal government assumed unprecedented responsibility for the social and economic life of the country. In public health the pendulum swung even further away from private funding, as the Public Health Service took over many of the functions once performed by philanthropy. Congress considered legislation on national health insurance and federal support for the nation's hospitals. In North Carolina, medical educators and politicians debated the merits of a four-year medical school at Chapel Hill and an expanded system of hospitals for the state.

The School of Public Health's first postwar initiative involved the creation of a Department of Health Education at the North Carolina College for Negroes (NCC) in nearby Durham. Chartered in 1910 as the National Religious Training School and Chautauqua under the leadership of Dr. James E. Shepard, NCC had become one of the nation's outstanding black colleges by the 1940s. After meeting Dr. Rosenau, Shepard wrote the General Education Board about the need for "trained health personnel. . . for the Negro people" and his idea for establishing a school of public health for blacks at NCC. The board took preliminary steps in that direction by supporting a summer institute for teachers and health workers and later establishing a student health service at the college. But Shepard pressed for at least a graduate program in health education. Finally, with Rosenau's support, Dr. Lucy Morgan agreed to assess the feasibility of such a program.[2]

When the Mississippi State Board of Health asked the School of Public Health to train eight black students in 1945, Shepard and Rosenau decided to go ahead with the program at NCC. A curriculum modeled after the one at Chapel Hill quickly took shape, with UNC professors providing the instruction. "They were willing to teach," Lucy Morgan remembered, "and it paid nothing but a pittance, but they went over

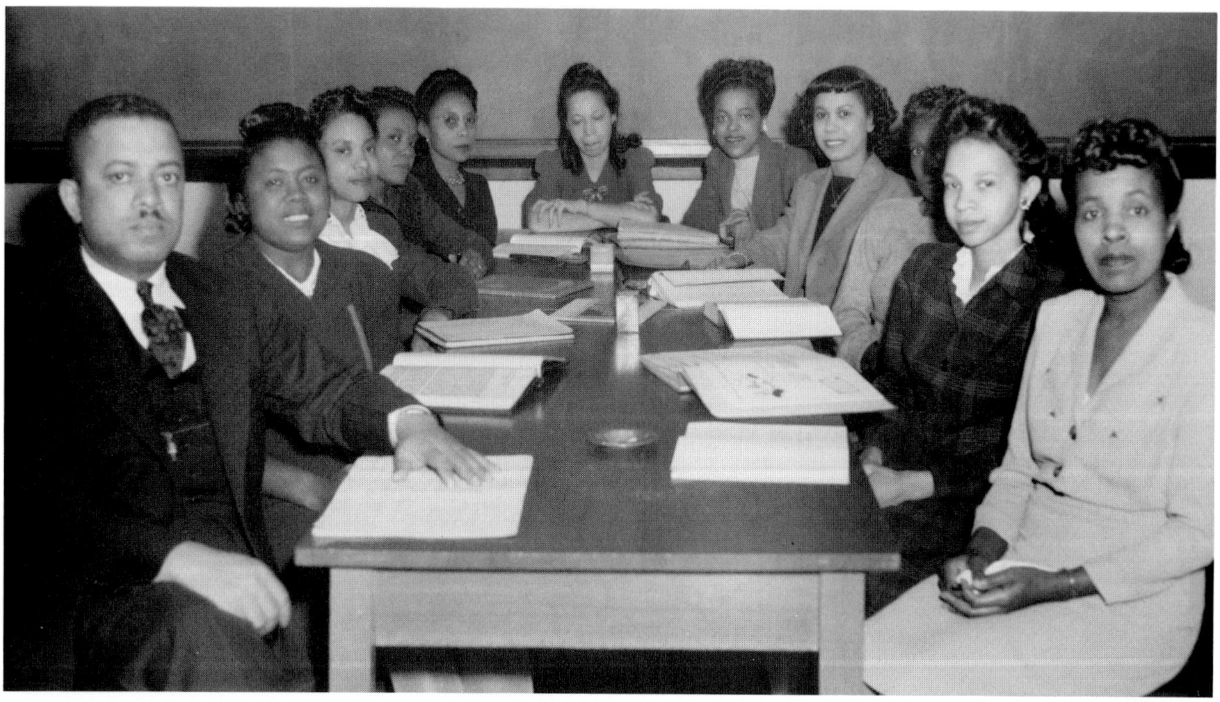

The first public health education class, North Carolina College for Negroes, 1945–46.

and taught the same classes that they did at Chapel Hill." John Larsh, for instance, taught his introductory course, "Parasitism in Human Disease." "They were very good students," he recalled. "Howard Barnhill, [Howard] Fitts, were very eager." Gradually students trained at NCC took over some of the teaching responsibilities.[3]

The Department of Public Health Nursing assisted in a similar program beginning in 1946. North Carolina College had a nursing program, so Ruth Hay and Margaret Blee served as consultants and taught courses in public health nursing. The program continued until 1956, and Chapel Hill professors taught a course in public health nursing at NCC until 1963.[4]

Dr. E. W. McHenry of the School of Hygiene at the University of Toronto visited a class at NCC in the spring of 1946. "The ten persons in the class," he reported, "gave a very fine impression. . . . This project to provide well-trained health educators is one of the most hopeful undertakings I have seen in the South."[5]

The black community certainly needed health educators, as well as doctors, hospitals, and health facilities of all kinds. Life expectancy was much lower for blacks than whites, and infant mortality rates were much higher. Nutritional problems abounded. The over one hundred health educators trained at NCC between 1945 and 1960 could not negate the years of neglect. But the lessons they learned and applied in their local communities helped gradually to improve the health status of the black population.[6]

The program at NCC was a progressive step in other ways. Jim Crow still reigned in the South, even in Chapel Hill, the bastion of southern progressivism. There was little effort on the part of the university or its faculty to reach out to blacks. "Public health was upsetting the hell out of everything," John Larsh remembered. "Those people in South Building [the university administration], they couldn't understand. You weren't supposed to do things like that. It was frowned upon. But in public health we've always believed in helping people, and training people to get out there and do things, and you don't do that by being very conservative."[7]

In addition to providing the students with classroom opportunities NCC could not afford, the UNC-NCC Department of Public Health Education promoted interracial cooperation on a limited scale. Lucy

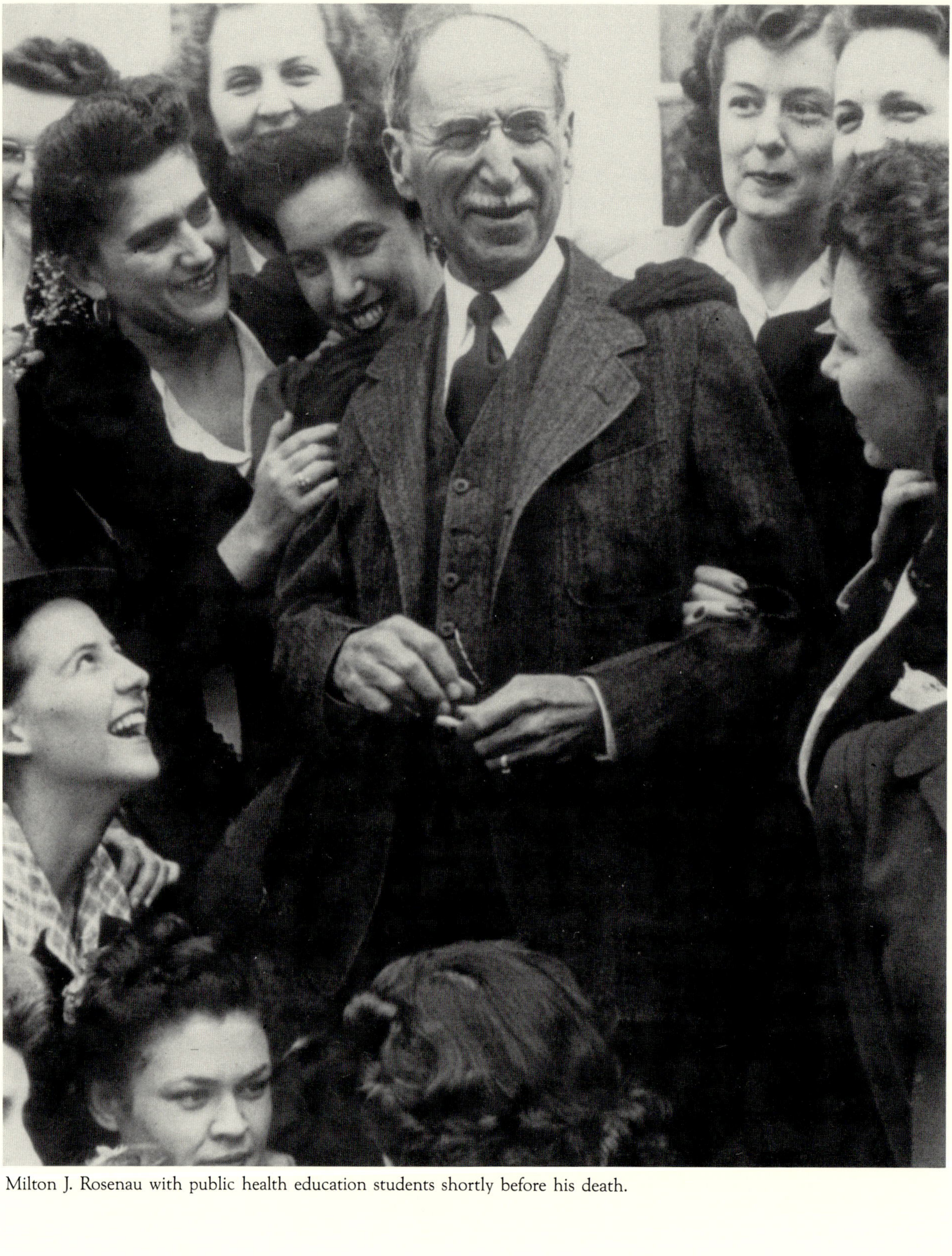

Milton J. Rosenau with public health education students shortly before his death.

Morgan recounted the efforts to bring black and white students together. "They had to be introduced to each other. They had never done that before. What we did was to have a journal club, and we met first over there [Durham] and then over at Chapel Hill. At that time you were not supposed to eat with blacks. So we always had refreshments at the meetings. We sent them together to the field, and then we had open houses when the people came in from the field, black and white together. Then it got bitter for a while, and we used to pull down the shades sometimes when we had meetings in Chapel Hill."[8]

Operating within the framework of "separate but equal," these efforts by public health educators highlighted the absurdity of the Jim Crow system. Yet at the same time the program's existence shored up a segregated system of higher education that remained blatantly unequal. For fifteen years NCC maintained a separate program. Only in 1960, as the civil rights movement pressed for an end to segregation, did the School of Public Health admit its first black students.

As the school began tackling some of the many health problems that faced the South in the postwar period, it lost its founding director. On April 9, 1946, at the age of seventy-six, Dr. Rosenau suffered a heart attack and died. In some respects Rosenau died at the height of his career. Only the year before, he had been elected president of the American Public Health Association, the final (and long overdue) tribute to one of the great leaders of the public health movement. Dr. Rosemary Kent, a student in Rosenau's last class and later a professor at the school, recalled the dean's last day in the classroom.

> Probably, short of construction blasts, nothing has ever rocked the building across the street [MacNider Building] as did the unaccustomed applause from the auditorium the day Rosenau closed the course in epidemiology in December 1945. On, on and on it thundered and rolled. Overcome at last, Dr. Rosenau turned to the stairs at the front of the room and slowly, quietly started down the long two flights to his office. And still the applause followed him every step of the way and could be heard by the staff on the ground floor. Only then, with damp eyes, did the class depart.... He knew, as did somehow the students upstairs, that he had just delivered his valedictory.[9]

Rosenau's death created many problems for the school and exposed the fragility of the enterprise. Still, the transition had been expected.

When Harold Brown resigned as dean in 1943, Rosenau had begun searching for a suitable replacement. He and Frank Graham seriously wooed General James S. Simmons, chief of preventive medicine in the office of the surgeon general. A native North Carolinian, Simmons liked the idea of moving to Chapel Hill but felt he was too old to set to work at a school that lacked financial security. Harvard also desired his services, and that school's endowment and the promise of more Rockefeller money enticed him to Cambridge.[10]

After Rosenau's death, John Wright and H. G. Baity assumed responsibility for running the school and looking for a new dean. But in the meantime there was much work to be done. Returning soldiers filled the classrooms, and replacements had to be found for the staff members who did not return after the war.

The school's first major step in the postwar period involved the establishment of a Department of Nutrition. Dr. Rosenau had begun the plans shortly before his death. "It is scarcely an overstatement," he wrote the General Education Board's A. R. Mann, "to say that nutrition is public health problem number one in the southern section of our country, and it is my opinion that the time has arrived to set up a Department of Nutrition in the School of Public Health." The decision by the Rockefeller Foundation's General Education Board to fund such a department made it possible for Wright and Baity to bring Rosenau's plans to fruition.[11]

The school hired Dr. A. Hughes Bryan to head the new Department of Public Health Nutrition. The son of a sugar chemist with the U. S. Department of Agriculture, Bryan studied chemistry at Harvard College and received his M.D. at Harvard Medical School. He taught and did research at the University of Chicago Medical School before joining the Public Health Service during the war. Dr. Bryan's most immediate task in his new assignment was to assemble laboratory equipment and plan renovations for his new home, Building C, a temporary structure located on the north side of MacNider Hall.[12]

Meanwhile, the search for a dean continued. After another candidate declined an offer to head the school, H. G. Baity issued words of warning to President Graham and Chancellor Robert House. The school's poor standing relative to the other schools of public health was undermining its recruitment efforts:

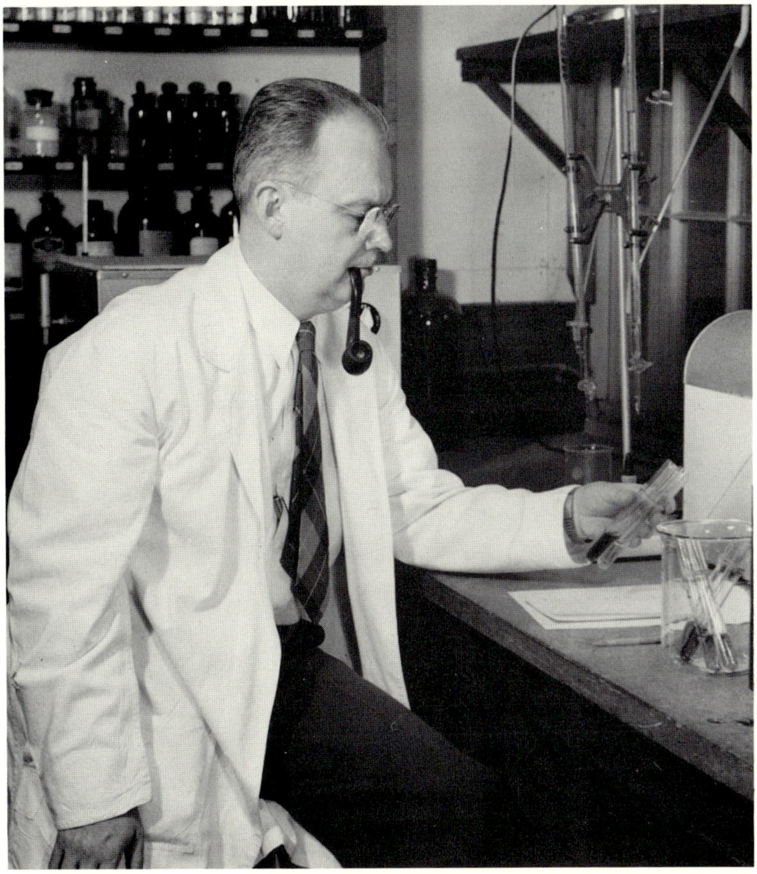

A. Hughes Bryan, first chair of the Department of Public Health Nutrition, at work in his laboratory.

> All of our eight competitors are institutions with great resources, stabilized budgets, excellent existing staffs, adequate physical facilities and good salary schedules with guaranteed tenure and attractive retirement allowances. In other words, they are going concerns which offer promise and opportunity.
>
> Here at Chapel Hill we can offer none of these things—only hope for the future and an abundant opportunity to better the health of our southern region. We have no stabilized budget, in fact no guarantee of existence beyond the coming year. We have little existing staff left to inspire newcomers. We have a low salary schedule, and have not been able to offer tenure. We are already so crowded in our physical facilities. . .that we are not only unable to accommodate the research activities of new staff members. . ., but we are actually unable to provide office space for the people we are trying to employ.
>
> If we cannot build a staff of first-rate people in key positions it would be better, I think, to discontinue the school.[13]

Not long after that, Baity began discussing the deanship with Dr. Edward G. McGavran, head of the Department of Public Health and

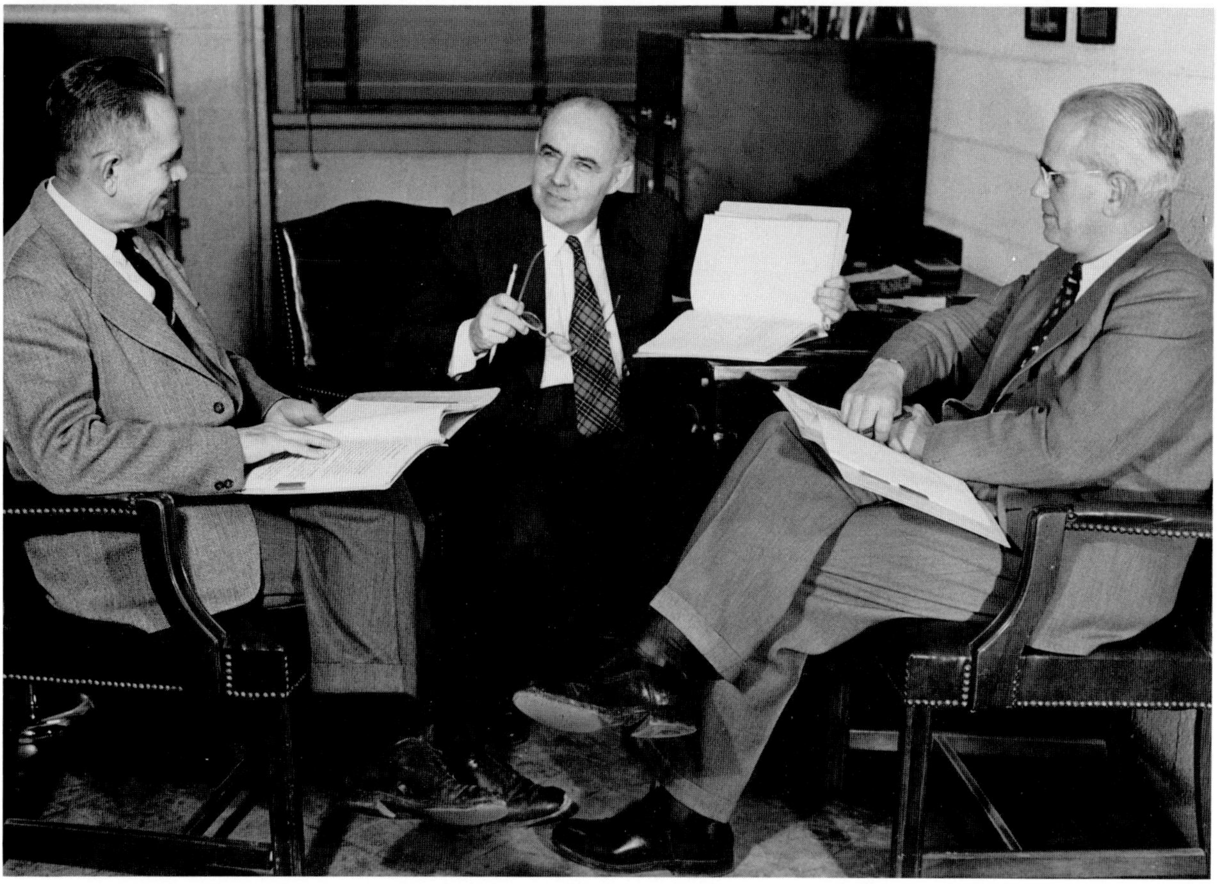

H. G. Baity, Edward G. McGavran, and John Wright working on the school's annual report.

Preventive Medicine at the University of Kansas Medical School. The job interested McGavran, but like the other candidates he found the lack of state funding to be a serious obstacle. After much discussion and persuasion, the North Carolina General Assembly agreed to provide token support for the school, the university allocated a limited number of tenure positions, and the Public Health Service agreed to supplement the new dean's salary. In April, 1947, McGavran accepted the university's offer. Baity was ecstatic. "I cannot begin to tell you how happy all of us are [at] the news that you have really decided to come with us as dean. . . . At long last I feel that we are on a solid fiscal foundation and are in position to establish ourselves among the leading public health institutions in the country."[14]

Like Rosenau, McGavran possessed extensive training and wide experience in public health. McGavran was born in India, where his parents were missionaries. An aunt who lived with them served as the town's only medical doctor, and her efforts to meet the almost unlimited needs of the community influenced his decision to go into medicine and public health. The family returned to the United States and settled in Indianapolis, where McGavran attended high school and college. After graduating from Harvard Medical School in 1928, McGavran spent four years in private practice before returning to Harvard to earn a master of public health degree. From 1934 to 1946 he served as a public health officer, first as director of the county health department in Hillside, Michigan, where he also administered the Kellogg Foundation project in field training, then as director of a training center in West Virginia, and finally as health commissioner of St. Louis County, Missouri. Shortly before taking the job at Chapel Hill, he had joined the faculty of the University of Kansas.[15]

McGavran saw himself primarily as an administrator whose job was to create an atmosphere where faculty, staff, and students could work and learn together. He described his philosophy in this way:

> The first step in accomplishing these objectives was to develop an organizational pattern within the faculty and a school philosophy. This was done by weekly formal staff meetings of the entire faculty with a carefully prepared agenda and subsequently approved minutes. All policy and most administrative matters were discussed in detail with the entire faculty and majority vote ruled. Time was set aside at each meeting for complete informational exchange between departments. Ad hoc committees were formed and appointed to study many specific problems, with the eventual development of standing committees within the faculty. The most desirable time of the week was set aside for these staff meetings; and neither classes nor commitments were permitted on Monday afternoons. These were strictly "Executive Sessions"—no holds were barred. Full expression and the privilege of dissension were encouraged.
>
> It thus became evident from action rather than by word alone that the new administration of the school was a democratic administration, informal, but firm in its purpose: to operate the School of Public Health as a team of professional equals who would determine policy, instruct the dean, and back him wholeheartedly in carrying out the school's wishes and desires.[16]

McGavran's presence had an immediate impact on the school. By the end of his first year, nine new faculty positions had been created, and the budget for research had increased from $75,710 to $230,710. Most of that growth came from two sources: the Kellogg Foundation's support for a Department of Field Training and the Public Health

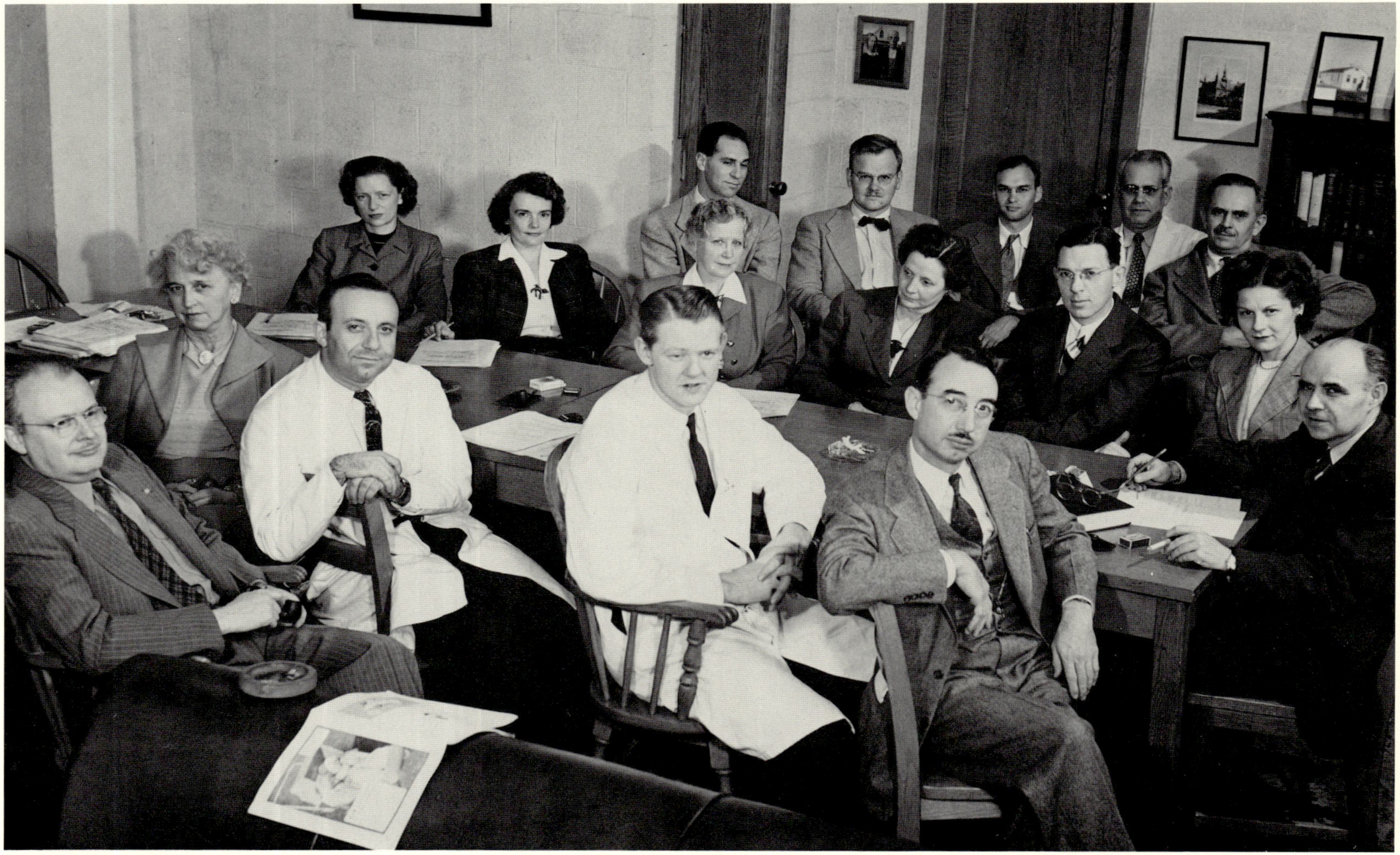

A meeting of the School of Public Health faculty, 1948.

Service's decision to move its Syphilis Experimental Laboratory to the school.

Field training had long been a staple of public health education. At the school, public health nurses and educators conducted field work in the spring quarter as part of their degree requirements. But soon after McGavran's arrival, the school submitted a proposal for a much more ambitious program to the W. K. Kellogg Foundation, where McGavran had worked earlier. Field training was crucial to McGavran's evolving notion of public health. He compared it to the clinical portion of medical education; to him, field training was equivalent to bedside practice. The proposal called for establishing a field training station in the Orange-Person-Chatham-Lee District, as well as improving local training sites throughout the South. This plan included short courses, in-service training, supervised field experience, apprenticeship training, and residency training. The Kellogg Foundation provided the initial funds for the program, and the State Board of Health provided additional money and personnel.[17]

Dr. William P. Richardson assumed the duties of head of the Department of Field Training on July 1, 1948. A graduate of Wake Forest College and the Medical College of Virginia, Richardson proved an ideal person for the job. He had rich experience as a local health officer (he had served as head of the Orange-Person-Chatham District Health Department from 1936 to 1944) and on the staff of the State Board of Health. In addition, the Public Health Service assigned a sanitary engineer and a public health nurse to the department.[18]

The school also became the site of the principal research laboratory of the Venereal Disease Division of the Public Health Service. In 1945 Dr. William L. Fleming resigned as director of the Reynolds Research Laboratory, and a year later the Z. Smith Reynolds Foundation withdrew its funding for venereal disease research in order to increase its contributions to Wake Forest College, then in the process of moving from Wake Forest to Winston-Salem. Dr. Harold Magnuson of the Public Health Service replaced Fleming, and the university, the State Board of Health, and the Public Health Service stepped in to support the laboratory. Meanwhile, The Johns Hopkins closed its Laboratory of Experimental Therapeutics, and the Public Health Service decided to relocate some of the laboratory's staff, equipment, and functions to Chapel Hill. The university agreed to construct a building to house a newly designated

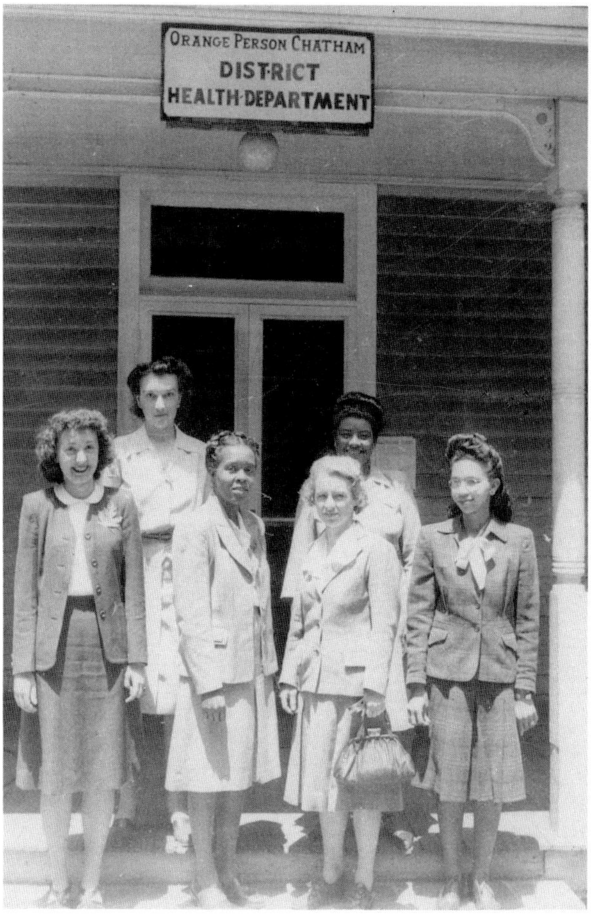

Public health educators from the North Carolina College for Negroes and the University of North Carolina at the field training center, 1946.

Syphilis Experimental Laboratory. The closing of another Public Health Service laboratory in 1949 brought additional equipment and personnel to Chapel Hill. While the Department of Experimental Medicine's primary concern was venereal disease, its research often had much broader applications. "We find ourselves engaged in a wide variety of projects," Magnuson wrote Dean McGavran, "involving chemotherapy, antibiotic therapy, bacterial metabolism and physiology, protein chemistry, and other areas that lie outside a narrowly defined venereal disease field."[19]

There was much excitement over all the changes at the school, but the daily demands of the classroom, the laboratory, and the field station kept everyone's feet on the ground. The school's most immediate problem was that it had no place to put the new people and programs. In a plea to Chancellor House to consider a new public health building as the university's number one priority, McGavran described the problems. "One department is housed in the old Water Works Building, halfway across the campus. Four temporary buildings have been put up and are full to overflowing. . . . Many workers are crowded into a single

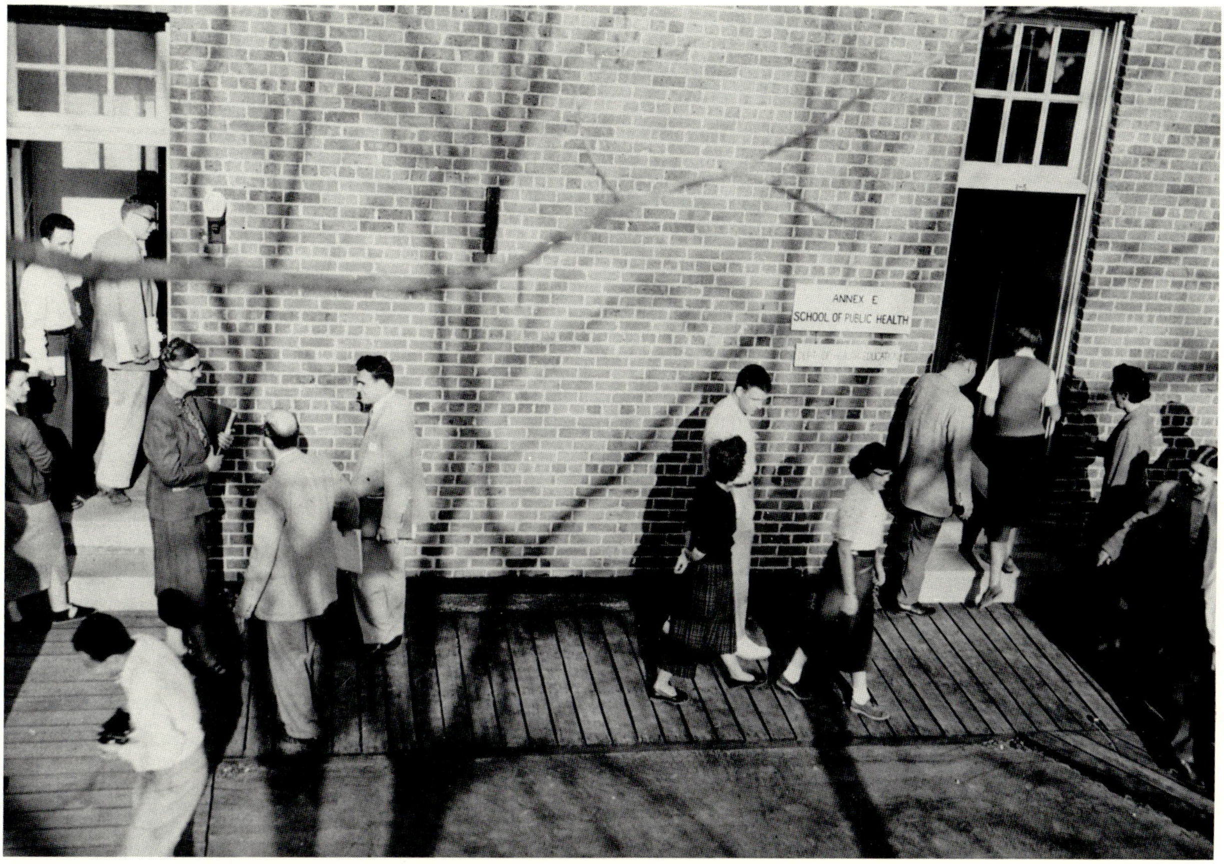

Many of the school's offices, classrooms, and laboratories were outside MacNider Hall in the 1950s. *Above,* the Department of Health Education's office in the old Water Works building on the main campus; *below,* the temporary buildings to the north of MacNider.

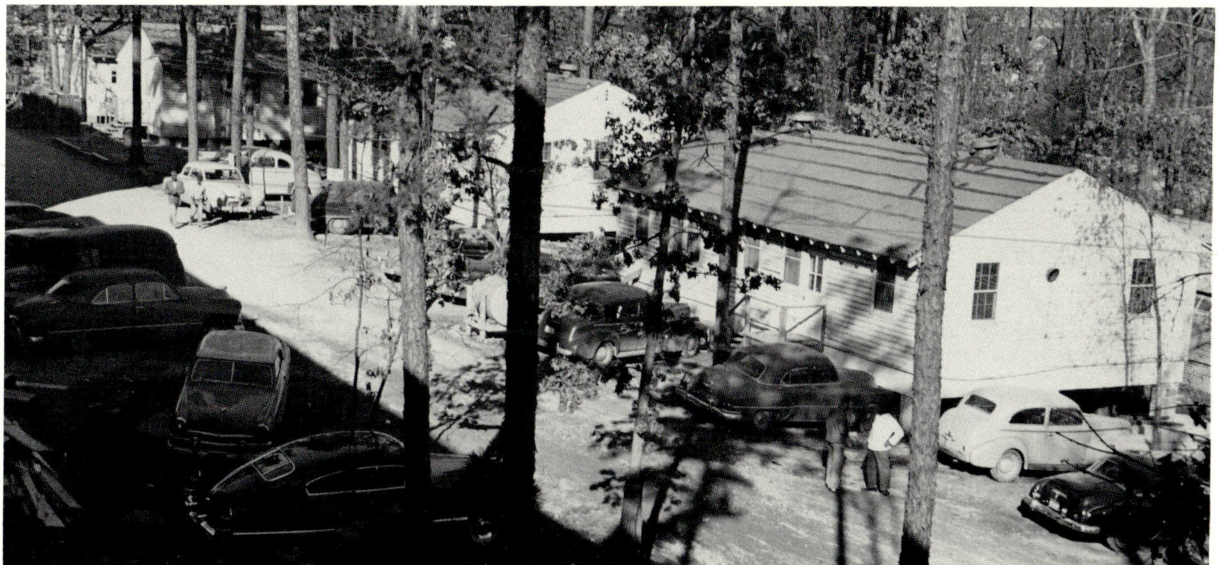

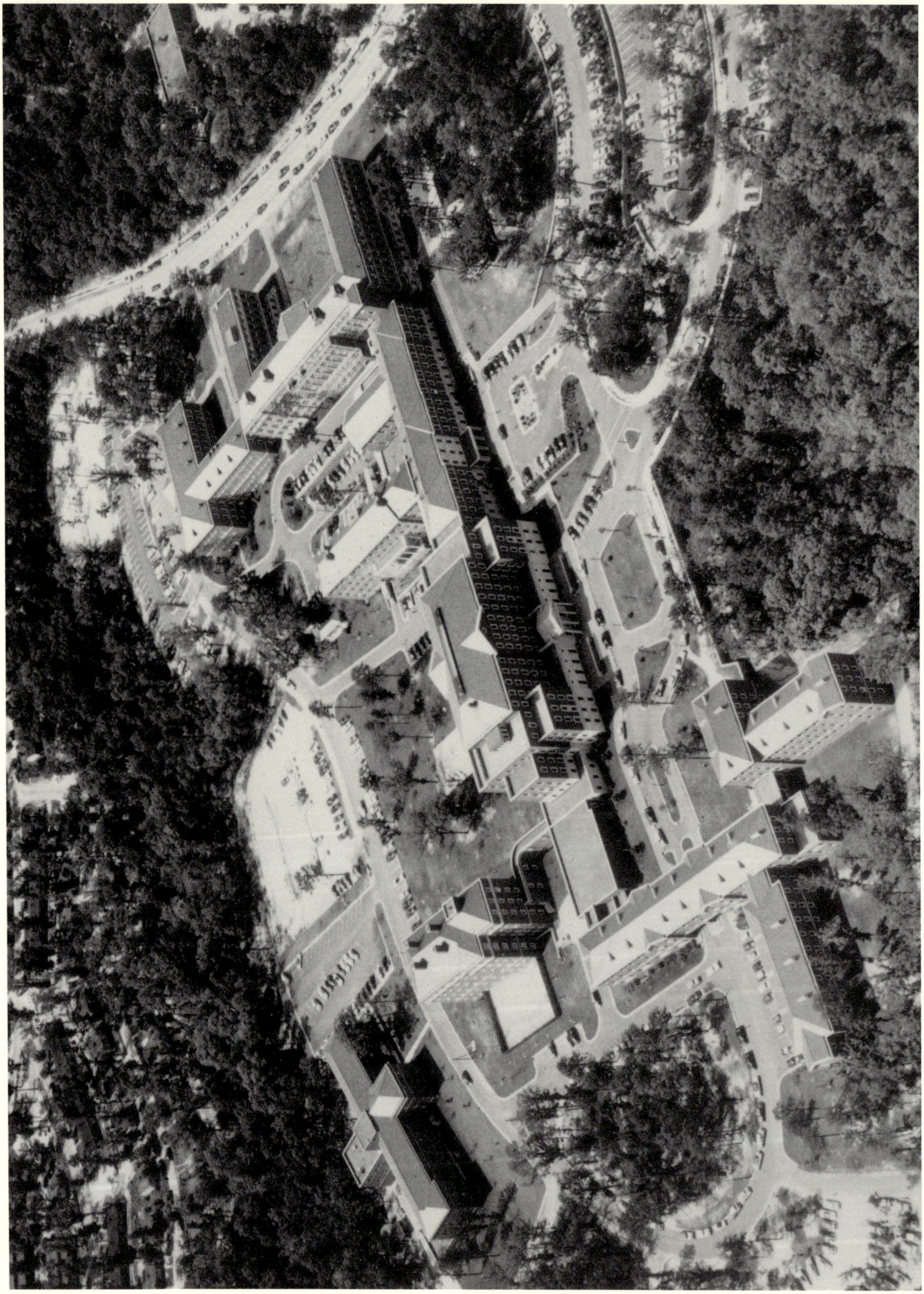

The medical complex at Chapel Hill in the early 1950s.

room or single laboratory meant for one person." Not only were present operations threatened, but the future of the school as well. Without additional space, there could be no expansion of the student body, no increase in foundation and federal funding. "The era of health interest and public support is here," the dean wrote House, "and we shall either be on the bandwagon or see the parade go by with other southern institutions taking the lead in public health development."[20]

The school's inability to secure funds for a new building would plague McGavran for the next decade. In part, the difficulty stemmed from the School of Public Health's multiple commitments. Was the school's primary constituency the university, the state of North Carolina, the southeastern region, the United States, or the foreign countries that increasingly sought its help? To McGavran, the health agencies that supplied student scholarships were the primary constituents. North Carolina's State Board of Health was one of these, but so were those of other southern states, foreign countries, and various federal agencies. The school saw itself as a regional, national, and international center, but unlike The Johns Hopkins and Harvard it had no endowment and so depended on the state for funds, especially for physical facilities. But the legislature was unwilling to use scarce resources for non-North Carolina students.[21]

The fact that the rapid growth of the school also coincided with a major expansion of medical services at the university also presented problems. In 1944 Governor J. Melville Broughton, at the urging of the North Carolina Medical Society, appointed a commission to study the hospital and health needs of the state. North Carolina's dubious distinction of having the highest rejection rate for draftees during the war prompted the decision, but it was also part of a nation-wide effort to increase the availability of hospitals. The commission called for the establishment of a four-year medical school at the university, the building of a teaching hospital in connection with the medical school, and the creation of hospitals and medical centers in parts of the state with inadequate facilities. Although many people supported the commission's recommendations, powerful figures in the legislature and the medical community opposed all or part of the report. Some felt the existing four-year schools at Duke University in Durham and Bowman Gray Hospital in Winston-Salem adequately met the state's needs. Others argued that such a school belonged in a major city, rather than on a college campus. Still others opposed the state-sponsored proliferation of

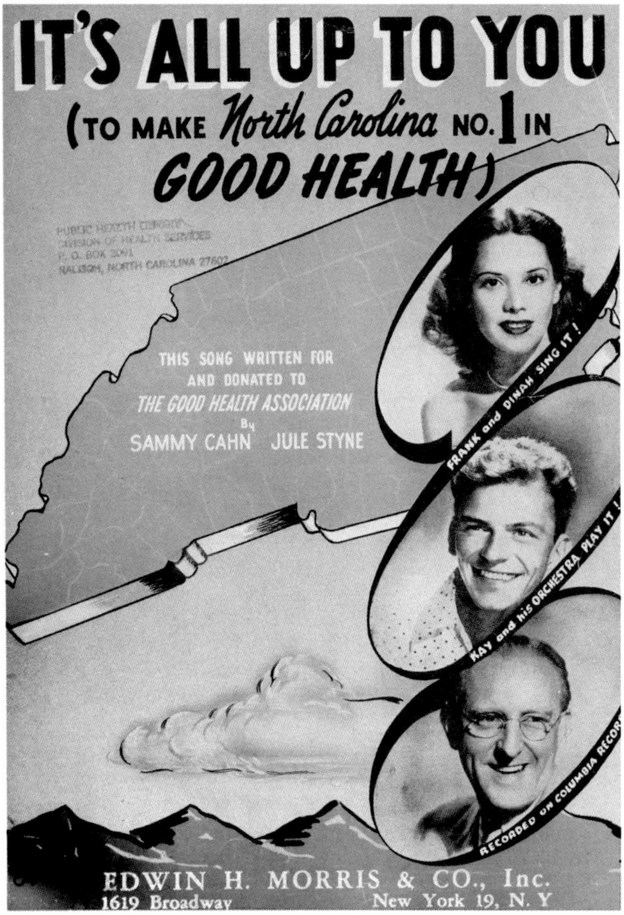

The Good Health Campaign was part of the post-World War II drive to upgrade medical facilities and improve the health of North Carolinians. The public relations effort, as represented by this song, were reminiscent of the State Board of Health's campaigns in the 1910s and 1920s. Department of Public Health Education students Ralph Boatman, Maisie Bookhardt, Mary-Elizabeth Gruwell, and Harriet Hylton Barr work on campaign.

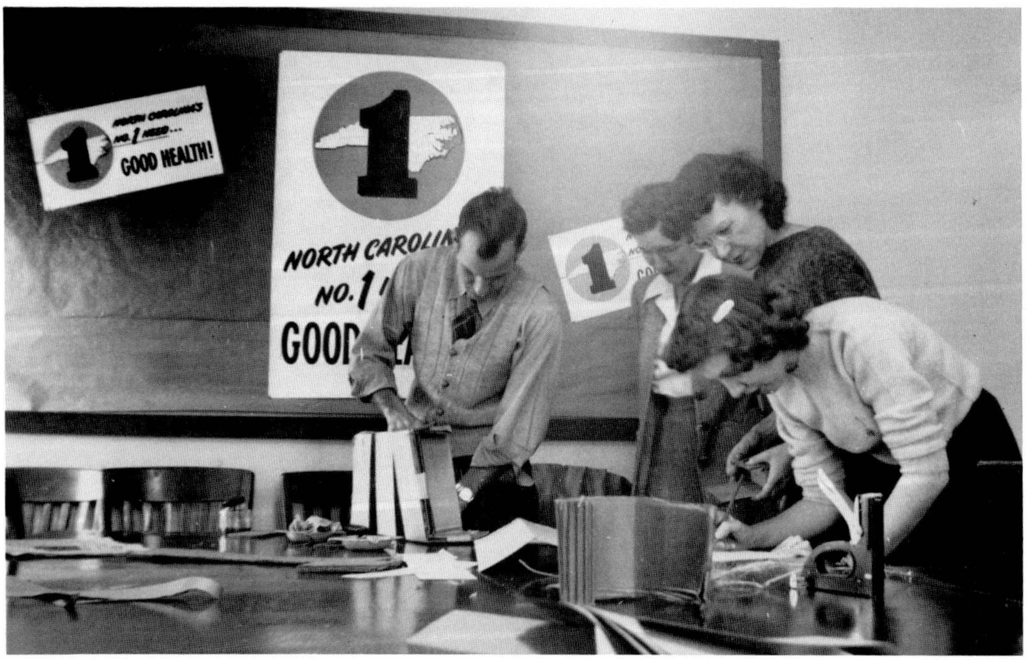

local hospitals. For the next few years politicians, university officers, and health officials debated the merits of the plan. In the end, the advocates of the North Carolina Medical Care Commission's recommendations prevailed, and in 1947 the General Assembly appropriated funds which, combined with federal support under the Hill-Burton Act, allowed for the building of a hospital at Chapel Hill and the expansion of the Medical School.[22]

Within a few years of these decisions, Chapel Hill had become a large regional medical center. The university added the Schools of Dentistry and Nursing and established a Division of Health Affairs to coordinate these new programs, as well as the Schools of Medicine, Pharmacy, and Public Health. Dr. McGavran strongly supported bringing the schools together in one administrative unit, hoping that such a move would foster cooperation between medicine and public health. He also agreed to serve as acting administrator of the division from March, 1949, until July, 1950. In his absence, John Wright served as acting dean of the School of Public Health. Finally, Dr. Henry Clark, Jr., took the assignment as head of the division and McGavran returned to the dean's office.[23]

These developments generated much discussion about the health needs of the state's citizens, but they had limited impact on the public health movement. The trajectory of postwar spending on health in the state and in the university clearly favored the medical profession and the hospital industry. The medical profession's ability to control postwar spending on health stemmed in part from public health's lack of a politically powerful constituency. Although efforts to eradicate communicable diseases, preserve clean air and water, and dispose of wastes benefited everyone, politicians often viewed public health as a welfare program for the less fortunate members of the society. People who benefited most visibly from public health services—blacks, the poor, the elderly, children—had little clout in the halls of power.[24]

The school also operated in a very different political environment from that of the early days of the public health movement. In the past, philanthropical foundations viewed a healthy population as good for the business interests they represented. Progressive Era and New Deal reformers sought to provide a safety net for those who lacked access to doctors and hospitals. But efforts to maintain or expand New Deal programs met stiff opposition after the war. President Harry Truman's proposal for national health insurance failed in Congress. The public health movement appeared at loggerheads with the conservative drift of the country.[25]

Dean McGavran hoped that legislators would see public health as an alternative to national health insurance. "It takes no political prophet," he wrote, "to see that the postwar conservative government will shy from the 'radical' medical care legislation and appropriations but cannot avoid fulfillment of some of its promises by public health and hospital support far in excess of anything heretofore proposed." McGavran was right about support for hospitals, but public health would have to wait.[26]

Despite these difficulties, the school continued to sink its roots deeper into the university community and reach out to the people of the state. "There is about the School of Public Health an interesting atmosphere of confident assurance," noted an official of the Commonwealth Fund. A major reason for this buoyancy was the creation of new departments and the arrival of new faculty members in the late 1940s and early 1950s, some of whom would play major roles in the future of the school and the university.[27]

Dr. Cecil G. Sheps joined the faculty as associate professor of public health administration in the fall of 1947. A native of Winnipeg, Canada, Sheps received his M.D. from the University of Manitoba and his M.P.H. from Yale University. His parents were Jewish socialists from the Ukraine, who immigrated to Canada after the 1905 revolution. Sheps initially considered law and politics as the proper sphere in which to fight for his notions of social justice, but a lecture on the triumphs of public health convinced him otherwise. "I was inspired by that lecture," he remembered, "and decided that I would go into medicine, that I could achieve my social objectives through medicine." After a few years of general practice, a stint in the Canadian Army, and a job in public health in Saskatchewan, Sheps accepted a fellowship to study medical care administration at Yale. From there he ventured to Chapel Hill to teach a summer session in epidemiology and biostatistics. Sheps's army experience in venereal disease control attracted the attention of John Wright, and Wright offered Sheps a job. Wright and Sheps began sifting through the data collected by the venereal disease project and published their findings in a number of papers.[28]

A future dean of the school, Dr. Bernard Greenberg, joined the faculty as chairman of the newly organized Department of Biostatistics in 1949. The lack of such a department had marked a serious weakness

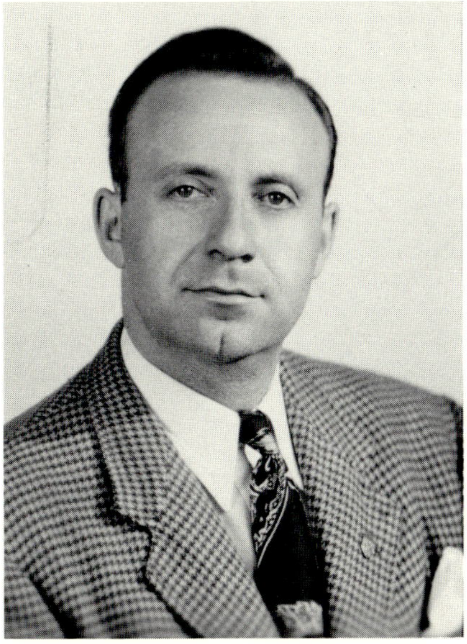

Cecil G. Sheps

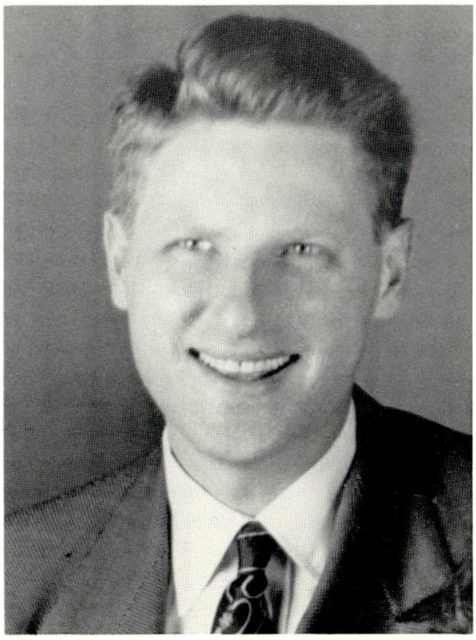

Bernard G. Greenberg

in the school's curriculum. Over the years various people had taught courses in biostatistics, and in 1945 the school began the search for someone to head a department. Greenberg established ties to the school in the fall of 1946, taking Dr. Baity's course in public health sanitation while a graduate student in experimental statistics at North Carolina State College in Raleigh.[29]

Biostatistics filled a critical hole in the school's offerings, but it took a while for faculty members to get over their initial skepticism about its relevance for their work. The Department of Public Health Nutrition provided Greenberg's first collaboration on a project studying the relationship between the physical measurements of school children and their diet. Before long, statistical methods became a vital tool in public health investigations.

The school established a Department of Maternal and Child Health in 1950 with funds from the U. S. Department of Labor's Children's Bureau. Since the passage of the Sheppard-Towner Act in 1921, the Children's Bureau had aided programs designed to reduce maternal and infant mortality. The expansion of these programs in the postwar era increased the demand for professionals in the field. Dean McGavran selected Dr. Sidney Shaw Chipman to head the department. A Canadian by birth, Chipman received his M.D. from McGill in 1928 and his M.P.H. from Yale in 1947. The maternal and child health team consisted of a physician, a nurse, and a medical social worker, and the Children's Bureau provided funds for all positions. In addition to Dr. Chipman, Jean Rebentisch joined the department in 1950 as associate professor of maternal and child health, and in 1953 Geraldine Gourley came on

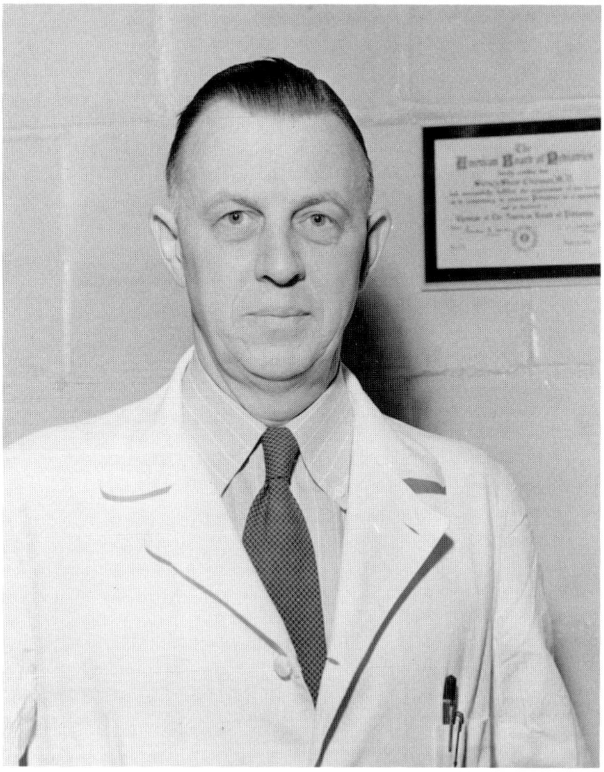

Sidney Chipman

board as associate professor of medical social work. The department developed a curriculum for students specializing in maternal and child health and more generally for all students in the school.[30]

The school had long been interested in providing instruction in mental health for its students, but lack of funds limited course work to a few lectures by visiting instructors. In 1952 a grant from the Public Health Service allowed the school to create a Department of Mental Health and to hire Dr. Roger Howell as its head. With Dr. Howell's arrival, students received more in-depth instruction in this area of growing concern. Howell also began developing a curriculum to train administrators for mental health centers.[31]

By 1952, all of the present-day departments had been organized. Rosenau, Baity, and McGavran had established a structure that fit the mission of the school and the personalities of the faculty. McGavran now had a tight-knit team of professionals ready to tackle the region's problems.

McGavran himself did much to create the sense of community that characterized the school in those days. "I liked the spirit of the

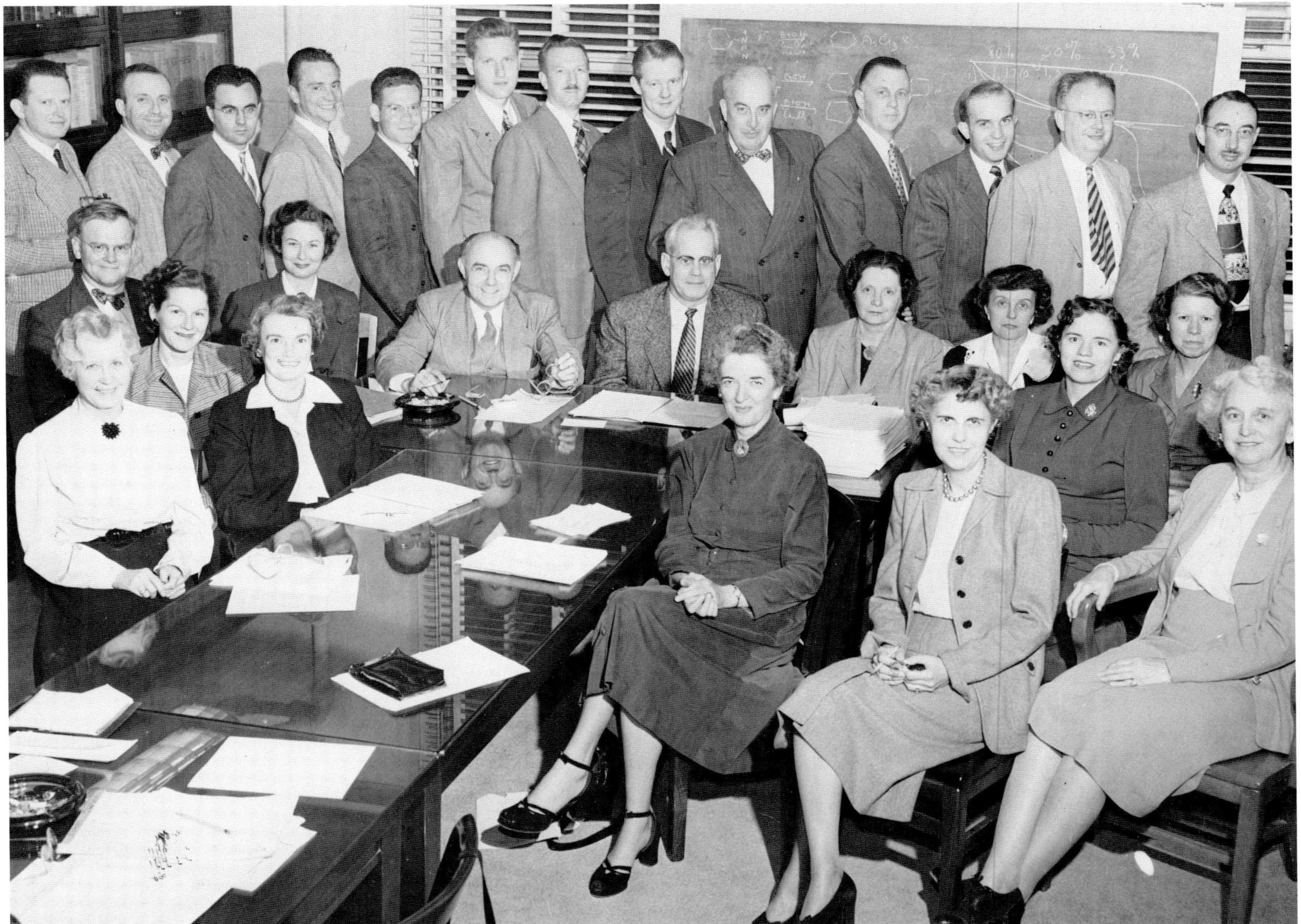

Faculty, School of Public Health, 1950.

whole thing," Rebecca Bryan, a student and later faculty member at the school, recalled. "The very first week we were here the McGavrans had all the student body come out to their house for a reception. Very soon after that they began inviting us in smaller groups for Boston baked beans and brown bread. We were really royally entertained." Members of the faculty also invited students to their homes. "We were all wet behind the ears," Bryan recalled, "so it was exciting and interesting to be able to sit down and share with somebody else what was going on in your state."[32]

Frances Gust, who joined the staff of the school as McGavran's administrative assistant in 1950, saw McGavran's sociability as central to his leadership style. "The students would marvel that Dr. McGavran's memory was so good that at these dinners he would always shake hands and call the students by name. But what they never knew was that he would bring in a list of who would be there Friday evening. We would get cards and if we could find a picture, we would put a picture on the

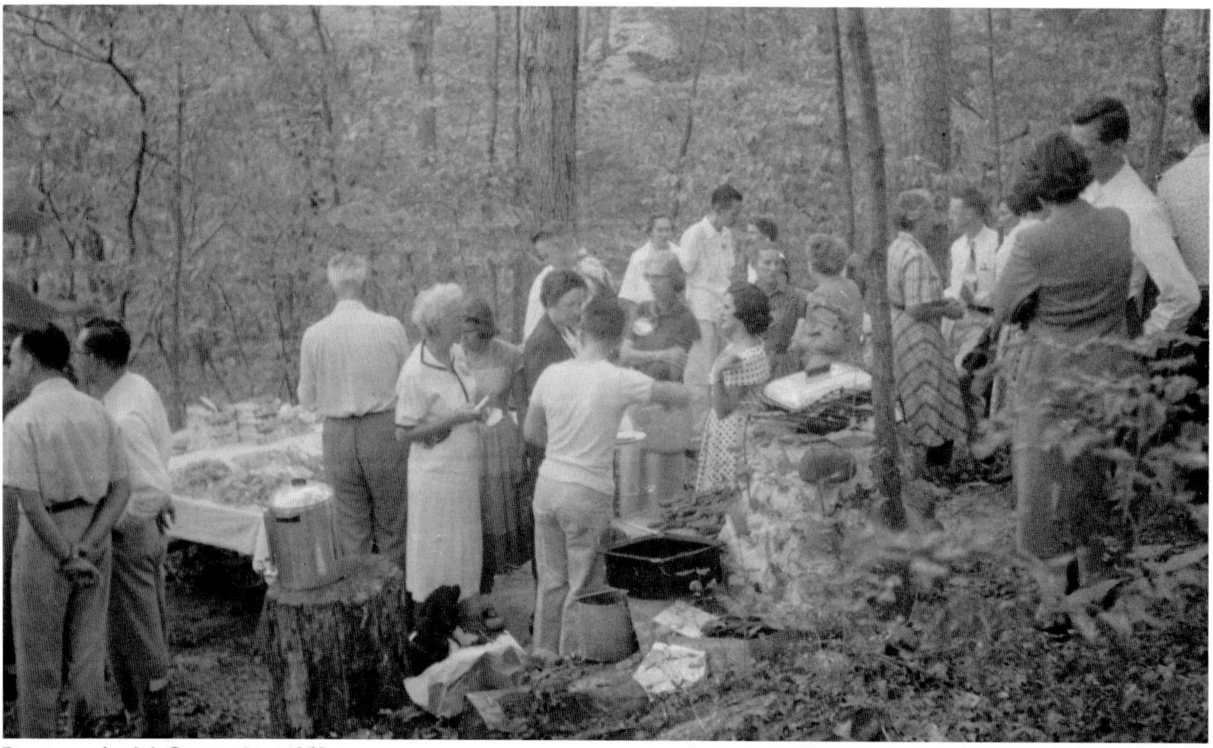

Picnic at the McGavrans' in 1953.

card, and if not we would describe the person. He played with these cards in advance and could say hello, how are you, and how are the people back in Abilene, Texas. We always chuckled over this, but we never gave away his secret."[33]

The school accepted increasing numbers of students from foreign countries in the 1950s, and McGavran wanted to establish the same sense of community among them. For many, adjusting to life in small-town America proved as difficult as the course work. Dean McGavran asked Geraldine Gourley to develop an orientation program for these students. "We got the sponsoring agencies to agree to the students' coming two weeks before school started," she remembered. "For students who needed it, we set up English classes. We had people who came in and talked to them and we had social things. Then we had field trips and went all over the state. We visited farms, sewage disposal systems, dairies, schools, and health departments. They knew the resources of the state better than the American students. They were much better able to fit into the academic part of the school. They had this time to get their feet on the ground."[34]

The highlight of this orientation program occurred in 1955, when Zebulon, a town of about fifteen hundred, hosted foreign students from Chapel Hill for a weekend. Civic clubs and church groups joined together for "THE WORLD IS COMING TO ZEBULON." The high school band and majorettes met the students at the town hall on Friday afternoon. Banquets, a dance at the high school gymnasium, a visit to a tobacco auction, and Cokes at the local drug store highlighted the weekend activities. "The students were astonished," Gourley recalled, "at seeing the mayor washing dishes and the head of the health department serving with an apron on. One of the things that surprised them the most was to find the farmers so prosperous and . . . people of authority. In many of their cultures farmers were very poor."[35]

Lucy Morgan created an equally strong esprit de corps among public health educators. Public Health Education remained one of the largest departments throughout the 1950s, and public health educators were among the most visible members of the school for many years. The philosophy that guided health educators defies simple explanation. More than anyone else, Lucy Morgan provided the intellectual and social rationale for the department, but other faculty members and hundreds of students also left their mark. The first issue of the department's publication, *Health Educators at Work*, defined the issues as the editors Lucy Morgan and Eunice Tyler saw them. Although the United States was the healthiest place in the world in which to live, serious health problems remained. Medical science had the ability to alleviate much of the suffering, but "ignorance, apathy, carelessness, and the high cost of medical care" too often kept scientific advances from the people. "Reducing this lag is one of the chief aims of health education," Morgan and Tyler explained. "Preaching the gospel of health is more than advocating the use of toothbrush and vitamin chart; it is more than teaching disease prevention. Health education implies a belief in the right of every person to be as healthy and safe as science plus human endeavor can make him and a belief in the necessity for informed opinion to gain this end."[36]

Morgan and her colleagues were most influenced by the teachings of Lucy's father, Harcourt A. Morgan, and the well-known public health advocate C.-E. A. Winslow. Harcourt Morgan grew up and received his education in Canada but spent most of his life in the southern United States, first as professor of entomology and horticulture at Louisiana State University, then as president of the University of Tennessee, and finally as chairman of the Tennessee Valley Authority. In the "Mooring

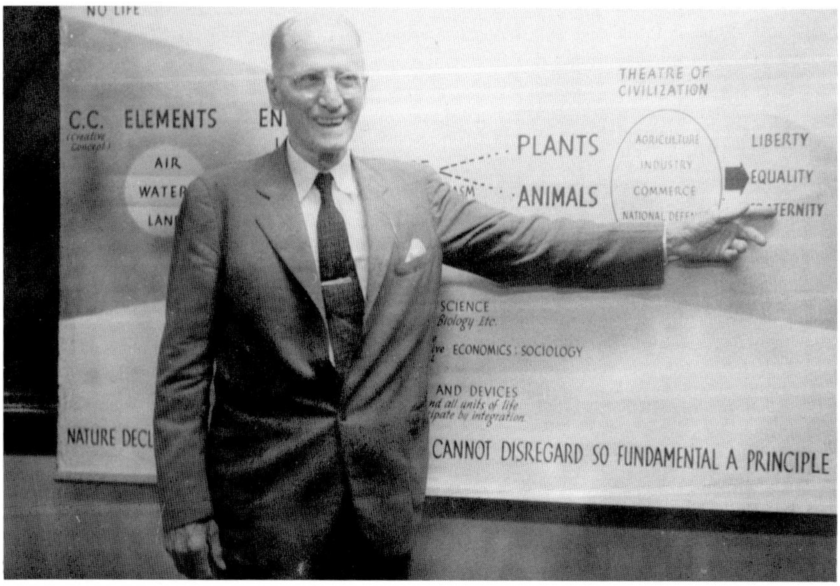

Harcourt A. Morgan

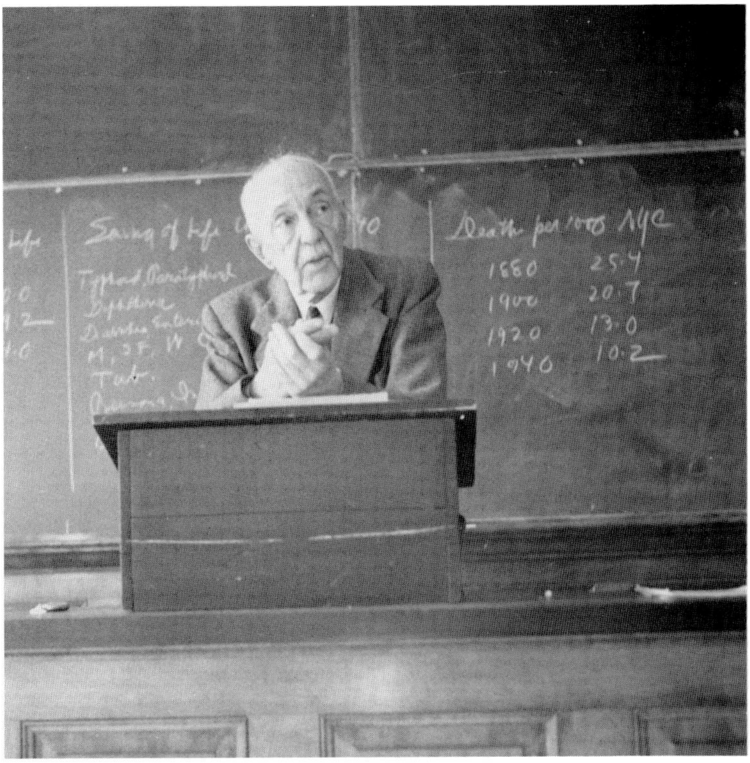

C.-E. A. Winslow, chairman of the Department of Public Health at Yale University School of Medicine. Winslow's expansive vision of public health, and especially his promotion of the role of education, made him a popular visitor to the school.

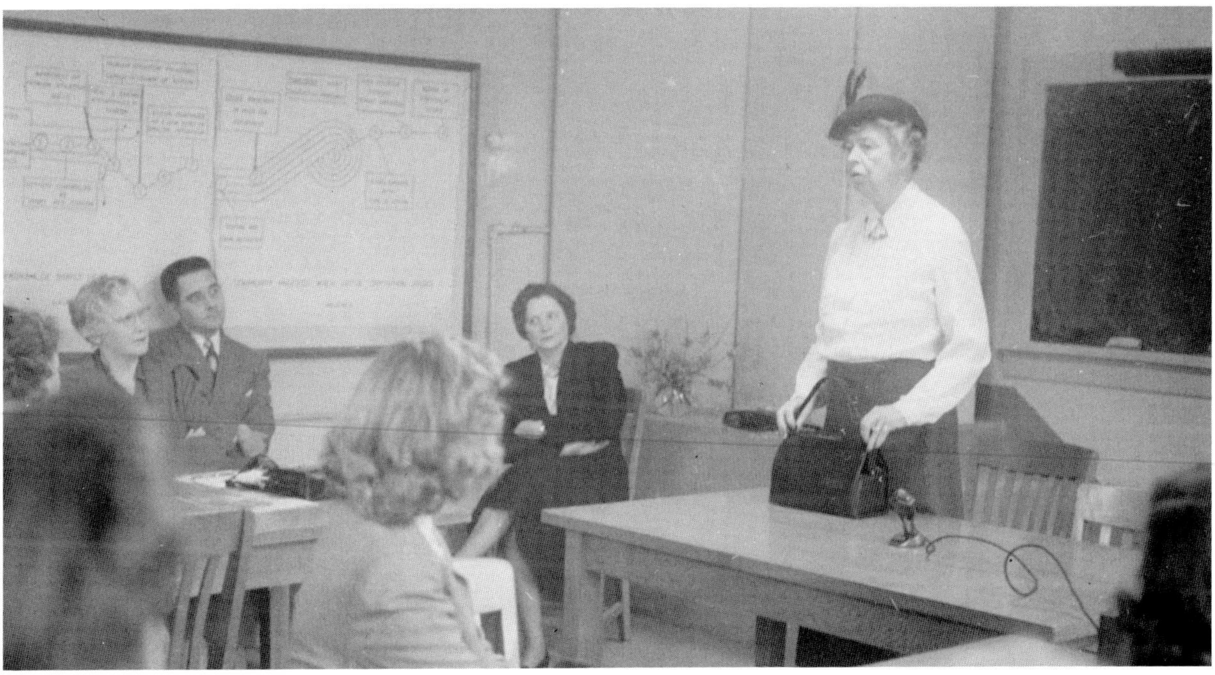

Eleanor Roosevelt addresses faculty and students in 1950. The school had the benefit of numerous presentations by distinguished visitors over the years.

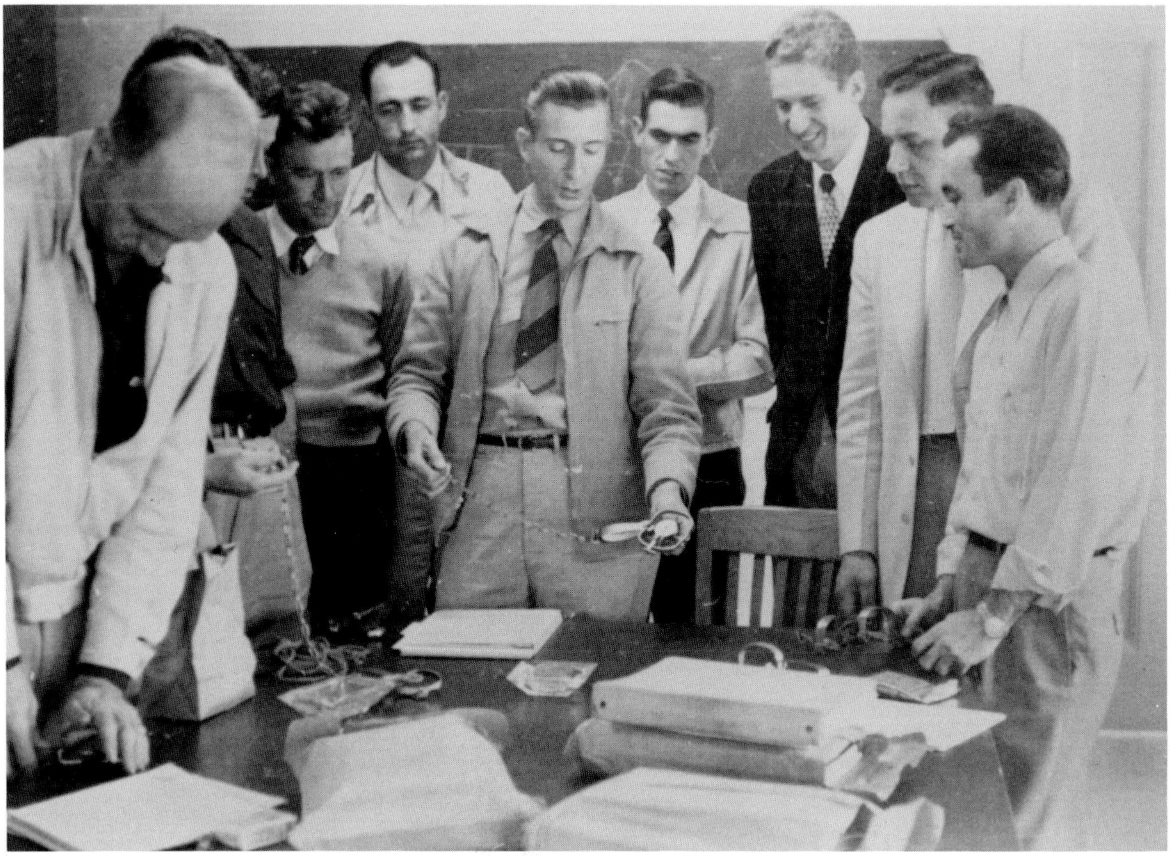

Don Ashton of the State Board of Health demonstrates the use of steel rat traps as part of a twelve-week short course for sanitarians, directed by the school's Department of Field Training, 1951.

Lecture Series," which he delivered at the School of Public Health from 1943 to 1950, Harcourt Morgan elaborated his philosophy of the interrelationship among minerals, plants, and animals, and related his holistic interpretation to social and economic as well as scientific problems.[37]

Despite the energy that seemed to drive the school in the early 1950s, significant problems remained. The school's annual report for 1951–52 listed five major needs: additional personnel, salary increases, a larger operating budget, increased support from federal and state agencies, and a new building. Personnel needs included administrative staff and teaching assistants, as well as additional faculty to meet the growing instructional demands. "Means must be found to provide more 'seconds in command,'" McGavran noted. "We are not propagating our own species. There is no replacement for too many of our key personnel." But even if the school could obtain additional faculty positions, low salaries prohibited the hiring of first-rate people, and there was a danger that present staff would leave. "Present key personnel in public health are not getting salaries commensurate with others of similar qualification, training, and experience in the Division of Health Affairs and are far below the 'market value' necessary to fill these positions," McGavran complained. Equally pressing was the lack of funds to support the school's expanding off-campus activities. "It should be borne in mind," McGavran argued, "that research in public health is largely field research, and though it does not require the university to provide expensive laboratory space and facilities, it does require equipment, secretarial help, and travel, far beyond the amount necessary for research conducted within the academic walls of the university. The 'field' is the laboratory and the bedside for public health research and teaching. Failure to provide or effort to curtail reaching this 'field' and using this 'field' is like locking the door of the laboratory, or closing the hospital and clinics to medical, dental, and nursing education."[38]

By the early 1950s, the frustrations associated with administering an ever more diversified school and trying to win support for that school in an increasingly hostile environment propelled McGavran into the role of public health evangelist. Although his ideas had been jelling for some years, they first saw print in 1953 in an article entitled "What Is Public Health?" At the time, McGavran declared, no clear definition of public health existed. "If this be true," he said, "it is no wonder that with the changing times there continues to be increased misunderstanding of public health by the organized medical profession; that there is apathy and indifference to public health on the part of the public and appropriating bodies of government; that there is lack of direction and planning among public health workers themselves; and that the recruitment and training of public health personnel lag far behind the needs in every county and clime."[39]

McGavran dismissed definitions that seemed too narrow—"public health is preventive medicine"—or too broad—"public health is the well-being of the people." The first definition intruded too often on the prerogatives of the physician, while the second necessitated knowledge beyond the possible scope of a public health practitioner. McGavran insisted, instead, that public health was a distinct profession with a "distinct body of knowledge that determines our competence without limiting our objectives." Expanding the medical model, he identified the community as the patient of public health, and the diagnosis and treatment of that patient as the profession's goal. According to McGavran, "Public health is, then, the scientific diagnosis and treatment of the body politic." He described how this self-understanding affected public health practice:

> Acceptance of this answer calls for a democratic team of professional equals. . . . It immediately becomes obvious and essential that many other professions with many other skills and knowledges must be integrated into scientific public health to obtain a diagnosis and plan of treatment for the body politic.
>
> To diagnose community ills we must have knowledge of community economy—the distinctive skills of the economist, a knowledge of the social structure of the community, and the impact upon their health practices of nutritional, . . . of recreational, religious, moral, and ethical patterns. . . .
>
> We must have knowledge and techniques of community organization, of the power structure of that community, of the political structure, of health laws and regulations, of attitudes that determine acceptance or rejection of change and development. We must have sophisticated knowledge of education and educational methods, of mores and morals that affect the growth and development of community consciousness and community action.
>
> We must have knowledge of community measurements, of the demographic characteristics of our patient—the age, sex, racial distribution, and the intricate ways in which this affects our patient's health; the biostatistical techniques of collection and analysis of the data that can determine mass phenomena of disease and health; the geographical base that determines isolation, transportation, and resources.
>
> We must have knowledge of sanitary science, the technical skills that can determine oxygen demand or biologic balance under widely varying circumstances. We must know the epidemiology of our patient, the community, and develop techniques to assess the symptoms of community illness, physical or mental. . . .
>
> All of this is nothing more or less than a scientific approach to the diagnosis and treatment of the body politic—the history, the physical examination, the tests, the analysis, the clinical judgment, and the prescription for treatment.[40]

It was bad enough that the medical profession, political leaders, and the general public misunderstood the role of public health, but McGavran also felt that the school's faculty lacked a clear sense of the movement's purpose. As a result the faculty spent the better part of the 1953 winter quarter discussing questions relating to the role of the school. "Before we can have a better understanding and appreciation among others," McGavran told his colleagues, "we must set our own

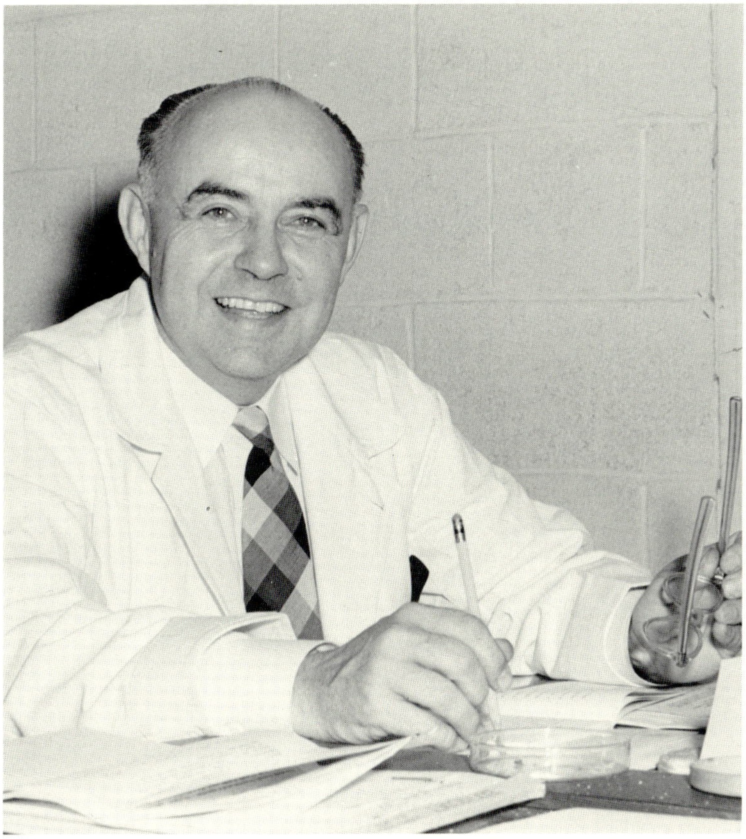

Dean Edward G. McGavran

house in order and have a better understanding and appreciation of public health ourselves." McGavran posed the following questions for the faculty to consider. "Are we a profession of public health or are we only a correlation of other professions, functioning in an indefinite area? Is there a body of knowledge, a discipline, which is distinctly public health? Is our loyalty primarily to public health or to the basic profession from which we have sprung? Can we define public health?" In general the faculty agreed that public health had some common body of knowledge, however nebulous. There was greater disagreement over the issue of a professional identity, with most wanting to maintain their identities as doctors, nurses, engineers, and so on. But in the context of the times, McGavran faced an uphill battle. The conservatism of the late 1940s and 1950s, the diversion of federal funds to the Korean war effort, and the increasing focus on scientific solutions to health problems limited the impact of his campaign.[41]

"The Body Politic" became the rallying cry of a campaign to win respectability for public health. Before his retirement in 1963, and afterward, McGavran spoke to many groups of people, and his speeches almost always included a variation on this theme.

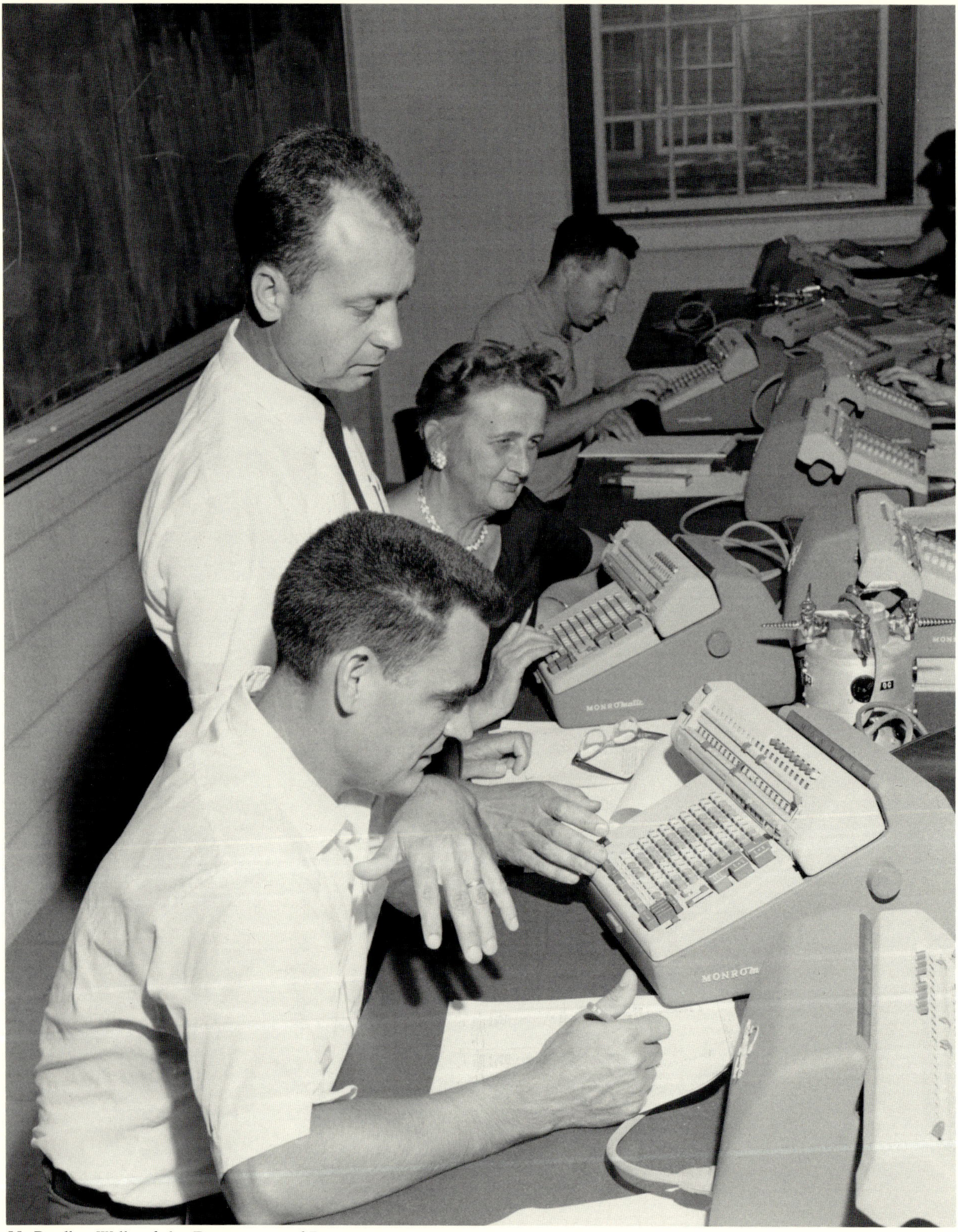

H. Bradley Wells of the Department of Biostatistics

Chapter 4

FOR SCIENCE AND SOCIETY

The funding crisis in public health began to abate by the mid-1950s. With the end of the police action in Korea, the federal government once again channeled funds into scientific and medical research. In the five short years between 1955 and 1960, the National Institutes of Health (NIH) budget increased from $81 million to $400 million. The successful Soviet launch of Sputnik stimulated the race for space and freed even more money for science and education. John Kennedy's election in 1960 focused attention on the problems of the developing world, and public health forces played an important role in new society programs such as the Peace Corps, the Alliance for Progress, and the Agency for International Development.[1]

Frustrated in their efforts to win adequate support from North Carolina sources, McGavran and his team set their sights elsewhere—on other states, the federal government, and countries in the developing world. Not everyone on the faculty shared McGavran's community-oriented philosophy of public health. But they were all ambitious, for themselves and the school, and a spirit of reform permeated their efforts.

The school's first major venture outside the United States involved assistance in establishing a sanitary engineering program at the National University of Engineering (UNI) in Lima, Peru. It was the first of Dan Okun's many successful educational advisory projects for the school. Dr. Daniel A. Okun, who would establish himself as one of the university's most dynamic faculty members over the next thirty years, replaced H. G. Baity as head of the Department of Sanitary Engineering in 1955. Born in Brooklyn, New York, Okun dated his interest in engineering to the time his father, an engineer for the city, took him

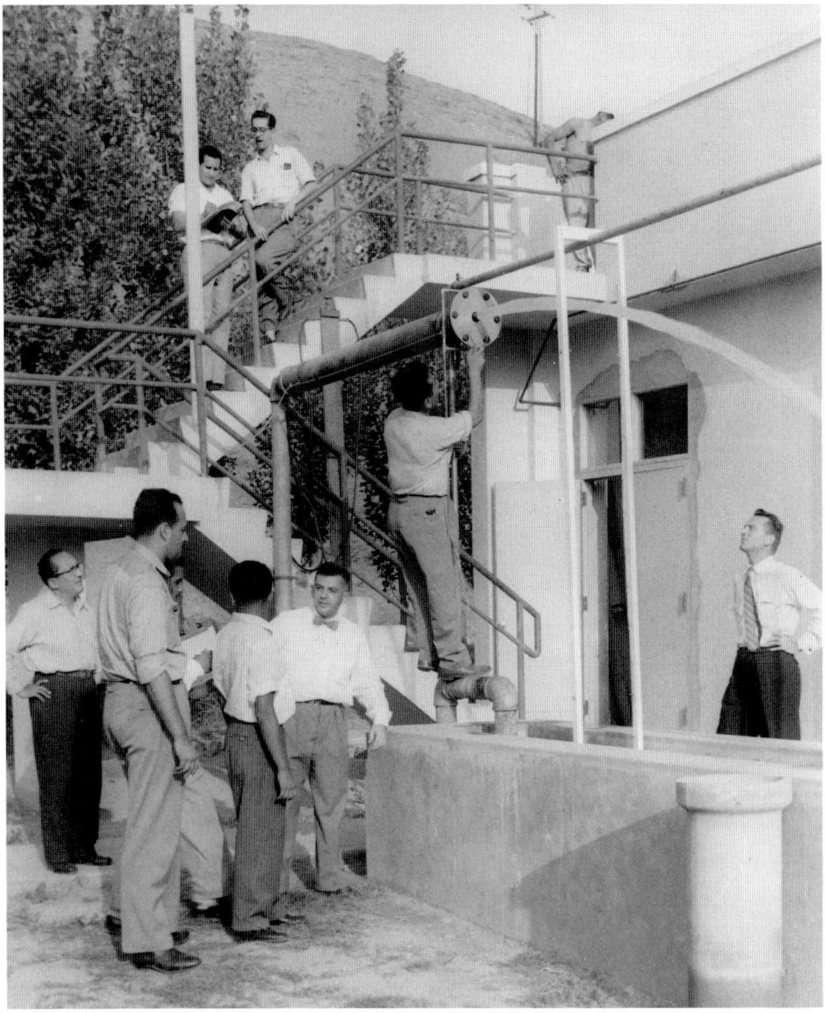

Marvin Granstrom (*far right*) at the National University of Engineering, Lima, Peru, 1956.

underground to see construction of the giant tunnel that would bring water to New York City. He took an undergraduate degree in civil engineering at Cooper Union and a master's degree at California Technical Institute before joining the Public Health Service, where he was introduced to the field of public health in a series of lectures by, among others, Dr. Edward McGavran. A stint in the army during World War II took him to Latin America, New Guinea, and the Philippines where he was exposed to the problems of the developing world. After the war, he studied with Gordon Fair at Harvard University, earning an Sc.D. in 1948. Okun worked for an engineering firm for a few years before coming to Chapel Hill as a temporary replacement for Baity. Baity, who had taken a leave in 1952 to work as the first director of environmental health for the World Health Organization (WHO) in Geneva, decided to stay in Switzerland, and Okun found teaching to his liking.[2]

Peru's water supply and waste disposal systems had not kept pace with urban and industrial growth. Less than 20 percent of the population received water from public supplies, and only a few larger cities had sewerage systems for human wastes. As a result, thousands of people suffered from diseases associated with contaminated food and water, such as typhoid, infectious hepatitis, hookworm, and dysentery. Ultimately, a massive program of education and public works would be necessary to control these problems. But before that could happen, Peru needed a trained core of sanitary engineers and related professionals. In the past, most of the country's sanitary engineers had received graduate training at North American universities, including the University of North Carolina. In 1940 Peru's National University of Engineering inaugurated an undergraduate degree program, but it was inadequate for the country's needs. One problem, according to Okun, was the lack of a "responsible core of full-time faculty." The UNI asked the International Cooperation Administration-Institute of Inter-American Affairs for technical assistance. The Administration-Institute, in turn, asked UNC's Department of Sanitary Engineering "to design, equip and supply laboratories, train personnel, assist in teaching procedures, set up extension courses and establish research."[3]

Dan Okun, Emil Chanlett, Marvin Granstrom, and Gilbert Kelso each spent a semester in Peru, while Ed McGavran, John Wright, and

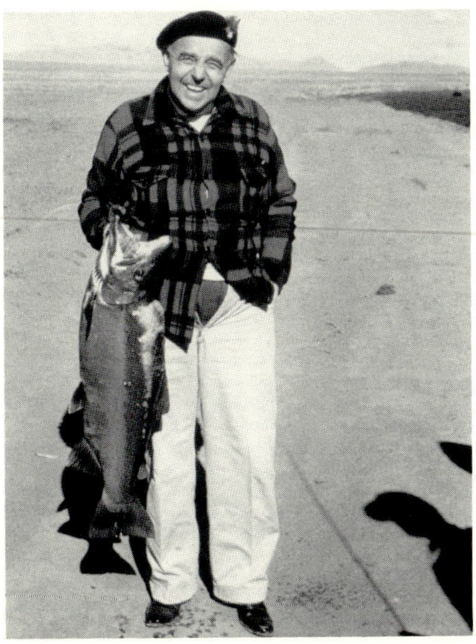

Dean McGavran displays a rainbow trout he caught in Lake Titicaca while on a trip to Peru.

John Larsh went for shorter periods to help with their specialties. Dr. Charles M. Weiss joined the department as a replacement for the faculty member stationed in Peru. Although the project was designed to last for only three years, a short period of time in which to launch an educational program, Okun felt the project accomplished most of its goals. The Peru project also proved valuable to the school's faculty. "They learned that the introduction of United States techniques alone is not enough. There must be a sympathetic discernment of the conditions and the customs, the patterns and the problems, the prides and the prejudices before sound progress can be made."[4]

The Department of Public Health Education also undertook a project far away from the Chapel Hill campus. In 1955 the department contracted with the Public Health Service to develop a multipurpose health education training program focused on the needs of American Indians. The health problems of native Americans were quite serious at the time, with many suffering from diseases long under control among other parts of the population. The project targeted western New Mexico

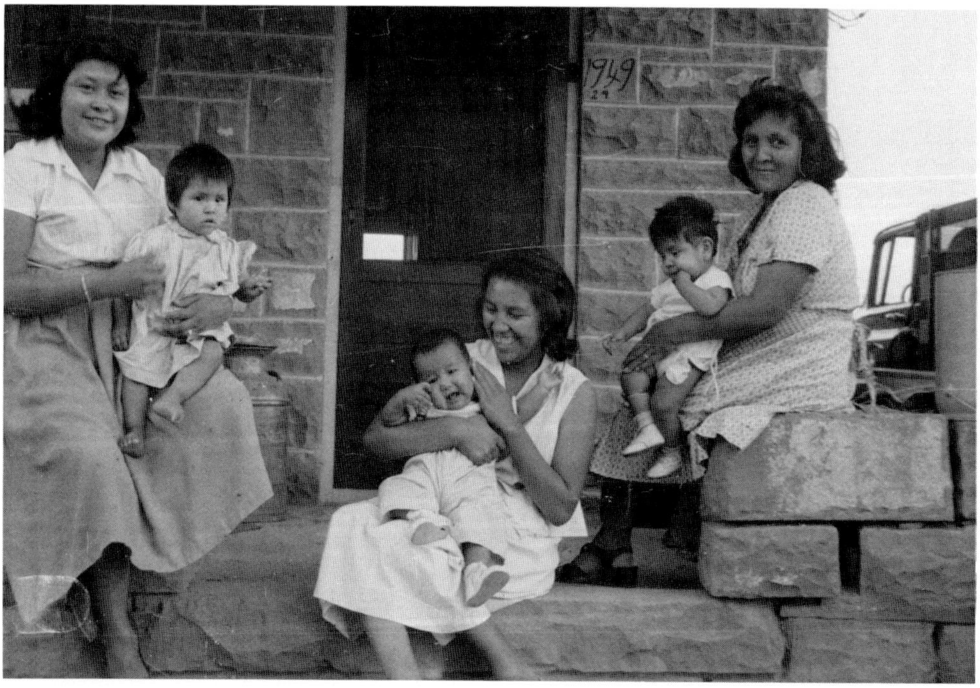

Indian mothers and children in New Mexico who benefited from the health education programs designed by the School of Public Health staff.

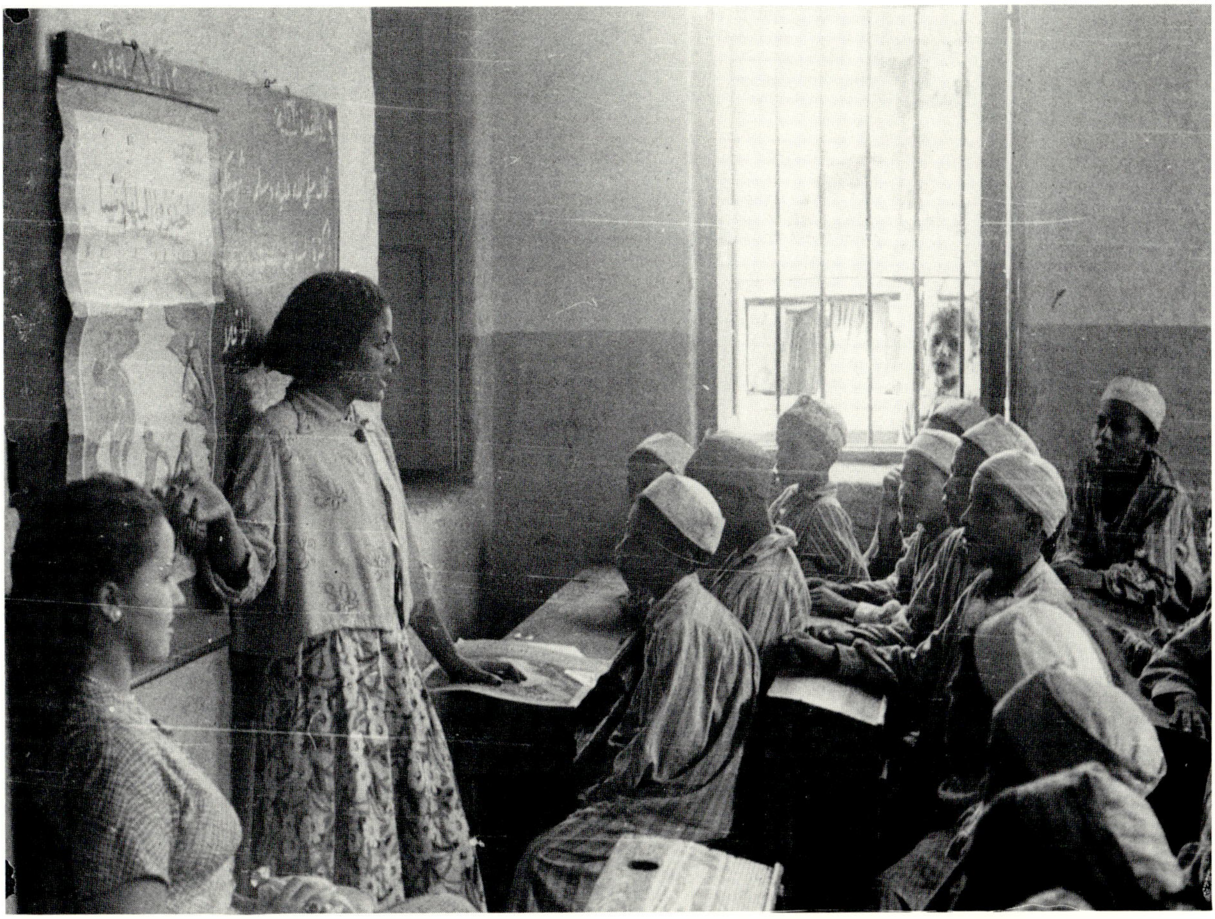

Health teaching in a Koranic school in Iran.

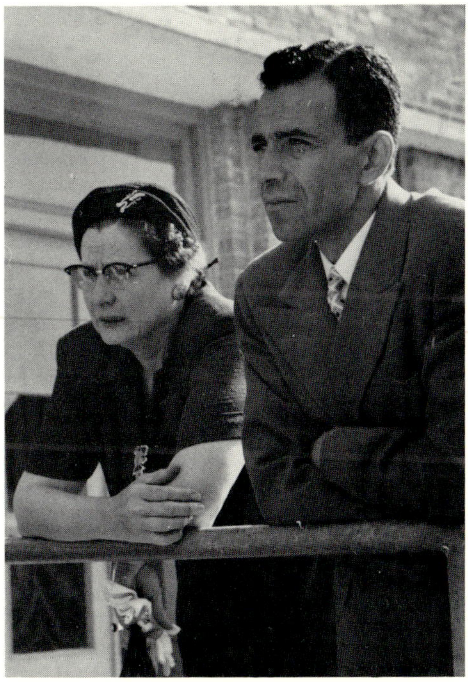

One of Lucy Morgan's efforts to "widen the circle" of understanding was her work as a consultant for the World Health Organization. Here, she is in Tehran, Iran, in 1956 with Akbar Moarefi, who received a Ph.D. from the school.

and southwestern Colorado. Pueblo tribes predominated, but the area also sustained Zuni, Apache, Ute, and Navaho peoples. Dr. Vaughn Smith served as the project's first director and was later replaced by Elta Mae Mast. Smith and Mast worked to develop health education programs on the reservations and to recruit and train community health workers who would stay on after the project ended. Faculty members provided on-site consultation, but among the project's most valuable resources were the foreign students who did their field training in the area. Their assignment to the project reflected the faculty's belief that the health problems facing American Indians closely resembled those in the students' native lands.[5]

Projects such as those in Peru and the Southwest—and there were many similar ones over the years—helped the school realize its commitment to better the health of all the world's peoples. Although it is difficult to measure the impact of such short-term training programs on the health of local populations, health education efforts among the Zuni Indian population produced some demonstrable results. Diarrhea was a major health problem, particularly among the newborn. In 1958 seven infants died of diarrhea. Health workers among the Zuni, along with School of Public Health students, devised an educational program for mothers, and the next year there were no deaths from the disease.[6]

But the very success of these projects began to undermine the unity that McGavran had tried so hard to create within the school. Individual departments had always had their own character and concerns, but the small size of the faculty and McGavran's insistence on the team concept had mitigated differences among them. By the mid-1950s, however, a perceptible tension between solidarity and individualism had begun to emerge. A number of factors contributed to this development. First, institutional growth naturally made it more difficult to maintain the cohesion of the earlier times. Second, many of the school's faculty had studied at Harvard and The Johns Hopkins, where strong departments were the rule, and they felt that the best contribution they could make was to build their own departments at Chapel Hill. Finally, the policies of federal funding agencies encouraged departmental divisions. The Public Health Service and the National Institutes of Health provided adequate categorical funding, which differentiated between disciplines, but very little funding for core public health activities. A grant might be available for an epidemiological study on cancer, but rarely did the federal government provide support for a broad-based study of cancer

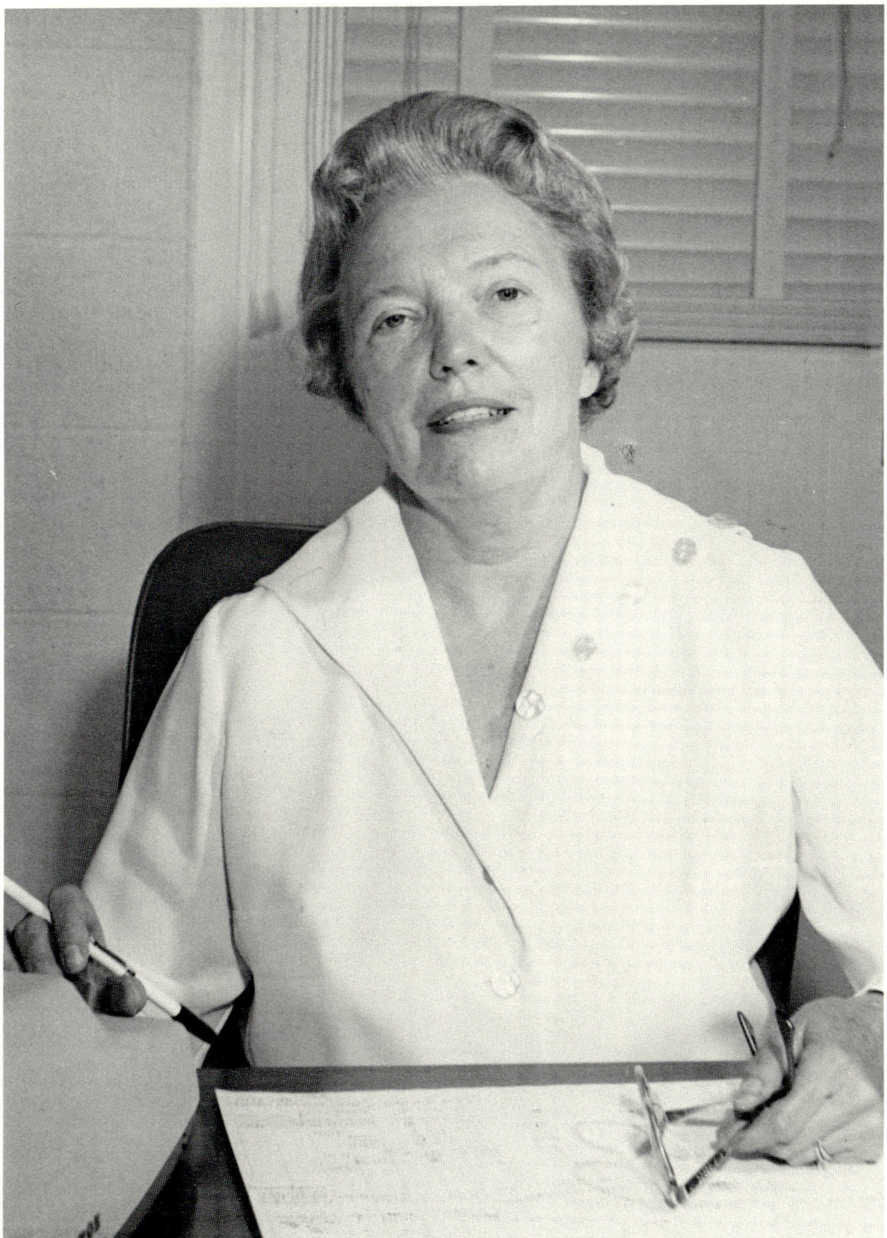

Frances Gust served as Administrative Assistant to Dean McGavran from 1950 to 1963. Her various skills as an administrator, diplomat, and advisor contributed greatly to the successful development of the school. She took courses to better understand the school and the faculty and eventually earned an M.P.H. degree.

that would involve the entire public health team. These patterns in federal spending meant that there was considerable money for scientific research and training but less for more programmatic endeavors.[7]

Despite these centrifugal tendencies, McGavran fought hard to maintain a sense of camaraderie at the school. He continued his practice of having the faculty meet in his office on Mondays for lunch, and during the football season, the men gathered to wager a dime on the weekend games. "He felt strongly about trying to create this integration," Hilton Goulson remembered, "to get people to talk across departmental lines." "He promoted this sense of togetherness and friendliness and a kind of informality," Rebecca Bryan recalled, "but he had high expectations of everyone, and there was no playing when you needed to be working."[8]

Biostatistics was one department that grew rapidly during the late 1950s as a result of increased federal funding. America's fascination with computers created a demand for statistical assistance in the School of Public Health, the Medical School, and the Public Health Service that quickly outstripped Bernie Greenberg's ability to supply. During his first flush of success in the early 1950s, Greenberg complained that "as additional burdens and responsibilities have mounted geometrically, there

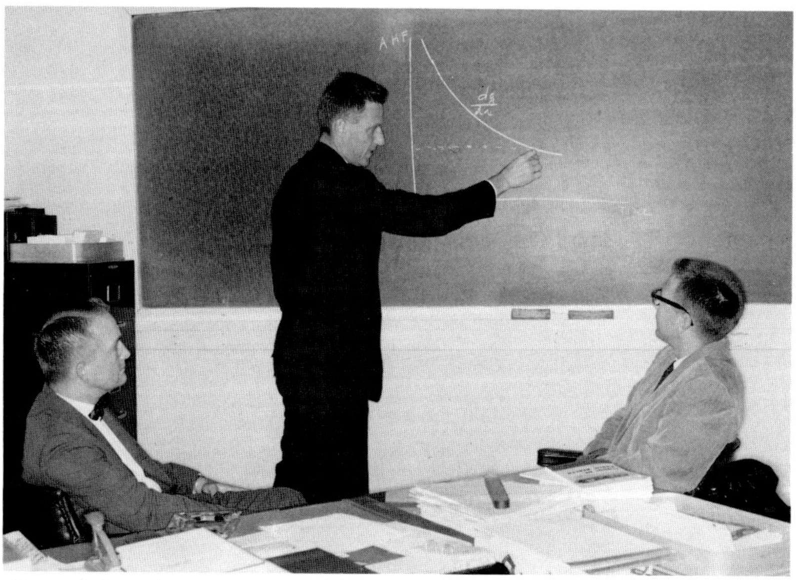

Bernard Greenberg *(center)* and James Grizzle *(right)* of the School of Public Health consulting with George Penick of the Medical School.

has been only an arithmetic increase in funds available for personnel." With hard money from the state in short supply, Greenberg had to look elsewhere. For most of the decade, training grants from the Public Health Service and research money from the American Public Health Association (APHA) paid the salaries of Greenberg's growing staff. The Public Health Service training grants supported fellows, who did both research and teaching.[9]

As with other departments, growth only increased the need for more space. Biostatistics started out in the annex known as Public Health Building A on the north side of MacNider Hall. "Inadequate housing and limitations in physical space are beyond the point where they are merely inconveniences," Greenberg wrote in 1951. "At the present time they are health hazards. Every one of the staff suffered an undue number of colds because of the lack of floor insulation, poor heating facilities, and drafts." The department obtained additional space in Annex B the next year, and the APHA project found offices in Miller Hall. By 1960 Greenberg reported that the department was spread out all over campus.[10]

In September, 1956, Biostatistics undertook its largest research project to date, a study for the APHA of factors influencing physicians to enter public health. The grant allowed Greenberg to hire a number of research associates, including Roy Kuebler, James Grizzle, and Bradley Wells, all of whom later joined the faculty.

Although research activities increased during the 1950s, teaching and service remained the mainstay of the school. Devising a curriculum for public health students required a great deal of discussion and experimentation. During the Rosenau years, individual faculty members taught courses in their specialties, while visiting instructors filled in the gaps. With the addition of new departments and faculty in the 1940s, McGavran pushed for a core curriculum. All M.P.H. and M.S.P.H. students were required to take Epidemiology, Public Health Administration, Public Health Statistics, Parasitism and Human Diseases, Principles of Sanitation, and Public Health Nursing. In 1950 the faculty began reevaluating that scheme. For two years, school and departmental committees discussed the appropriate body of knowledge required of public health practitioners. By 1952 and 1953 a revised curriculum was in place. Included were PH102, Principles and Practices of Public Health, and PH103, Applied Principles and Practices of Public Health.

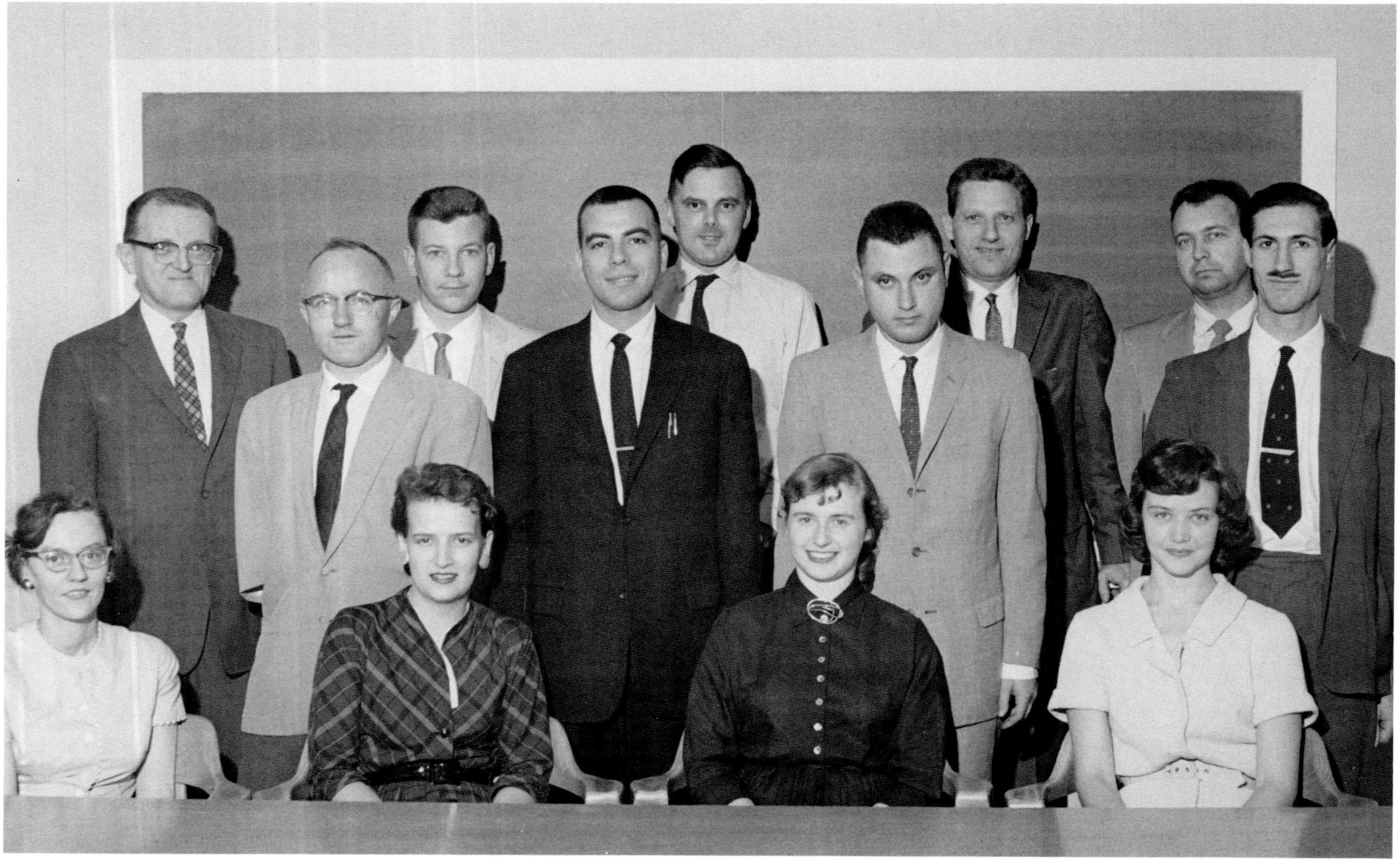

The Department of Biostatistics, 1960. *Seated, left to right:* Carol Stoeson, Benita McCarson, Ellen Kaplan, and Martha Farmer. *Standing, first row, left to right:* T. G. Donnelly, B. S. Pasternack, Alan Gross, and R. Elston. *Second row:* Roy Kuebler, Jr., James Grizzle, D. J. Newell, Bernard Greenberg, and Bradley Wells.

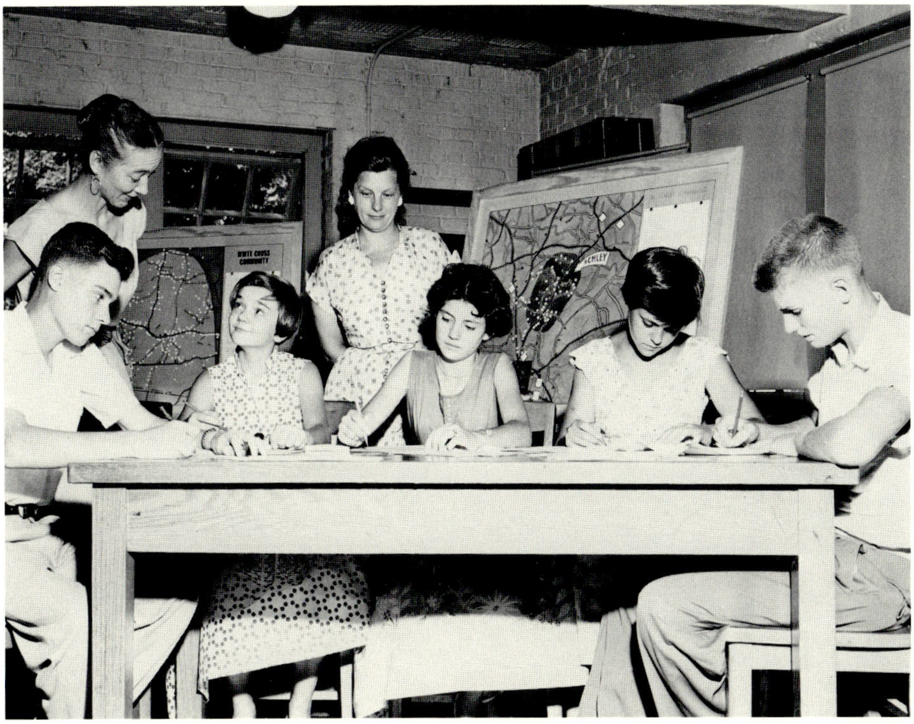

Rosemary Kent and Elta Mae Mast work with high school students in the Schley community.

For the field-oriented staff, PH103 "represented the peak in curriculum planning." Dean McGavran described the course:

> All departments were involved in this project. The total student body was enrolled in the course—all the faculty were participants and the total staff of the four field centers within a fifty-mile radius of Chapel Hill became the "clinical instructors." One day a week was set aside for this course from 7:00 a.m. to 7:00 p.m. Each faculty member took four or five students in his (or her) car and went to "his community patient." . . .These small groups "observed the patient" superficially—they gathered "patient opinion" on health matters—they studied the record—interviewed official and voluntary health and related agencies and individuals, observed schools, factories, facilities, and activities and functions of health departments and other agencies, and finally picked one particular. . .area for study in greater depth.

Although the students and faculty seemed to benefit from this hands-on learning, it was expensive and time-consuming. Soon many faculty members lost their enthusiasm and the course was phased out. "But it was a superb experiment," McGavran remembered, "and for two brief years the School of Public Health demonstrated to students, practitioners, and ourselves that there was a public health team."[11]

This team concept was applied more effectively when done voluntarily. Maternal and child health's Geraldine Gourley remembered that "during those times we did a lot of teaching in other departments. I taught interviewing in public health nursing and education, even in biostatistics. I taught health problems with special social implications." This kind of interdisciplinary cooperation extended outside the classroom. "I spent a lot of time with Roger Howell in the Department of Mental Health," Gourley recalled. "We went around all over the state with workshops for social workers, nurses, and various people around mental health issues."[12]

Epidemiology had been one of the original departments in the school, headed first by Rosenau and then by McGavran. But administrative responsibilities left little time for teaching or research by either of the deans. "The result," McGavran wrote in the 1953–54 annual report, "is that this department, which should be the strongest in the School of Public Health, is actually the weakest." That situation began to turn around in 1954 when McGavran obtained funds from the Public Health Service to start a Chronic Disease Section, for which he hired Dr. John Cassel. A native of South Africa, Cassel received his medical

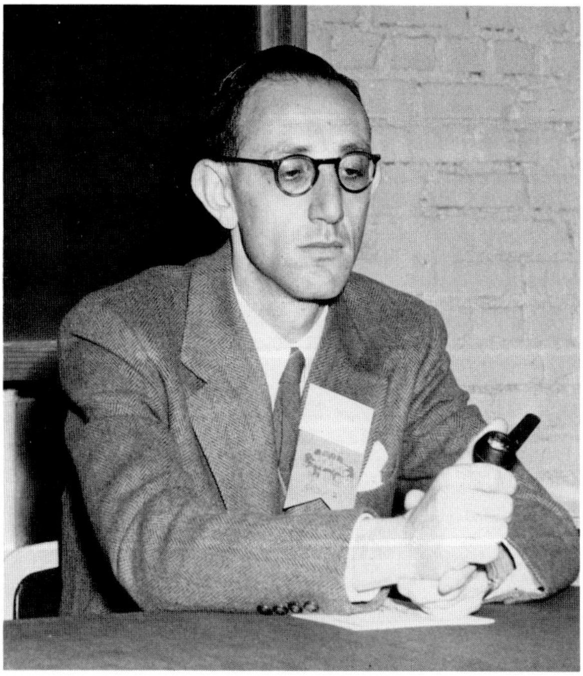

John Cassel

degree at the University of Witwatersrand. He won a Rockefeller Foundation fellowship to study at the School of Public Health in 1952, and after receiving his M.P.H. he returned to South Africa to work as a medical officer at a health center.[13]

Medical science had made such strides since the late nineteenth century that by 1950 there were effective cures for most infectious diseases. But scientific understanding of chronic maladies such as cancer, mental illness, and heart disease was still rather primitive, and investigations of these illnesses dominated the medical research agenda. Cassel's job was to provide instruction in the treatment of cancer and other chronic diseases to public health students and to conduct epidemiological research on such ailments. Cassel quickly established a reputation as an excellent teacher and researcher and within a few years had received attractive offers from both The Johns Hopkins and Harvard.[14]

Epidemiology grew dramatically in 1958 with the addition of three new faculty members paid by training grants from the Public Health Service and NIH. McGavran wanted an experienced, well-known person for the job of chairman and, through John Cassel, contacted Dr. Sidney Kark. Kark was professor of social, preventive, and family medicine at the University of Natal in South Africa, but prior to his academic appointment had had extensive experience as a public health officer and as a research epidemiologist. Kark was at the time pursuing a job with the World Health Organization (WHO), but McGavran offered him a one-year contract to help direct the growth and reorganization of the department.[15]

Kark left after a year to be WHO professor of public health and social medicine at the Hebrew University in Jerusalem. McGavran recommended John Cassel as Kark's replacement. A few years later McGavran wrote to Kark, "I am sure you would be proud to see how well John Cassel has continued and developed your good work here in establishing a dynamic Department of Epidemiology. John is a jewel and is gaining more and more national recognition. His department is stimulating to students and faculty alike and intensely loyal to John. I think we have a new and fresh approach to the teaching of epidemiology which is going to make its mark."[16]

That fresh approach involved a focus on the social causes of disease. Michel Ibrahim, another future dean, came to study at the school in 1960. He spent one year in biostatistics, but a desire to use his medical

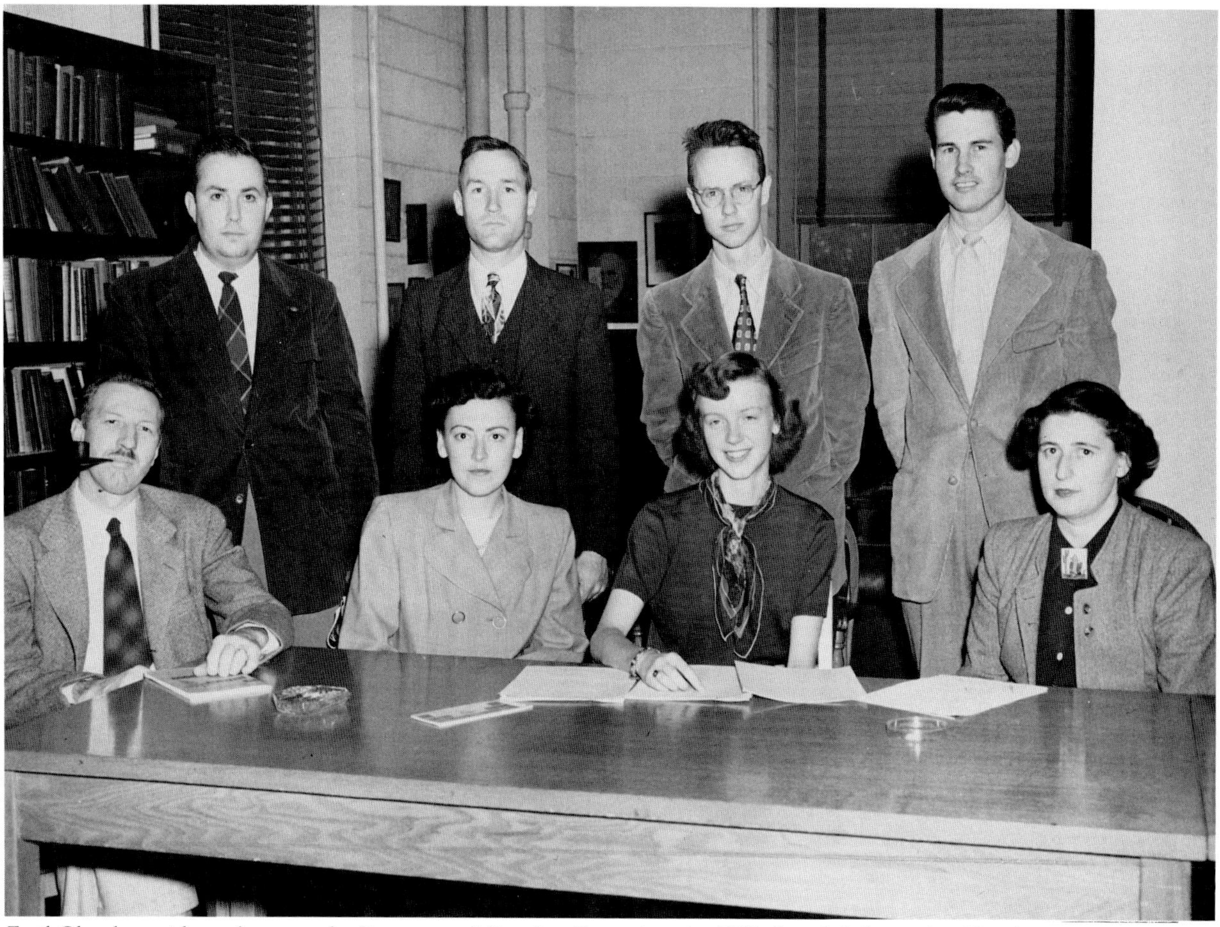

Emil Chanlett with students on the Program and Steering Committee in 1950. *Seated, left to right:* Chanlett, Barbara Adams, Mary-Katherine Rellahan, Ruth Richards. *Standing:* Wayne Messick, Alfred Fletcher, Eugene Taylor, Charles Campbell.

background led him to transfer to epidemiology. Ibrahim described the insights that propelled Cassel's research and teaching: "Most of medicine was very biologically oriented. We thought in terms of germs and degenerative diseases. He advanced the theory—he did not invent it, but he pushed it very hard—that social and psychological factors affect people's health. [He was concerned with] cultural values, societal values and stress and how they related to illness."[17]

While biostatistics and epidemiology flourished in the 1950s, the Department of Mental Health hung on for dear life. The initial funding from the Public Health Service proved inadequate to support Dr. Roger Howell, the department's only faculty member, on a full-time basis, so he also served as acting director of the Mental Health Section of the State Board of Health. Dr. Howell spent many hours in the field, working with local agencies and talking to civic groups about mental health, a new and sometimes difficult subject for Americans in the 1950s.

Howell resigned in 1957 to accept a position as director of the Division of Preventive Psychiatry at the Lafayette Clinic in Detroit, Michigan. His reasons for leaving indicate some of the problems the school faced in those years:

> Probably the greatest reason for my change concerns the promise of being able to do research. Being a one-man department, with rather demanding administrative responsibilities as well as teaching and field activities, seems to make impossible any consideration of spending time on research, which is much needed in the field of mental health. The policy of having to obtain outside funds to support the department, and to make possible personnel additions so that research is forthcoming, is rather short-sighted for a progressive university, interested in advancing the body of knowledge which will bring greater happiness and health to the people of its state.[18]

For a year and a half the department had no faculty members. Finally the school hired Dr. John Filley as assistant professor and head in the fall of 1958.

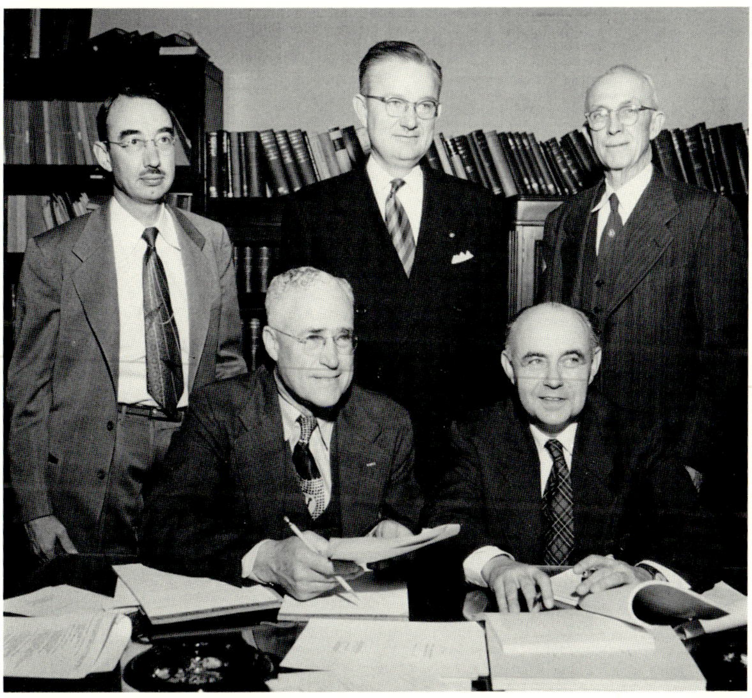

State Health Officer J. Roy Norton with Dean McGavran in 1951. Norton served on the faculty in the late 1930s and again in the 1960s. In 1963 he was president of the American Public Health Association.

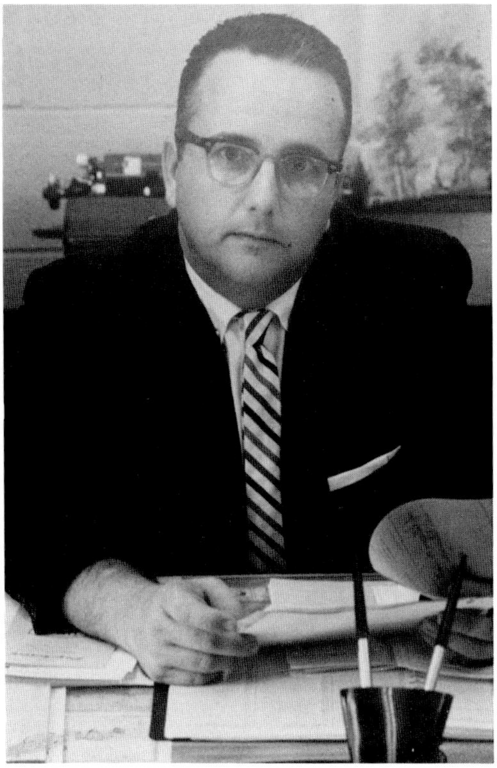

Charles M. Cameron, Jr.

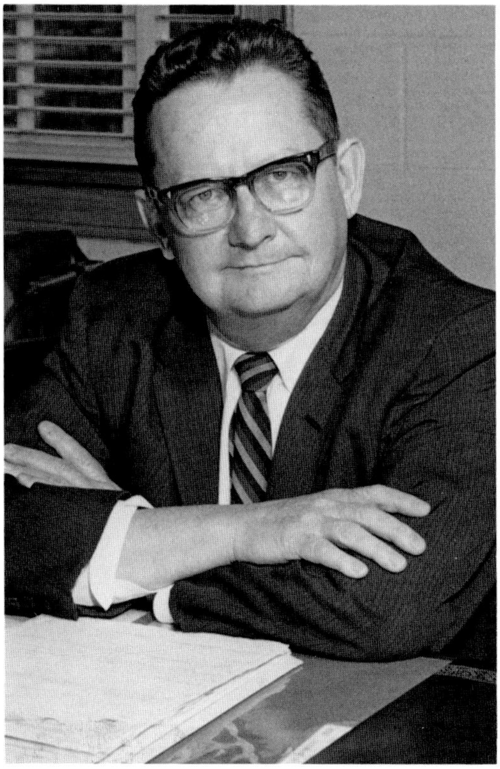

Robert E. Coker, Jr.

With Cecil Sheps's resignation in 1952 to become director of program planning in the Division of Health Affairs, the Department of Public Health Administration lost its most dynamic young professor. John Wright and a series of visiting professors carried on for the next few years, but most of Wright's time was taken up with his responsibilities to the school, the university, and the state. In 1955 Dr. Charles M. Cameron, Jr., joined the faculty. Another of the school's Vanderbilt-trained physicians, Cameron had served as a health officer in Tennessee, as a commissioned officer in the Public Health Service, and with the North Carolina State Board of Health. In 1954 he had received an M.P.H. from the School of Public Health. Much of his work at the State Board of Health and at the school dealt with accident prevention. Dr. Robert E. Coker, Jr., came on board a few years later. The department focused mostly on teaching and service, and by the end of the decade the three professors were on scores of boards and committees.

The Department of Public Health Nursing continued to attract large numbers of students throughout the 1950s. Ruth Hay and Margaret Blee remained the mainstays of the department, both as teachers and consultants. In 1954 the members of that year's class in public health nursing presented a portrait of Professor Hay to the school. "It is hoped," the students wrote, "that the portrait may be an inspiration to all nurses

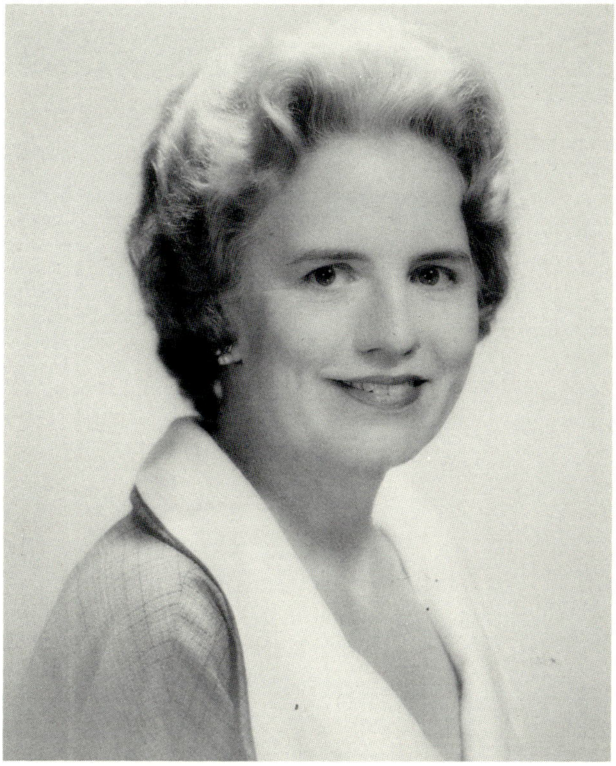

Margaret Dolan

in the field of public health, and will serve as a constant reminder to us in fulfilling the challenge Miss Hay had instilled in us."[19]

In 1950 a new person who would become a national figure in public health joined the department. Margaret Dolan came from an old North Carolina family with strong ties to the university. She received a nursing degree from Georgetown University and served for a number of years as an epidemiological nurse, first with the Public Health Service and then with the Greensboro, North Carolina, City Health Department. In 1944 she returned to the university and received her B.S. from the School of Public Health in public health nursing. She also received an M.A. from Columbia University in 1953. Margaret Dolan had an immediate impact, both as a teacher and as an ambassador for the school. By the mid-1950s she served on boards and committees of state and national nursing and public health associations. In 1959 she succeeded Ruth Hay as head of the department.[20]

The Department of Public Health Nutrition grew more slowly during the 1950s. In 1949 Frances MacKinnon, a nutritionist and dietitian with rich experience in public health practice and teaching, joined the faculty, bringing a clinician's perspective to the department. The next year the department enrolled its first M.P.H. students. Rebecca Broach Bryan was a student during the 1951–52 academic year. Like so

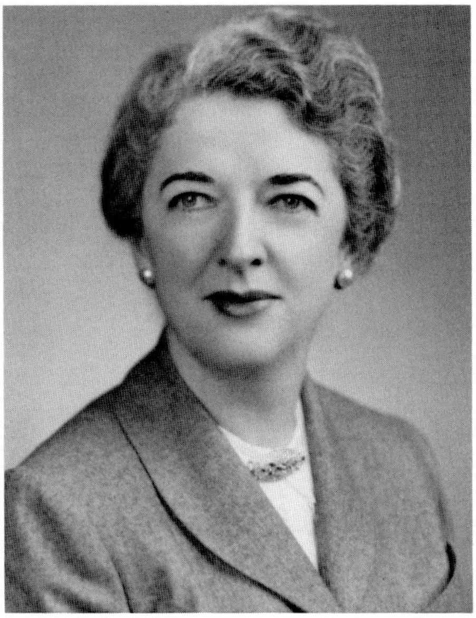

Frances MacKinnon

Faculty and students in the Department of Public Health Nutrition, 1958. Rebecca Broach Bryan is third from left in back row. Hughes Bryan is far right.

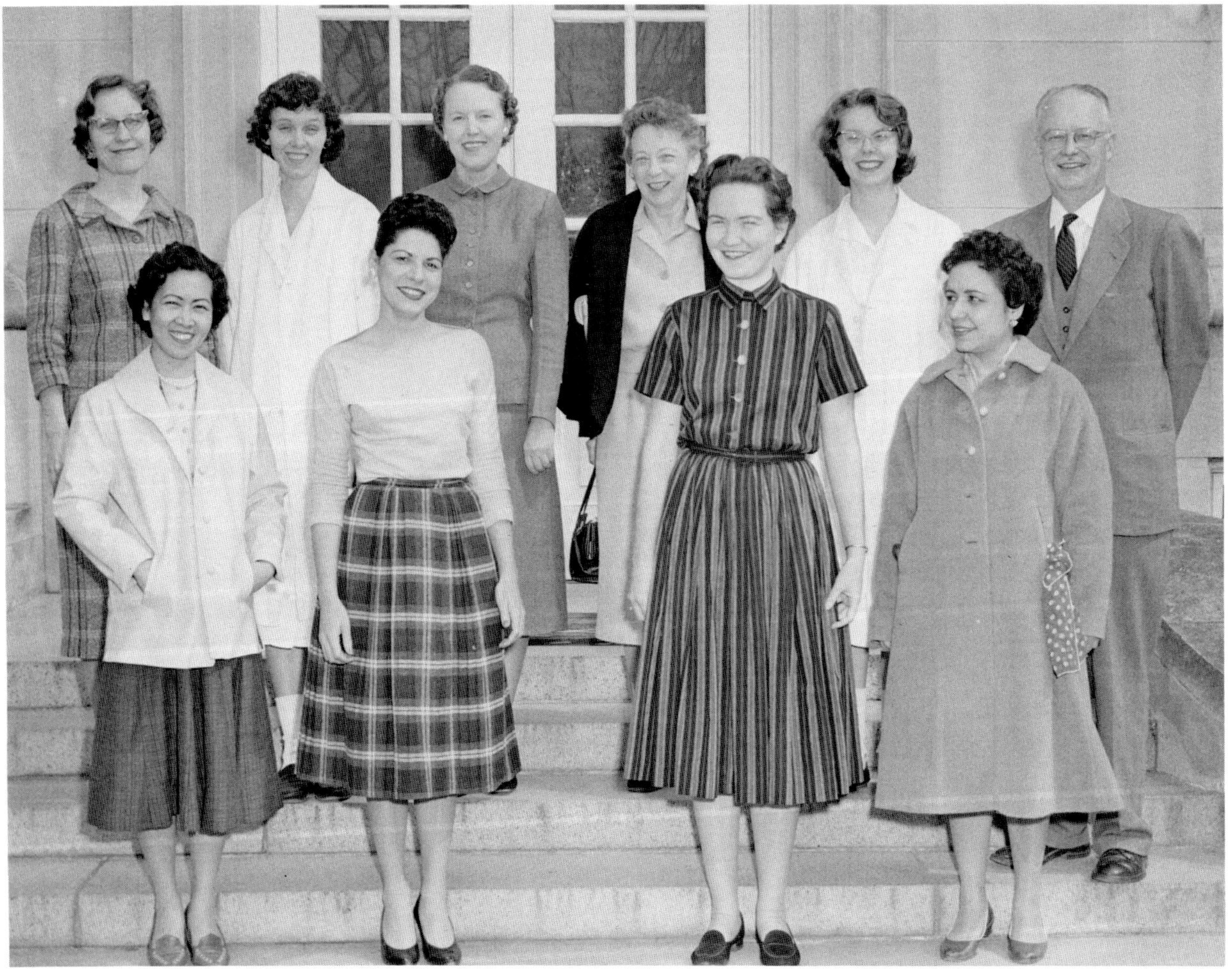

many other students in that period, she brought valuable experience as a public health worker to the classroom. "I had a feeling," she remembered, "that the faculty felt they were learning as much from the students as we were from them, and they probably were. The department was being funded by the Children's Bureau, and most students were here on Children's Bureau scholarships. When the visiting chiefs from Washington came, we were a part of the thinking. I felt I had my thinking stretched a mile."[21]

The Department of Public Health Nutrition's strength lay in teaching and service, but Dr. Hughes Bryan continued to do both laboratory and field research. He began a study with Dr. Greenberg in the early 1950s on the growth of school age children and, with money from the Public Health Service, expanded the project in 1955 to look more closely at the relation of diet to growth patterns. Like other members of the school, Bryan repeatedly complained that the lack of space prevented him from undertaking any larger research projects.

By the mid-1950s, John Larsh had become something of a senior citizen in the school, although he was still in his late thirties. His reputation as a teacher and a stickler for academic excellence won him praise from his students and colleagues. Hilton Goulson came to the school in 1952 from Luther College in Decorah, Iowa, one of a long line of students from that college who studied with Larsh. "He was one of the most amazing teachers that I have ever known," remembered Goulson. "Completely organized. He would come into a room and be ready to go, no notes, just a piece of chalk. He would start writing and talking at the same time, so you'd have to get that knack of listening and being able to write down what he writes on the board and hope the lead in your pencil doesn't break. When you got through for the day, or for the week, or for the semester you had a complete outline of the subject." "Teaching was my number one love," Larsh recalled. "The idea that I knew something that I could pass on to someone else was the greatest thrill I ever had."[22]

Although Larsh firmly believed in the primacy of teaching, his ever-present white lab coat indicated his continuing connection to research. Larsh's research concerned *Trichinella spiralis*, the agent of trichinosis, and some of his students expanded on his early findings. "The main thrust of our research at that time was trichinella paralysis in the white mouse," Goulson remembered. Larsh worked closely with these students. "In the early days I'd have one or two working under me, and I could have time to teach them some techniques. How do you estimate the number of worms in an animal you have infected? How do you look at malaria parasites and get the density? I had a policy that everyone who finished his Ph.D. would publish at least one full-length paper in which only his name was on it. I felt that was the way to launch somebody into research. Go through all the facets, show exactly how it is done. You get the data, but the data is no good if you don't publish it."[23]

The role of research in the school was a matter of contention during the whole of McGavran's tenure as dean. John Larsh remembered his first interview after McGavran arrived in Chapel Hill:

> I'll never forget how disappointed I was with him. I thought I would impress him with how much research I had got done. He says, "Well, if you want to do it, that's all right, but that's not helping the school." I thought, my god, if research doesn't help the school, why do we do research? He didn't clip anybody's wings, it was just his blunt way of saying, well, I'm not interested in that. I'm interested in the school making a reputation as being a resource for the community.
>
> See, Dr. McGavran was a dyed-in-the-wool field man. Rosenau had no experience out in the field. Rosenau I picture as more of an intramural type. He wrote his famous textbook, he was a researcher at the National Hygienic Laboratory, and he taught. But he did not go out and see how public health really worked out in the field, but that's what McGavran did.[24]

Although Larsh was more committed to teaching and research than to field work, he supported McGavran's notion that the primary responsibility of a school of public health was to train practitioners. "You are not trying to train research people," he said, "you are training people that know the value of research."[25]

The Department of Experimental Medicine, however, was one area in which pure research held sway. In looking back, McGavran acknowledged the department's contributions (not the least of which were the funds it received from the Public Health Service) but felt he had set a dangerous precedent. The department, in his opinion, "remained an 'institute of research' housed in the School of Public Health—separate and distinct in every regard. . . . The only excuse for research in an edu-

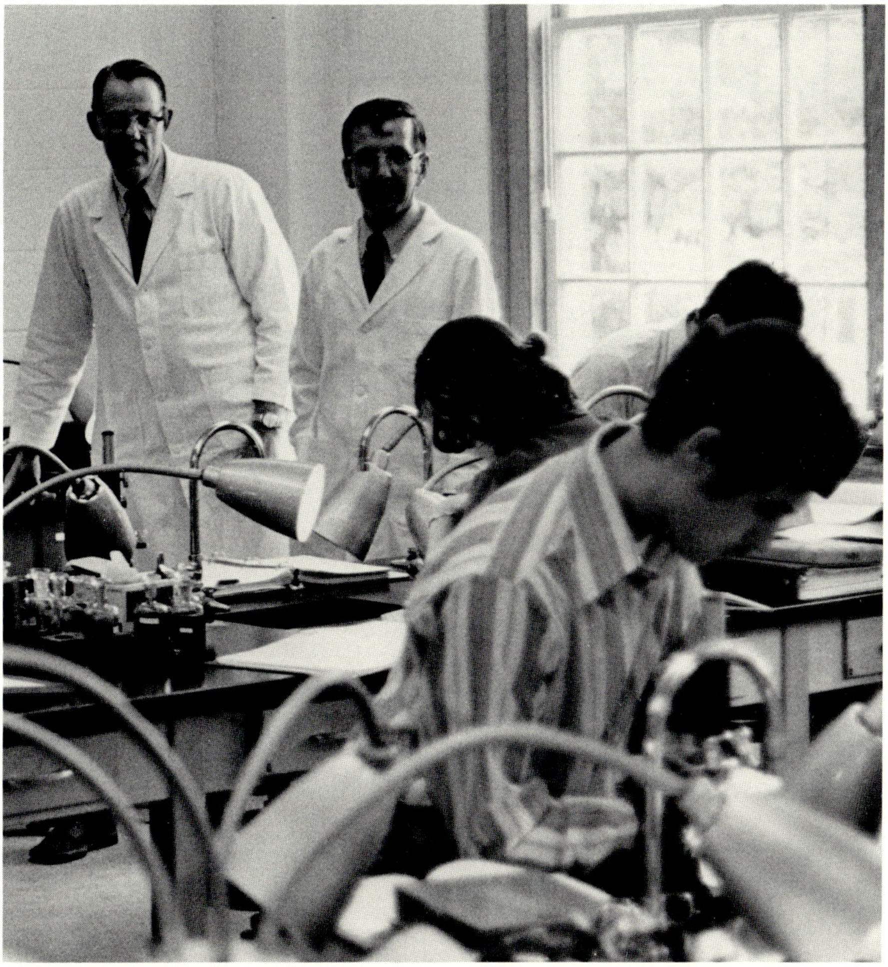

John Larsh and Hilton Goulson working with students in the Department of Parasitology.

cational institution," McGavran wrote, "is that it becomes part of the teaching and learning process and not an end in itself; that it enriches and strengthens education, faculty and students alike. This does not (and did not) happen when the research is conducted in a separate institute—call it a department or what have you. This research institute is the 'European pattern,' which has been followed by too many institutions in this country."[26]

Dan Okun, on the other hand, believed that "teaching and service is best done when built on a research foundation."

> In the early days of the school there was no research going on. McGavran was for teaching, improving everybody. My feeling has always been that there are some functions that could be better served by some of the other schools [in the state]. We shouldn't occupy space here to do only what McGavran wanted to do, take someone from this level and raise them to that level. That was an

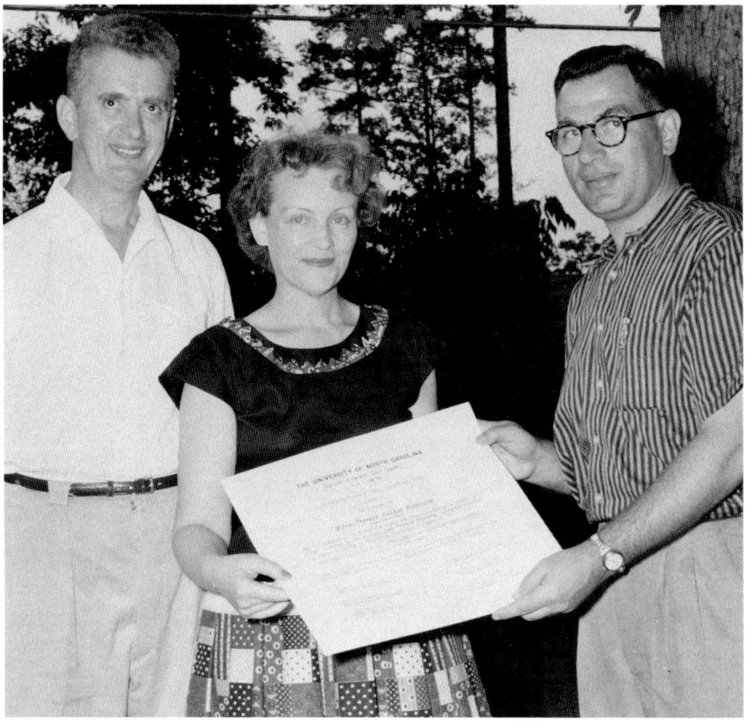

Daniel Okun presents an "honorary degree" from the Department of Sanitary Engineering to Marie-Therese Francotte for her support of her husband, Francois, while a student at the school. Attitudes about female roles varied widely at the school since departments were largely segregated along gender lines.

> academic service obligation, but one that could be met by other institutions. We had big fights about it and most of the rest of the faculty in the School of Public Health—when I came here—did not agree with me.[27]

In any case, by the late 1950s, federal funding policies were making McGavran's priorities increasingly difficult to sustain. Federal research money became more plentiful, while money for teaching and operating expenses remained in short supply. The school, however, did receive a needed shot in the arm in 1958 with the passage of the Hill-Rhodes Act. The bill allocated a million dollars annually to the nation's eleven schools of public health based on the number of federally sponsored students they admitted. Unfortunately, Congress did not appropriate money until the next year, and even then the funds did not cover the cost of educating the students. Nevertheless, McGavran called it a "step in the right direction." "If continued," he said, "it will assist the schools materially in improving and expanding the amount and caliber of education in public health."[28]

The people of North Carolina also seemed more receptive to the school's needs. On October 27, 1959, voters approved a bond issue for

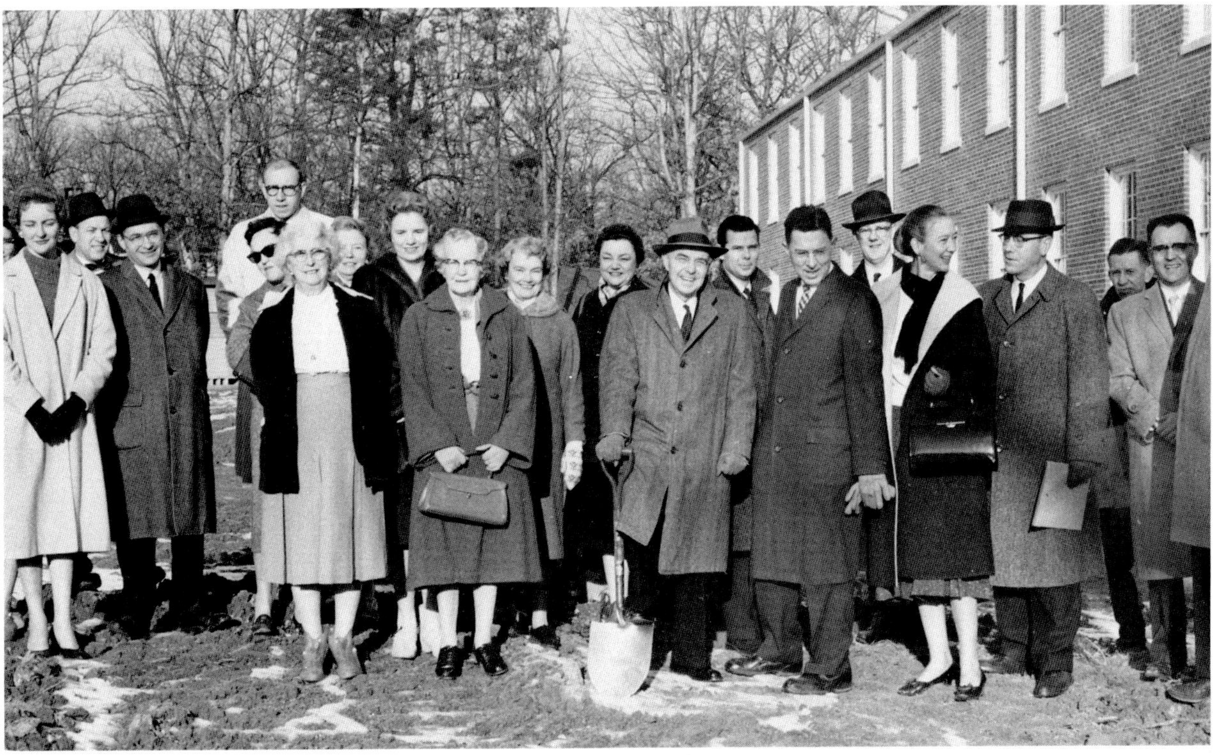

Faculty and staff at the ground-breaking ceremonies for Rosenau Hall, February 6, 1961.

capital improvements for state institutions and agencies, which included a million dollars for a new building for the school. School of Public Health alumni and staff played an important role in securing the favorable bond vote through their involvement in the North Carolina Public Health Association. The association sent letters to its 1200 members asking them to promote the bond in their communities. The association's successful promotion of the bond drive was one indication of the school's growing influence. As more and more graduates took positions in local health departments, they used their training to spread the school's philosophy throughout the state.[29]

School officials appreciated the support of the people of North Carolina, but a million dollars was far short of the needed funds. Fortunately, Congress directed construction funds under the Grant and Research Facilities Act to the Public Health Service, which in turn provided $700,000 in matching funds to the school.[30]

Ground-breaking ceremonies for the new building took place on January 16, 1961. The dean posed with shovel in hand, and the faculty and staff huddled around him on a cold and snowy day. On another cold day that January, President John F. Kennedy, enjoined his fellow Americans, "Ask not what your country can do for you, but what you can do for your country." Kennedy's rhetoric of self-sacrifice resonated deeply with those who had already devoted themselves to furthering the cause of public health, and public health leaders looked forward to help from the new administration.

Kennedy's domestic policy, as it turned out, offered few new proposals on health care, although it did support additional money for construction of health facilities and scholarships. The thrust of his legislative efforts was the Democratic Party's continuing fight for the addition of hospital insurance to Social Security. In May, 1961, Dean McGavran testified before the U. S. House of Representatives on a bill "to expand and improve community services and facilities for the health care of the aged and chronically ill." McGavran spoke forcefully for the bill, but he also offered two amendments on behalf of the American College of Preventive Medicine that would remove the ceilings on grants for schools of public health. If additional funds for training were not also made available, he argued, new services would only aggravate the shortage of trained personnel.[31]

The construction of a new building and the inauguration of a new young president portended a new era at the school. Soon the torch would be passed to a new generation. Ruth Hay and Margaret Blee were the first of the "old guard" to retire. In 1960 they started serving on a half-time basis, and in 1962 took full retirement. That same year Lucy Morgan turned over the chair in public health education to Ralph Boatman. Dean McGavran also announced his retirement.

Such transitions provide institutions with an opportunity for reflection, and the school cast its eye backward on a number of occasions in the early 1960s. Dr. Rosemary Kent undertook a history of the school in 1962. For many months she and other members of her committee searched the university archives, examined records in the Dean's Office, and corresponded with old friends of the school. The eventual publication provided only a sketch of the early years, but the effort generated great interest in the school's past and preserved many important documents.[32]

The school also participated in a university-wide self-study in 1962. The report presented the state of the school on the eve of Dean McGavran's retirement. Growth was the key word. Enrollments were on the rise. Research funds were increasing. The faculty was not only growing, but salaries and benefits were beginning to catch up with those of other schools.

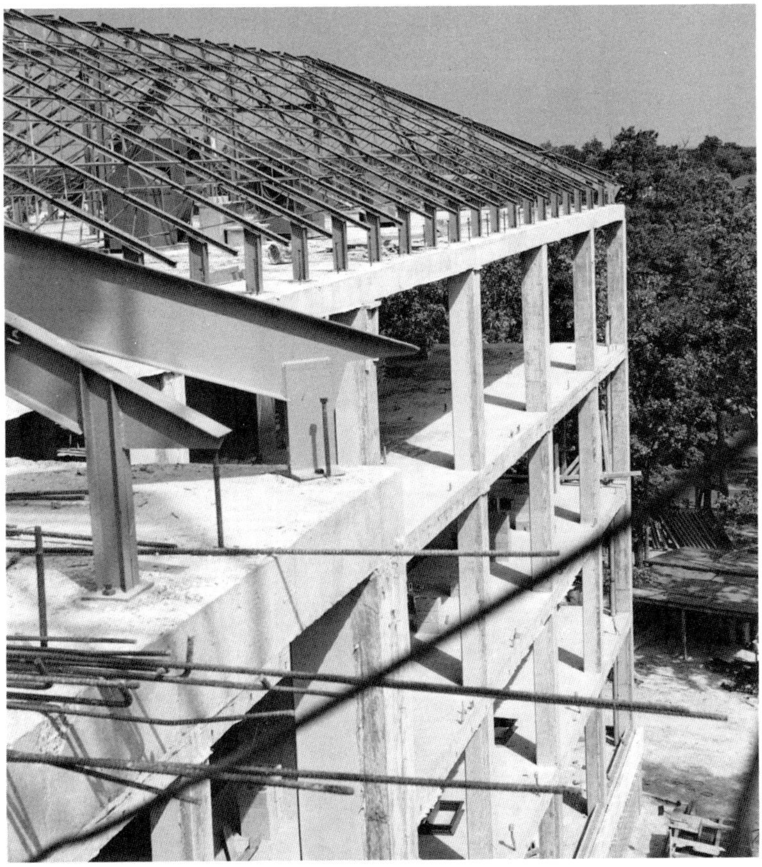

Construction of the new School of Public Health building.

Below, Retirement dinner for Ruth Hay and Margaret Blee at the Carolina Inn on the Chapel Hill campus. School of Public Health faculty have probably eaten more meals per capita at the Carolina Inn than any group on campus.

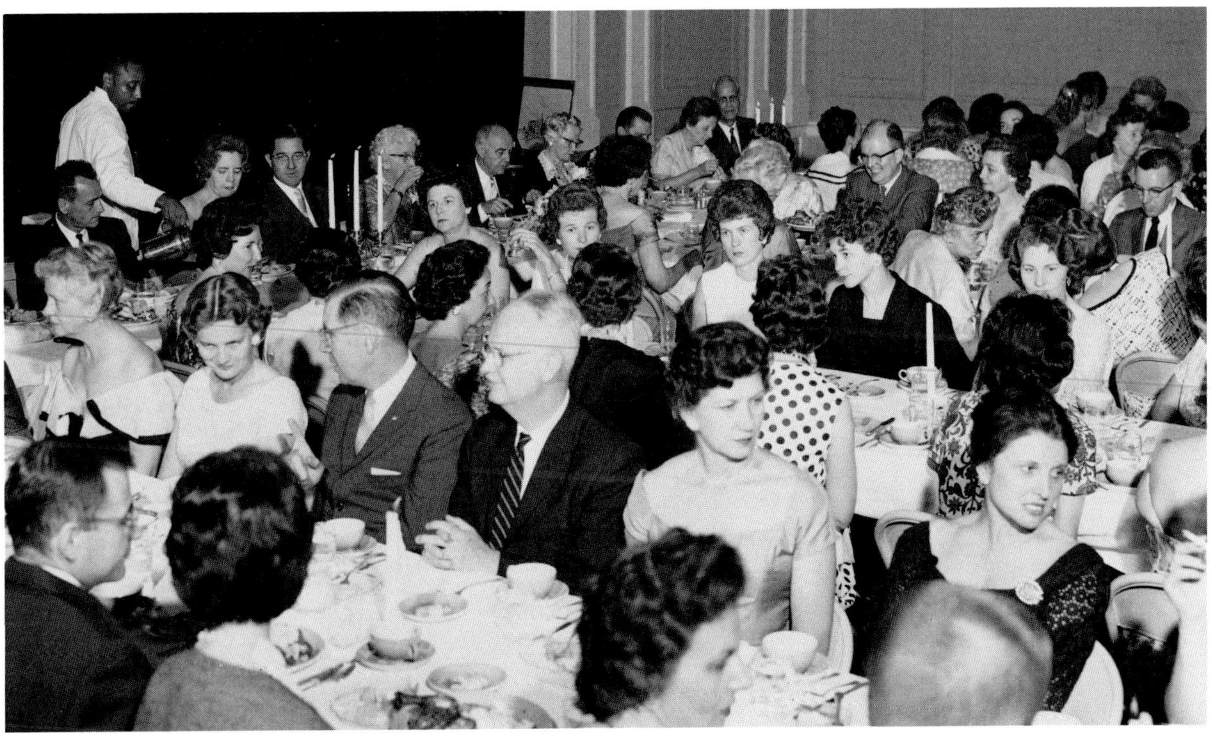

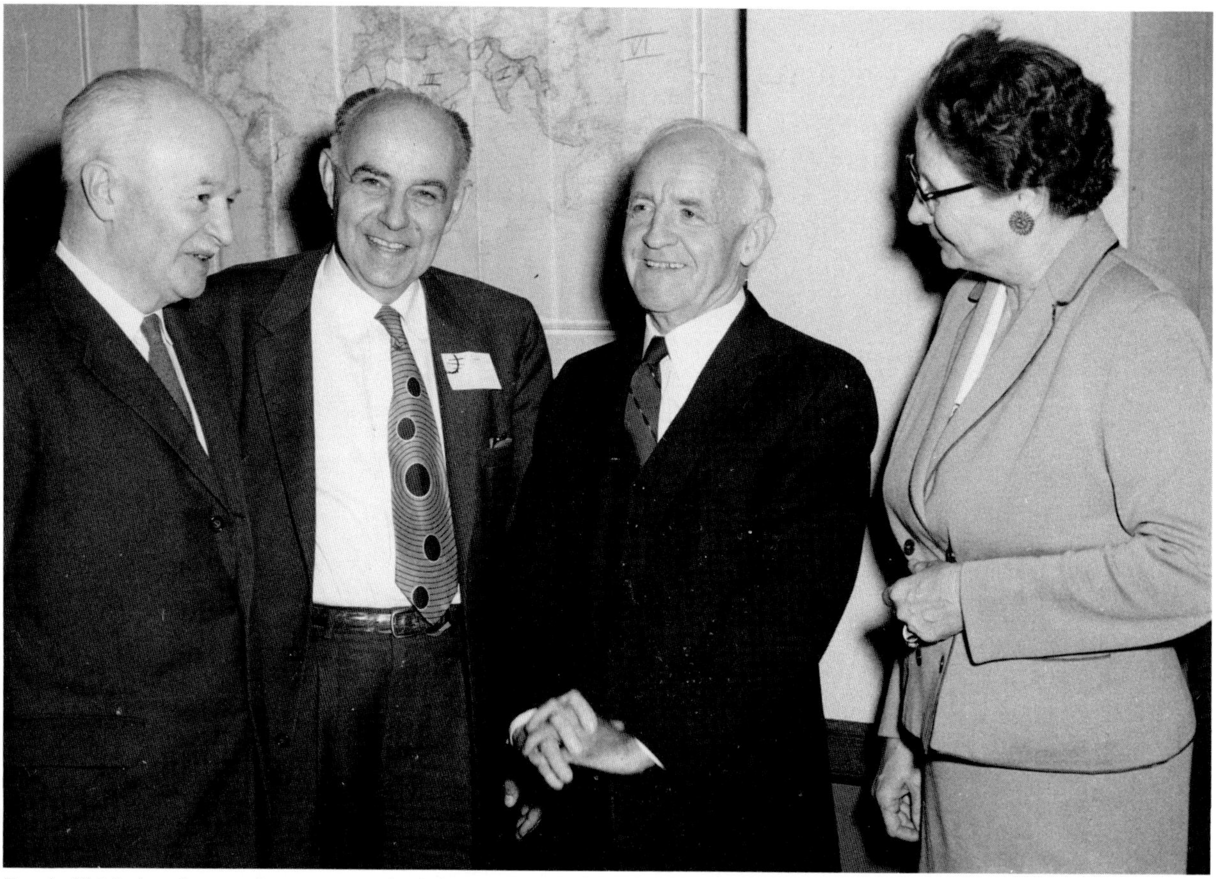

Brock Chisholm, former director-general of the World Health Organization, discusses international health issues with Dean McGavran, Frank Graham, and Lucy Morgan.

Any academic institution's reputation is based on the reputation of its individual faculty members. Research and teaching are the primary criteria for judging an individual's standing in the profession, but in a service-oriented field like public health, activities outside the classroom and the laboratory are also crucial to the individual's and the school's reputation. From working with local schools and health departments to consulting with the World Health Organization in various parts of the world, the school's staff spent thousands of hours dealing with practical health problems. "This leadership role," the self-study committee reported, "is more than a prestige factor in the School of Public Health. It provides for better student recruitment and selection, better learning and teaching situations, revitalization of research, and closer correlation with community need and educational effort. Good performance here is to the School of Public Health what good performance in patient care is to the Medical School."[33]

There was a momentum in public health that the 1963 self-study report very accurately predicted. The committee foresaw growth in the number of students and federal money and in the diversity of educational programs. "In all these things," the committee wrote, "we shall either move ahead with the tide or be left behind in the wash; there is no halfway alternative." The waves of the future, according to the committee, were health care, environmental health, and international health. Who or what determined the destiny of public health, the committee did not say. The issue was not why, but how.[34]

The development of new programs and the addition of more faculty members entailed some administrative changes that ran counter to McGavran's "town meeting" vision. In 1952 an Executive Faculty Committee, made up mostly of department heads, replaced the general faculty as the policy-making body of the school. Then in 1959 McGavran appointed his first assistant dean, Dr. Millard Bethel. Dean McGavran, in a confidential comment included in his "Report to the Faculty," warned his colleagues about the consequences of continued growth.

> None of the faculty will probably wish to change the democratic administrative approach to the organization and operation of the School of Public Health, but the change may come anyway. Increasingly in the past year, the executive faculty had insisted upon the Dean's Office assuming more and more of the functions which in past years have been carried on by faculty individuals and through committees. These have been called administrative details; for example, the preparation of the catalogs, much of the administrative activity, and scheduling of classes.
>
> Admittedly, these activities are time consuming functions that remove faculty "from departmental activity, from important teaching, research, and services," but I warn you that you can't "have your cake and eat it." The incoming dean (as I would) will no doubt bow to these faculty pressures and even welcome more administrative control unhampered by the democratic process, but what will be the net result? Be sure you want to lose control before you dump "chores." There are few schools with faculties that have the responsibilities and opportunities to guide their school that you have earned. Responsibilities with subsequent opportunities are easier to keep than to get.[35]

To the end McGavran tried to forge the unity he felt was necessary for a successful public health team. "One of the last things he did," Hilton Goulson recalled, "and one that I remember so vividly, was to walk through the entire building making certain that there were no

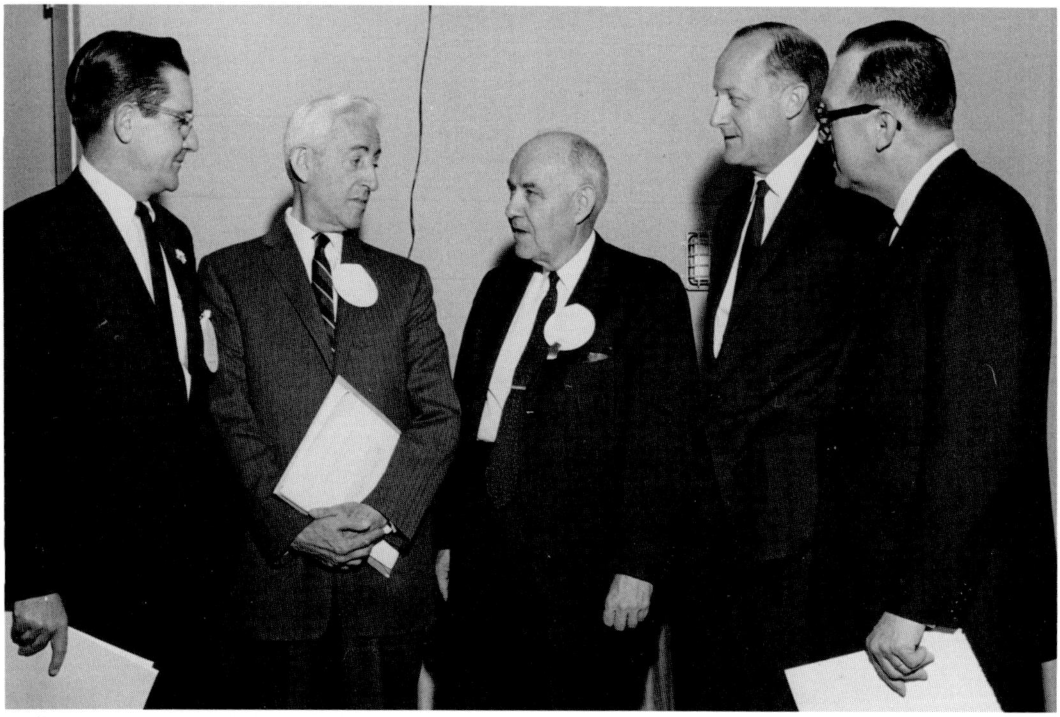

William Friday, Abel Wolman, Dean McGavran, Henry Clark, and Hugh Holman.

coffee pots. Coffee pots were not allowed because he had a coffee room down on the first floor, and everybody was supposed to come down there and drink coffee." Soon after McGavran left, however, the room became a laboratory.[36]

By the spring of 1963, the School of Public Health had much to be proud of. The student-faculty ratio had declined dramatically, state appropriations had increased steadily, and research funds supported many important projects. The dedication of the new School of Public Health Building (the building was not officially named for Dr. Rosenau until 1965) brought hundreds of people to Chapel Hill for two days of speeches, discussion, and socializing. Some of public health's most notable personages graced the stage of the new auditorium. On Saturday morning, April 6, 1963, Dr. Abel Wolman, professor emeritus of sanitary engineering at The Johns Hopkins, presented the opening address. That afternoon four group sessions discussed the past, present, and future of public health. A speech by the school's most senior supporter, Frank Porter Graham, highlighted the evening activities. On Sunday morning John Wright planted a southern magnolia in memory of Milton J. Rosenau, and that afternoon North Carolina Governor Terry Sanford dedicated the building. The future seemed so promising that nostalgia for the past was fleeting. Dr. and Mrs. McGavran were headed to India; the school had a new home and soon would have a new dean.[37]

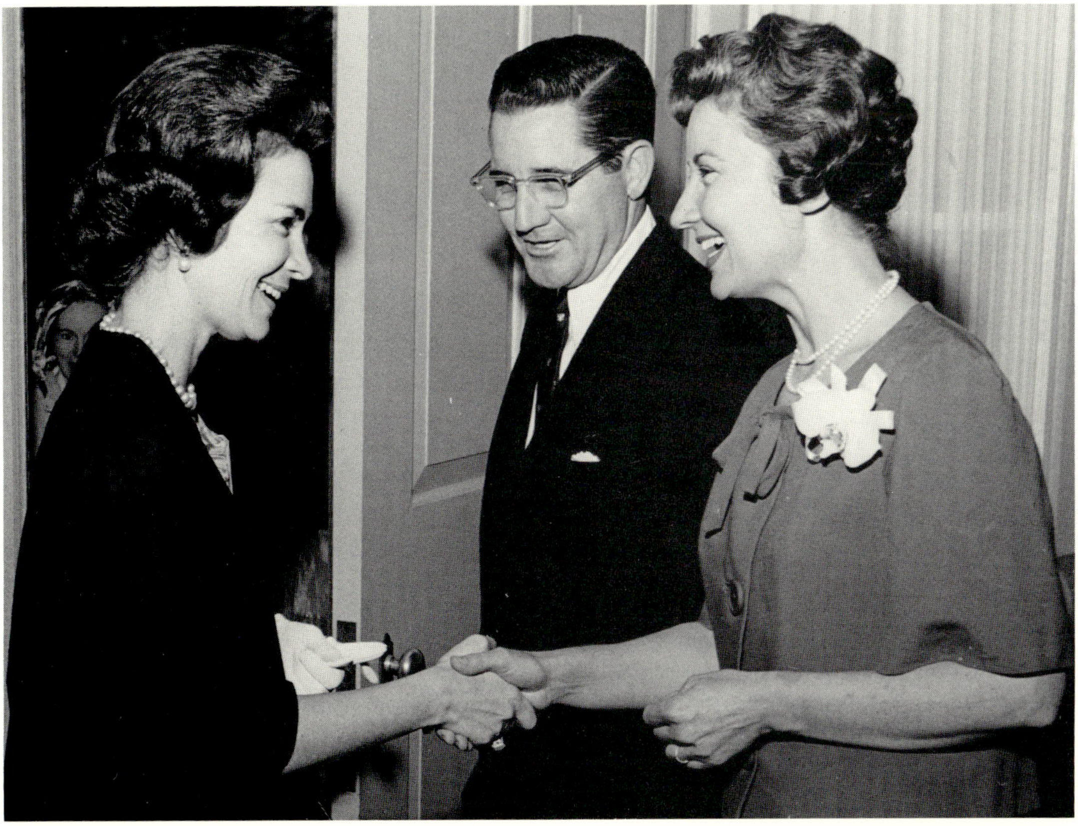

William Friday, president of the University of North Carolina, and Ida Friday, a former student and instructor in the Department of Public Health Education, both long-time supporters of the school, greet Leila Morgan at a reception during the dedication.

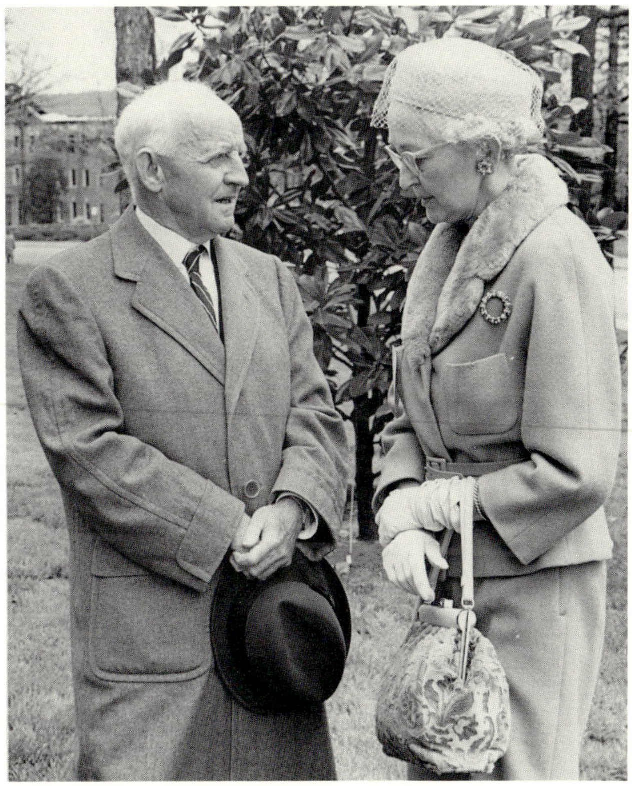

Frank Porter Graham and Miss Ruby Ross, Dr. Rosenau's secretary, exchange greetings at the dedication ceremonies.

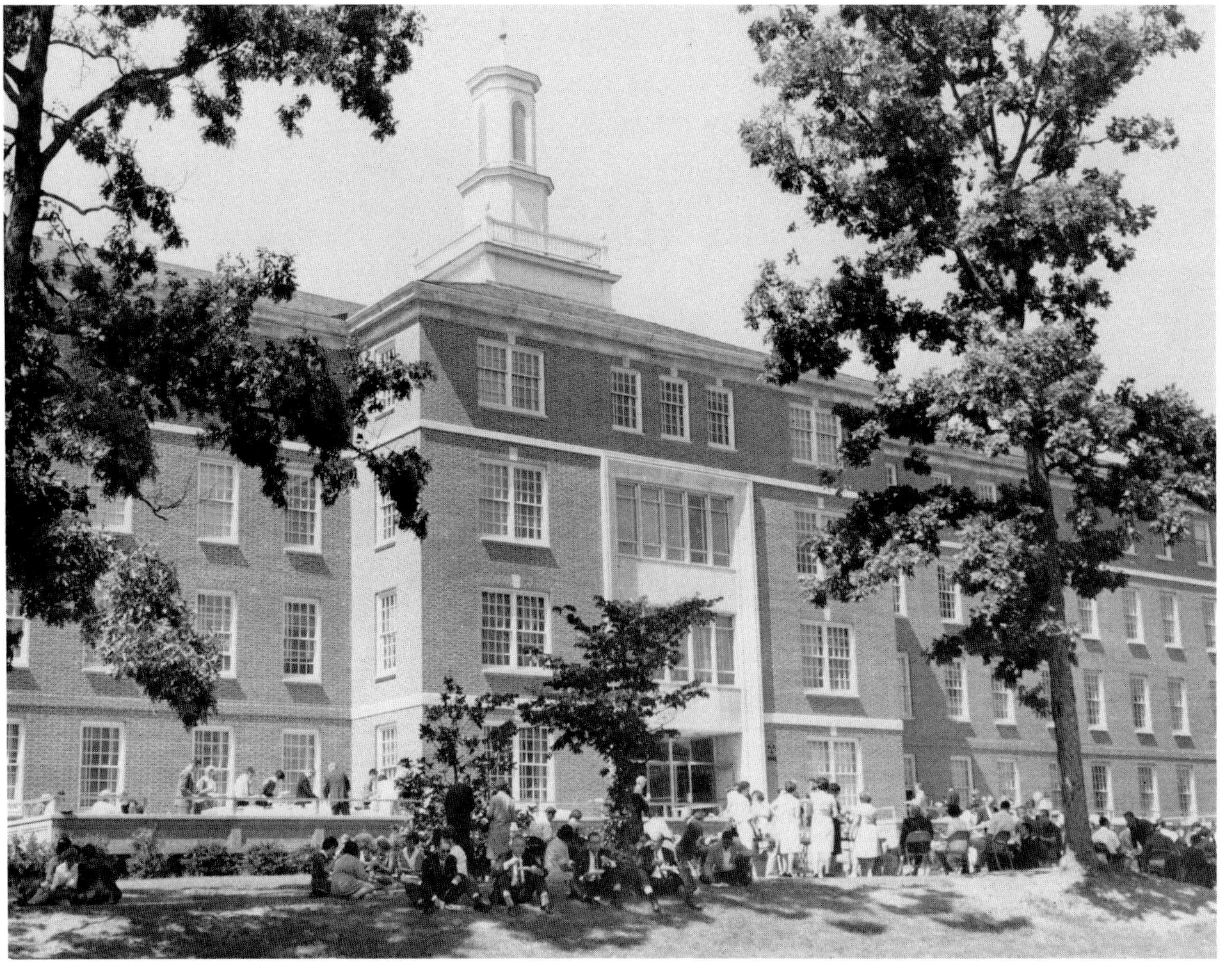
Rosenau Hall

Chapter 5

CONFLICT AND CHANGE

The 1960s was among the most tumultuous decades in American history. The civil rights movement, student protests against the war in Vietnam, and women's demands for equality helped define the times. The assassination of President John F. Kennedy rocked the nation in 1963, and within five years assassins' bullets had killed Malcolm X, Martin Luther King, Jr., and Robert Kennedy. Violence broke out in urban ghettos, in small southern towns, and on college campuses, as the struggle for justice and equality tested the mettle of the nation. In an effort to confront some of the republic's more obvious problems, Congress passed civil rights laws and channeled millions of dollars into social programs. This search for the good society ended with the expansion of the war in Vietnam and Richard Nixon's election in 1968.

The decade represented something of a golden age for the public health movement. Medicare and Medicaid were the centerpieces of President Lyndon Johnson's "Great Society" programs. But smaller measures also left their mark. Particular programs sought to increase medical research, reduce barriers to health care for the poor, develop treatments for chronic diseases, and reduce the gap between scientific knowledge and available health care. During Johnson's administration, Congress passed over forty pieces of health care legislation, and millions of dollars became available for research and training.[1]

At the School of Public Health, the search for a new dean began shortly after Dr. McGavran announced his retirement in 1962. A search committee chaired by John Wright considered dozens of candidates. Many were unavailable at the time, and philosophical differences among committee members eliminated others from consideration. In the end

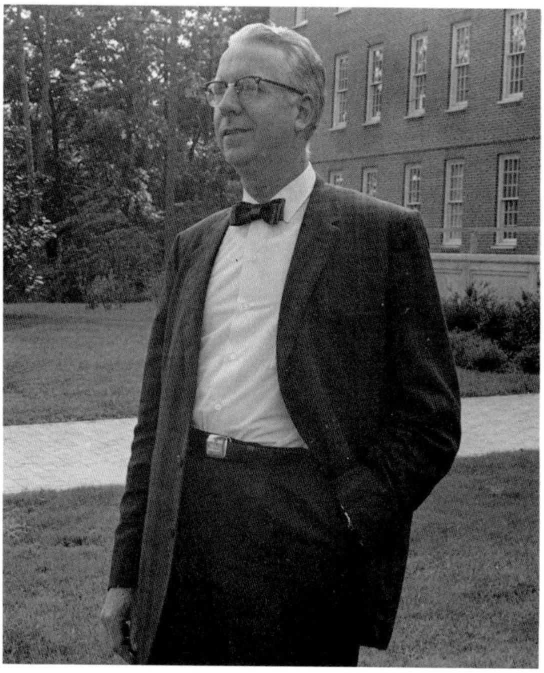

Dean William Fred Mayes

the committee nominated Dr. William Fred Mayes, a choice strongly supported by McGavran.[2]

Fred Mayes had a varied background as a public health teacher and practitioner. He received both his B.S. and M.D. from the University of Kansas, where he also did his residency in pediatrics. Mayes worked as a local and state health officer in Kansas before taking an M.P.H. at Harvard in 1948. After that he served as health director for the town of Brookline, Massachusetts, and as a professor at the Harvard School of Public Health. A two-year stint as a U.S. health adviser in Pakistan preceded his move to Washington to join the Public Health Service. When he accepted the job at Chapel Hill, he was directing the agency's Division of Research Grants in the Bureau of State Services.[3]

The new dean barely had time to unpack before a series of national and international events intruded on the quiet village of Chapel Hill. John Kennedy's assassination, civil rights protests along Franklin Street, and the speaker ban controversy (an attempted legislative mandate to require advance approval of all campus speakers) shook the university community. More profoundly transformative, however, were the explosions of knowledge and population that characterized the period, and both had major implications for public health. On the one hand, investments in education begun in the 1950s paid off in the 1960s with major advances in the biological, physical, and social sciences. On the other, the baby boom of the 1940s sent student enrollments skyrocketing while the rising birthrates in underdeveloped countries presented public health professionals with new challenges.

The School of Public Health grew tremendously, and both the administration and the faculty deserved much of the credit for its success. But dollars from Washington and Bethesda (the home of the National Institutes of Health) fired the engines of growth. In 1962 the school had a budget of almost $2 million, with just over $1 million coming from the Public Health Service. By 1972 the service contributed $3.5 million out of an $8.3 million budget.[4]

The Department of Environmental Sciences and Engineering set the pace in the 1960s. The economic boom of the post-World War II years provided Americans with the highest standard of living in the world, but the affluent society generated many potential dangers to the environment and to the public's health. Chemicals, radioactive wastes, and contaminated water were just a few of the by-products of development.

In the late 1950s, Dan Okun acquired funding from the Public Health Service and enlarged the department's mission to include the study of these new environmental dangers. Lyman Ripperton in air hygiene, David Fraser in industrial hygiene, and Donald Johnson in sanitary chemistry came aboard, bringing their expertise in these new fields. In 1962 the department changed its name from Sanitary Engineering to Environmental Sciences and Engineering and organized its courses into five program areas to allow students the opportunity for specialization: sanitary engineering and water resources, environmental chemistry and biology, environmental and food sanitation, air and industrial hygiene, and radiological hygiene.[5]

Okun and his colleagues recognized that environmental issues increasingly demanded interdisciplinary research and teaching. In the early 1960s, they set up two joint training programs with North Carolina State University. The Public Health Service saw merit in this approach and provided funds to create an Institute for Environmental Health Studies (now the Institute for Environmental Studies), with Okun serving as director. The institute brought together faculty from the Departments of Biostatistics, Botany, Chemistry, City and Regional Planning, Environmental Sciences and Engineering, Epidemiology, Geology, and Zoology at Chapel Hill, along with the Department of Food Science at North Carolina State. Dr. Stanley Weidenkopf, the deputy director, oversaw

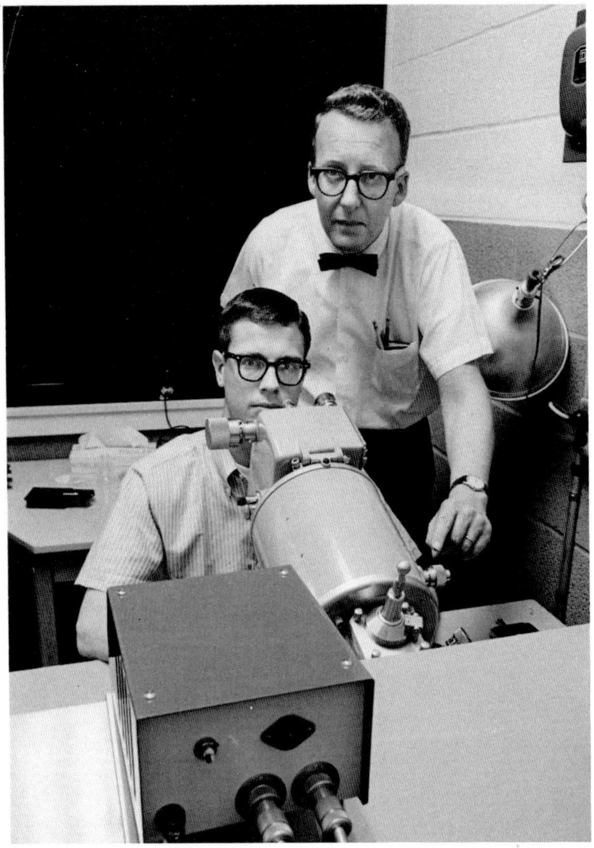

David Fraser instructs a student in the use of an electron microscope.

Otto White, Jr., and Harvey Jeffries prepare experiments for their joint technical paper in the M.S.P.H. program.

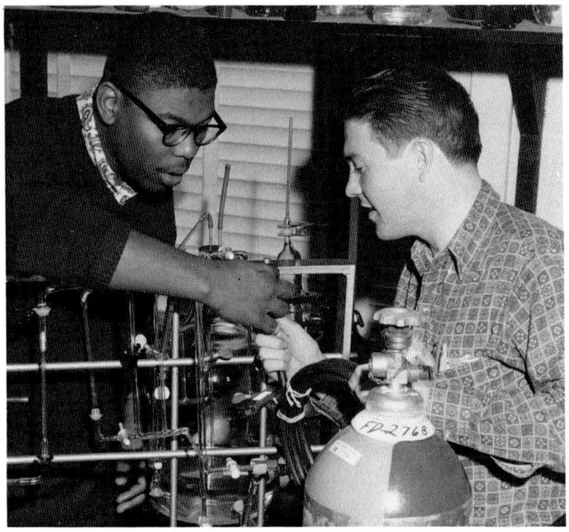

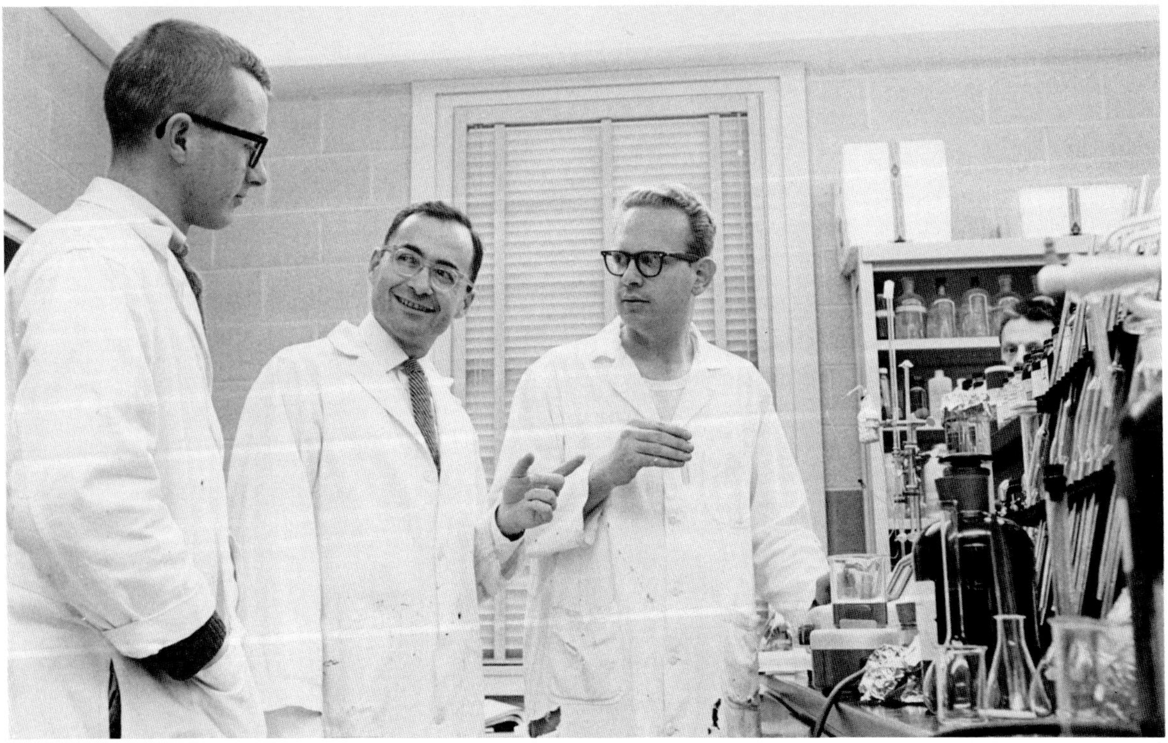

Charles Weiss *(center)* at work in the lab with graduate students Frank Wilkes *(left)* and Alan Rubin *(right)*.

the day-to-day operations of the institute, which prepared pre- and postdoctoral students for careers in environmental health.[6]

The Department of Environmental Sciences and Engineering established a quarterly newsletter, *ESE Notes*, to communicate the results of its expanding research program. *ESE Notes* featured short, technical articles about ongoing projects, as well as reports on student and faculty activities. Early titles included "Ozone in the Atmosphere Over the Southern Appalachians," "Biological Monitoring of Exposure to Low Level Air Pollution," and "Phosphate Concentrations and Marine Algal Ecology."[7]

The department's expansion can be attributed to a number of factors. It had an illustrious history, going back to the early 1920s under the nationally known engineer Thorndike Saville, and continuing in the 1930s and 1940s as H. G. Baity established a worldwide reputation as a teacher and a sanitary engineer. Dan Okun built on this foundation by widening the scope of the department's research and teaching, hiring excellent faculty, and recruiting good students. The department was in a perfect position to ride the wave of concern for environmental issues that appeared in the 1960s.

The Department of Biostatistics also grew rapidly in the 1960s. Here too, the presence of an ambitious, nationally known chair and an expanding federal budget contributed to the department's success. Bernard G. Greenberg began building the Biostatistics Department in the late 1950s with government and foundation money, most of which went to research. Although Greenberg and his colleagues did a great deal of teaching in the School of Public Health, as well as in the Schools of Medicine, Nursing, and Dentistry, the department had few students of its own. Still, Greenberg and his colleagues found many ways to serve. "Statistical advice on design of experiments and interpretations of data," an anonymous faculty member wrote, "is dispensed with a lavish hand to those who seek it." Slowly, the department's reputation and the availability of fellowship money attracted more and better students. By 1967 the department had a strong doctoral program that included specializations in biometry, demography, genetics, and computer sciences.[8]

For a time the new space in Rosenau Hall adequately served the needs of the Biostatistics Department. There were individual study spaces equipped with electric desk calculating machines for each student.

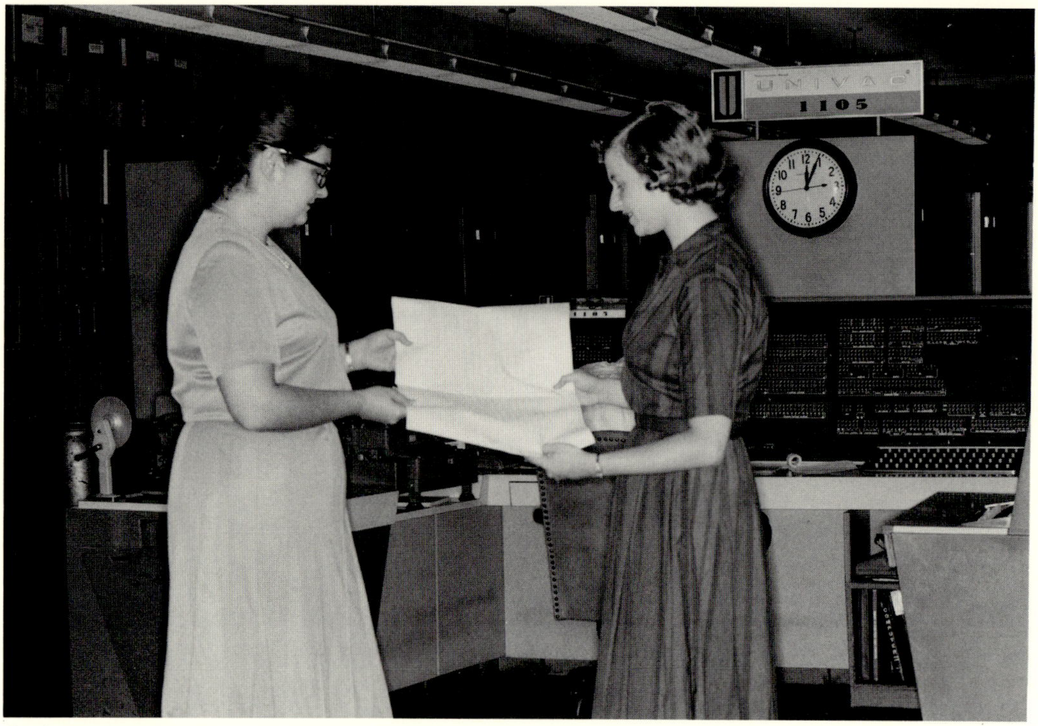

Ruth Stephenson Hassanein and Ellen Kaplan, research associates in biostatistics, examine data from the Univac computer in the early 1960s. Biostatistics was one of the first departments on campus to use computer technology.

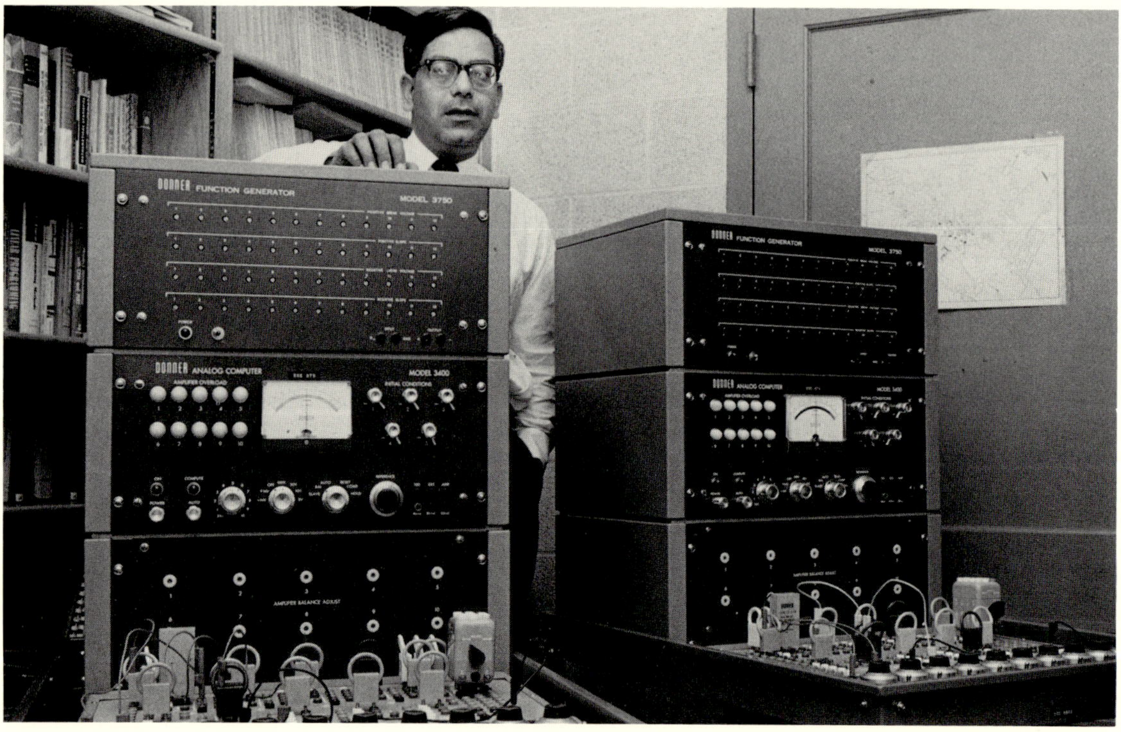

Jabbar Sherwani of the Department of Environmental Sciences and Engineering displays an analog computer used for ground-water studies in eastern North Carolina.

There were laboratory rooms with IBM punch card machines and a Friden Flexowriter for punching paper tape to be used in the university's Univac computer. But another growth spurt in 1965 quickly filled the available rooms in Rosenau. Once again the department found it necessary to move faculty and staff into temporary space, in this case the Drane Cottage and Drane House behind the school on Pittsboro Street.[9]

Perhaps the department's most enduring contribution during this period lay in establishing the Carolina Population Center. The school began discussing the possibility of creating a center for population studies in 1964. The idea was to coordinate ongoing research and teaching on population issues, to expand consulting services to state and local health agencies as well as to foreign countries, and to increase theoretical research on population at the university. The Carolina Population Center was set up in 1966, with Moye Freymann as director. The scope and urgency of population problems in developing countries, along with financial support from the Ford Foundation, resulted in an early concentration on international issues. In North Carolina, the center worked with local agencies to develop a comprehensive family planning program.[10]

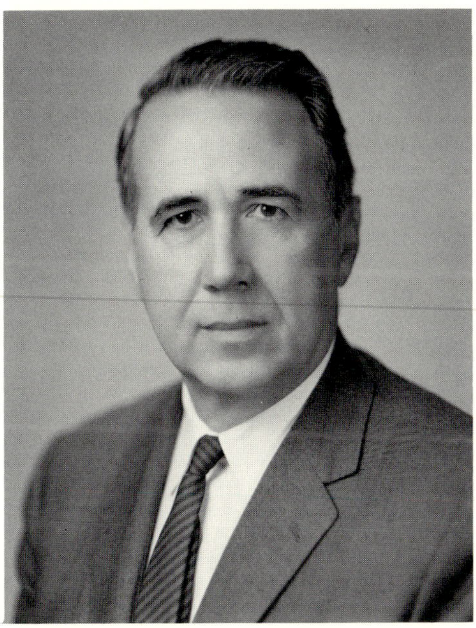

Forrest E. Linder, professor of biostatistics and founder of the Poplab, an agency that helped other countries develop better demographic statistics for population study and planning.

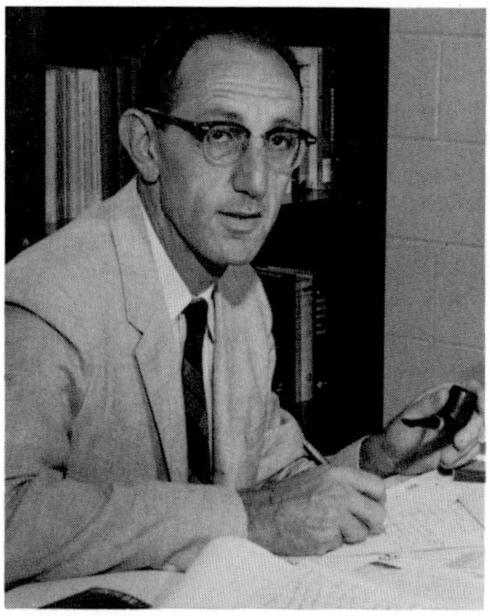

John Cassel

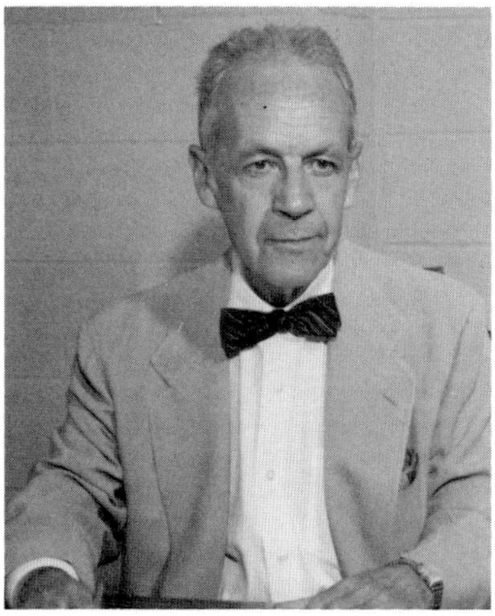

John Fulton

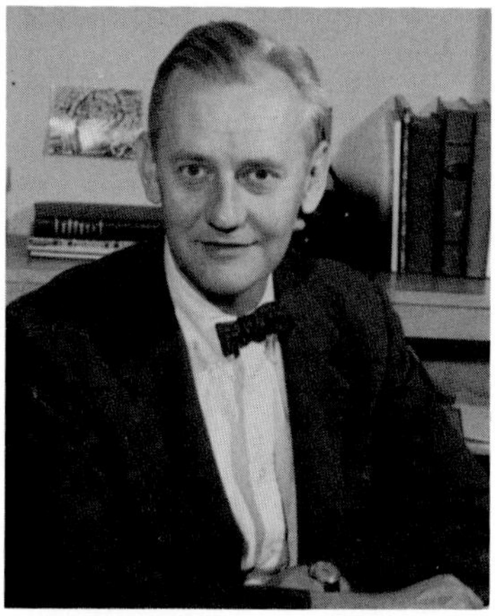

Ralph Patrick

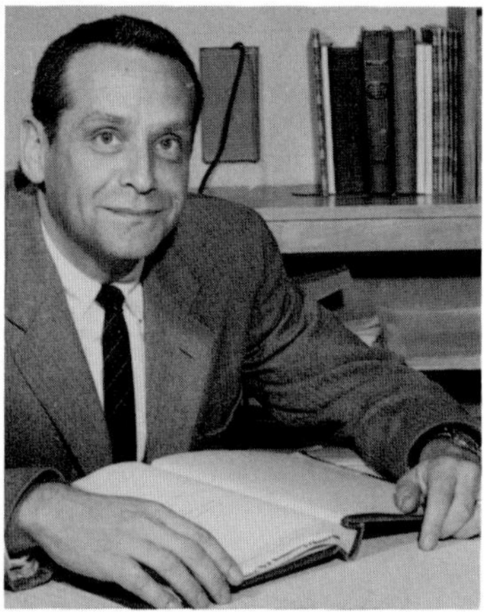

Herman Tyroler

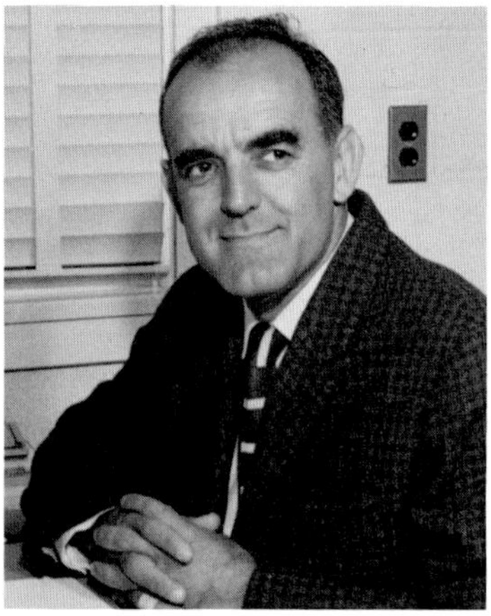

Cecil Slome

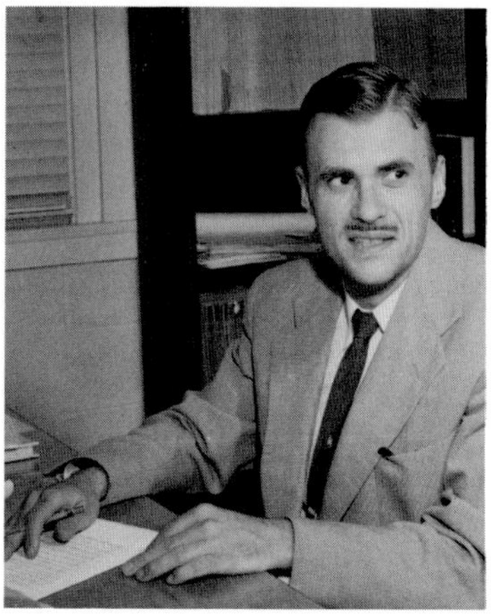

David Jenkins

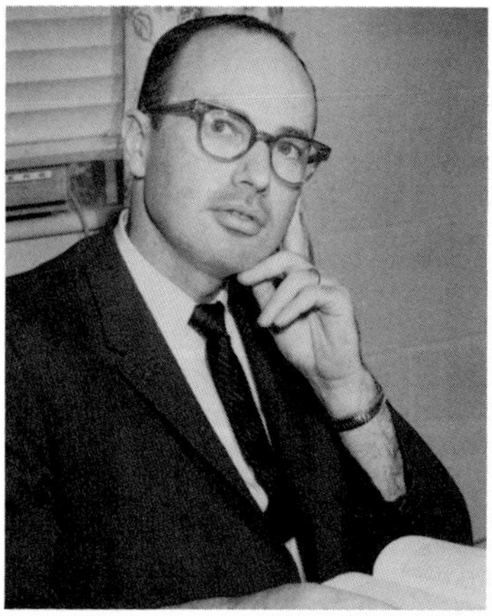

Bert Kaplan

Some members of the Department of Epidemiology faculty during the early 1960s.

The other bright star in Dean Mayes's "constellation" was the Department of Epidemiology. The department undertook numerous studies in the 1960s, but the Evans County Cardiovascular and Cerebrovascular Epidemiologic Study drew the most attention. Evans was a small Georgia county about sixty miles inland from Savannah. Dr. Curtis Hames, a local physician in Claxton, noticed in the 1950s that the black patients he treated seemed to have a lower incidence of coronary heart disease than whites. He contacted the Public Health Service about the possibility of doing a study in Evans County to see if his clinical observations were correct, and if so what the explanation might be. The Public Health Service suggested that Hames contact the Department of Biostatistics at Chapel Hill for help in designing the program. Bernie Greenberg remembered the occasion:

> The Public Health Service asked me to evaluate a research project proposed by a solo medical practitioner in private practice in Claxton, Georgia. I visited there for a few days with this physician but returned with serious doubts about the project's feasibility.
>
> Nevertheless, I persuaded John Cassel to go back to Georgia with me a few weeks later to meet Dr. Curtis Hames in order to take a closer look at this project. I was still skeptical when we got on the plane to go there, but by the time we came home, John and I were thoroughly convinced that this project represented a unique epidemiological potential.[11]

Between 1960 and 1962, 92% of Evans County's population over the age of forty underwent medical examinations and laboratory tests. The results confirmed Hames's observation. Black males suffered heart disease at half the rate of white men. More surprising, however, was the fact that white men in lower socioeconomic groups had rates comparable to blacks. When the investigators studied the population again between 1967 and 1969, there was less difference among white men. "The only circumstances in which white men had as low rates as blacks," John Cassel reported, "was when they were both sharecroppers. The only relevant difference between white sharecroppers and all other white men that could be invoked to explain this finding was the high level of physical activity in sharecropping." Hames and the school's epidemiologists concluded that psychosocial experiences and genetics might be contributing factors, but that levels of physical activity were primarily responsible:[12]

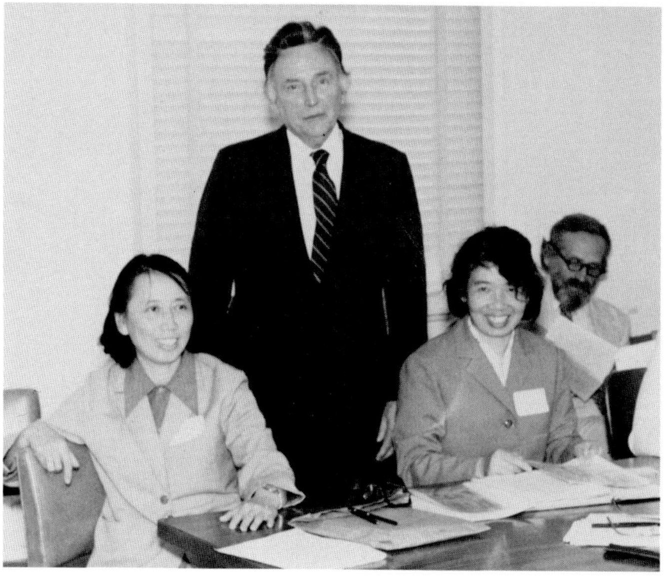

Curtis Hames *(standing)* and Herman Tyroler with delegation from the People's Republic of China.

> That study grew exactly as John [Cassel] had predicted. Today it is the most famous nongovernmentally-administered cardiovascular study in the world. Dr. Curtis Hames turned out to have the medical and managerial capability that John had seen in him, and the Evans County project became a uniquely comprehensive field of study of heart disease in a natural, rural setting.
>
> The project had given rise to hundreds of manuscripts, dozens of doctoral dissertations, and best of all, to some of the most important discoveries ever made about the precursors of coronary thrombosis, hypertension, and myocardial infarction.[13]

The rapid expansion of the Departments of Environmental Sciences and Engineering, Biostatistics, and Epidemiology caused concern among some members of the faculty. The increasing emphasis on research was one issue, but, in addition, not everyone supported the strategy of building the school on soft money supplied by the federal government. "I didn't believe in being paid to do research," John Larsh, head of the Department of Parasitology, said. "It rubbed me the wrong way. A lot of my good friends, Bernie Greenberg, Dan Okun, and a lot of them, they took every damn grant that came along. Soft money, that's the way you expand. My point was that larger was not necessarily better." Hilton Goulson explained:

> John Larsh's philosophy was let's develop a department on solid ground and to him solid ground meant state appropriations. He would build the department by developing faculty positions with state moneys. He was not as enthusiastic about federal dollars. The department would literally get calls from NIH, "We've got this grant

program, wouldn't you like to apply?" Money was available for the asking. His philosophy was we are primarily here as teachers, but we will do research as we can budget out time.[14]

Everyone on the faculty understood that long-term security depended on appropriations from Raleigh, but some, like Dan Okun, saw the pursuit of federal grants as the most effective short-run strategy. "We didn't grow out of state money," Okun explained, "we grew on soft money. The state money followed the soft money. We would get a project and hire someone on soft money. We'd have a guy and we'd say, 'Look, you're coming here but your staying depends on your being productive.' So we'd try to find someone who would be productive, get research grants. The next time there was state money, we said, 'Look, we've got this guy already here.' It was a tactic which was useful at the time."[15]

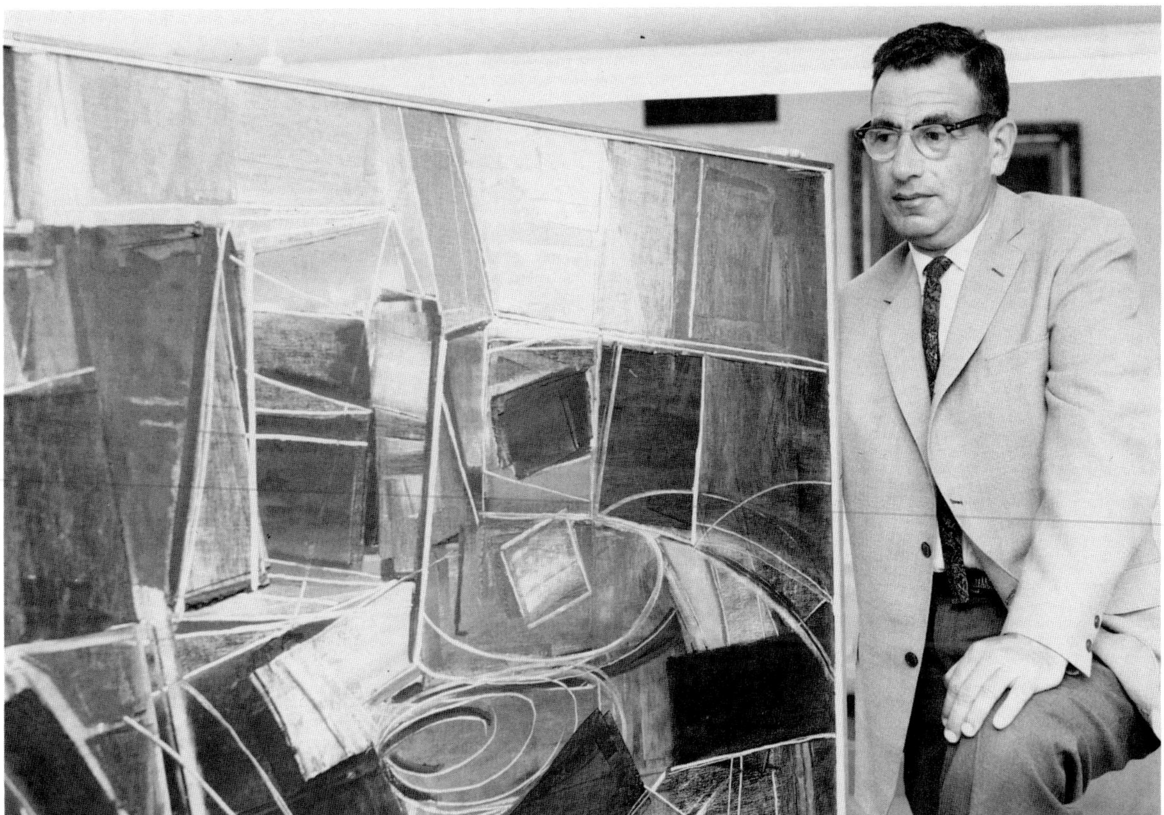

Daniel Okun with 1965 purchase award, "September Party" by George Kachergis, at the School of Public Health Annual Art Exhibition. Dr. Okun got the idea for displaying and purchasing work by local artists while in the Netherlands, where art is used extensively in public buildings.

Not everyone appreciated Okun's ability to bring money into the school. "There was a lot of tension," Okun remembered. "We were thorns in everybody's side. The problem in our department was always space. We needed laboratory space, not space for offices. There was a laboratory above us in [the Department of] Nutrition. They weren't doing any research work at the time, so we made a deal to use their laboratory space. I went up and asked if we could [also] use their desks. [The department head] said 'You're a cancer in the school.' This is the way we were perceived because we were growing. We had needs for everything [because] we were getting research grants. So there was a lot of tension. I won some battles but felt I may have lost the war."[16]

During McGavran's time Okun may have suffered some setbacks, but by the mid-1960s the research-oriented departments exercised considerable influence in the school. Although Dean Mayes had initially been seen as a strong defender of an older community-service orientation, under his leadership the school's focus clearly shifted to research. William Herzog, a student and faculty member at the school, witnessed the change. "Mayes came in at a time when three of the four horsemen who were most influential in the school, Dan Okun, Bernie Greenberg, and John Cassel [Margaret Dolan being the fourth], were very strong research people. To be credible as dean, Mayes became more supportive of the research-oriented departments. That was quite a disenchantment [for some people], in some sense a betrayal. We went from the idea of the community as the focus of the school to research as the focus."[17]

The issue, however, was not merely research versus teaching and service, but what kind of research and for whose benefit? Any research effort that relied on funding from government agencies and private foundations ran the risk of tailoring its agenda to fit the fashions of the day. Earlier public health activities in underdeveloped countries, for instance, mixed humanitarianism with political and economic motivations. During the 1960s, the federal government's interest in finding cures for chronic diseases often precluded funding vital research on prevention.[18]

The rapid influx of money, faculty, staff, and students required changes in the school's administrative structure. Dean Mayes, in his first address to the faculty in 1963, outlined his administrative principles. These included "an appropriate division of labor among administrative, professional, technical, clerical, and other fellow workers," the delegation of authority to people in responsible positions, and autonomy for department heads.[19]

The most noticeable administrative reform involved the expansion of the Dean's Office. Soon after his arrival, Mayes appointed John Larsh as assistant dean for academic programs, a position, as Mayes acknowledged, that Larsh had informally held for a number of years. William S. Flash joined the school as assistant dean for administration and associate professor of public health administration; John Gentry became assistant dean for program development; and Harry Spense assumed a position as a consultant on international health programs. In 1967 Charles Harper took Flash's job as assistant dean, and Robert Moorhead became an assistant to the dean.

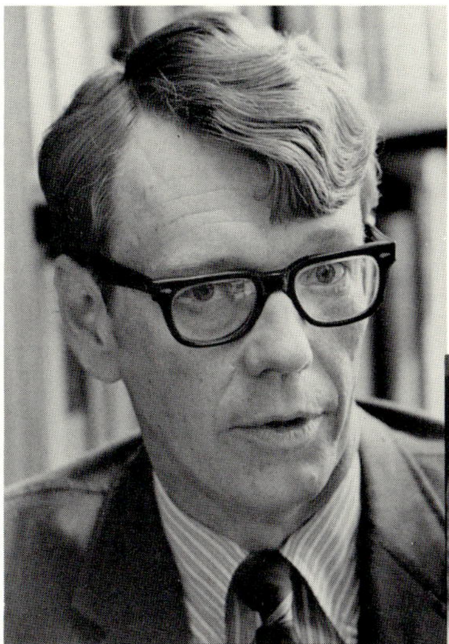

Robert Moorhead

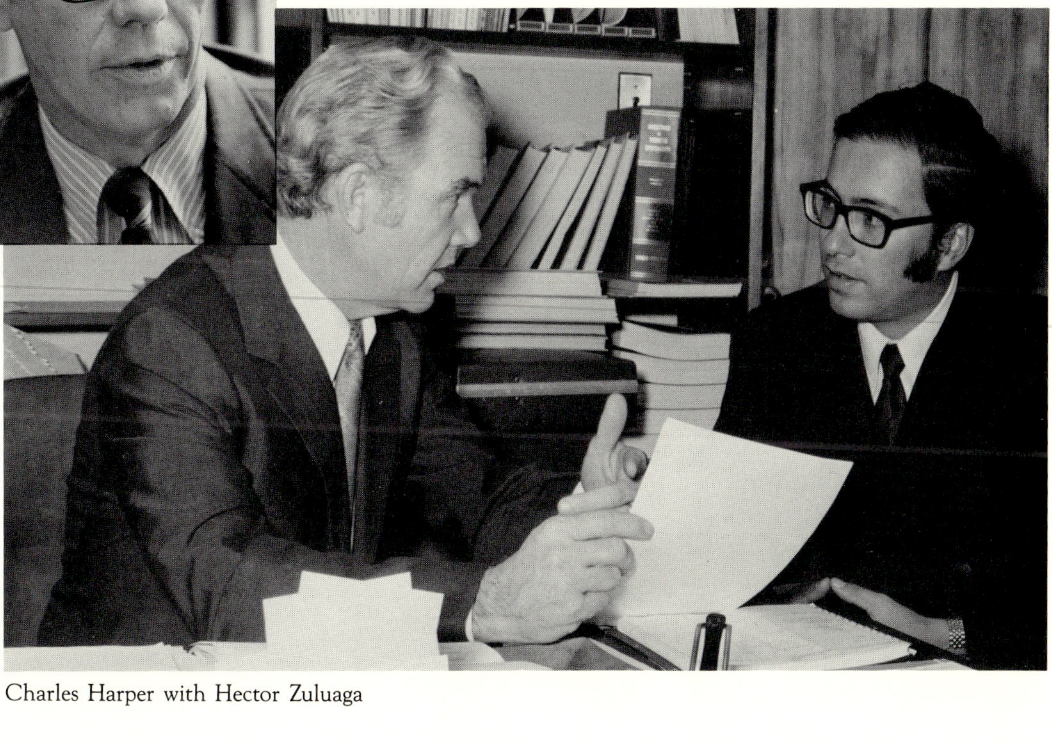

Charles Harper with Hector Zuluaga

Unlike Ed McGavran, Fred Mayes saw himself as more than the executive secretary of the faculty. "The leadership responsibilities of the dean require going far beyond [that] role," he said. The dean served as the school's spokesman to the university and the outside world and held responsibility for safeguarding the long-term interests of the school and its faculty. Mayes took Harry Truman's motto as his administrative principle: "The buck stops here." Consistent with the dean's more exalted role was the decision to rename the Executive Faculty (the heads of all the departments) the Dean's Cabinet (which included some administrators, and later, some students as nonvoting members).[20]

Expansion of the administrative structure of the school was unavoidable, given the number of people involved. Gone were the days when the faculty could sit around a table in the dean's office and make decisions. A stronger central administration was also necessary to balance the growing inequalities among the different departments. But administration was also Dean Mayes's strong suit, and that is where he decided to put his efforts.[21]

Lucy Morgan, for one, was uncomfortable with this new administrative style. In retrospect, she felt that the school was being "ruled by fiat." The participatory democracy she saw as essential to public health, whether at the school or in the community was giving way to bureaucracy. The consensus style of decision making that had been a distinguishing feature of the school was being replaced by more hierarchical forms. But underlying Morgan's concerns were other serious problems in the relationship between the Dean's Office and the Department of Public Health Education, in fact, between the Dean's Office and all the nonresearch-oriented departments.[22]

The retirement of Lucy Morgan and Eunice Tyler in 1966 left the Department of Public Health Education understaffed and somewhat uncertain of its future. When Department Chair Ralph Boatman and Dean Mayes asked Elta Mae Mast to rejoin the faculty, Chancellor Carlyle Sitterson questioned the appointment. His primary concern was "the problem of academic inbreeding. A department the size of health education which has on its staff no person with graduate training outside its own program presents real problems." Mayes admitted that the department needed to hire someone from outside, but since the school trained roughly 50 percent of the people in the field of public health education, it was not easy to do so. In any case, Mayes defended Mast

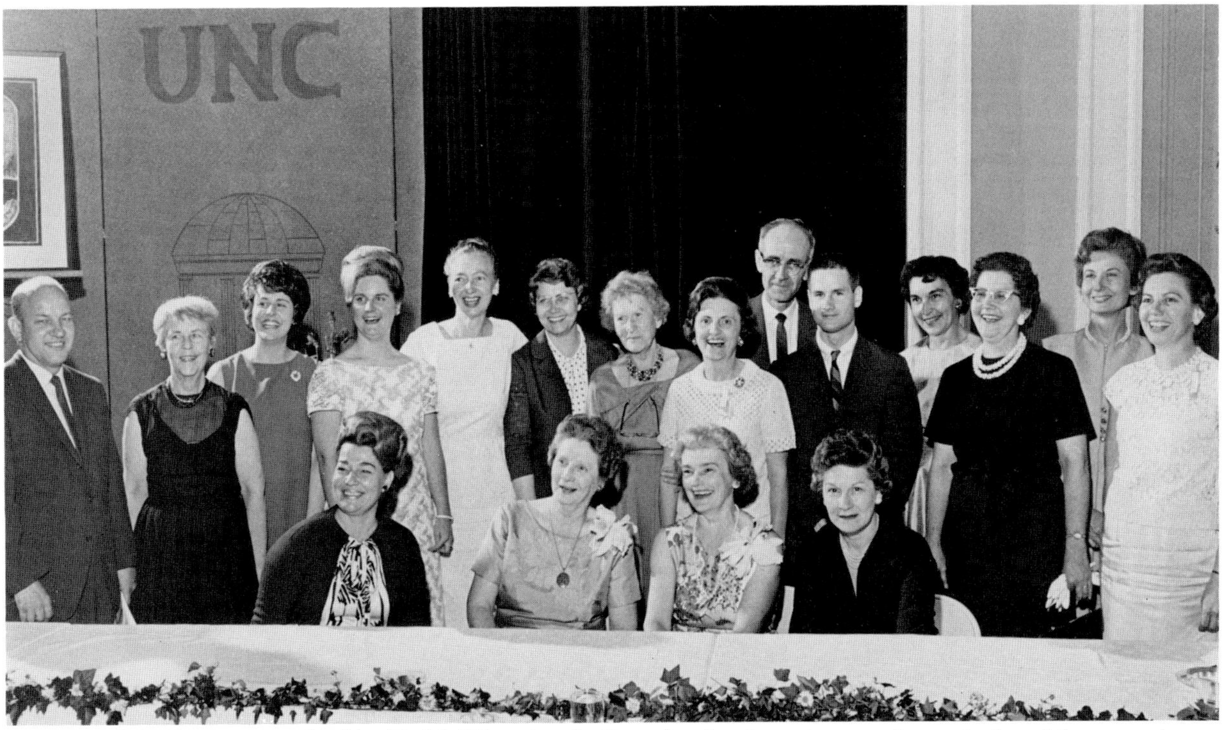

Members of the Department of Public Health Education family gather for the retirement dinner for Lucy Morgan and Eunice Tyler.

as an excellent choice. "Her value as a very able teacher has previously been demonstrated."[23]

Meanwhile, Mayes had instituted a wide-ranging assessment of the school, beginning with the Department of Public Health Education. The dean appointed an external committee to make recommendations to him and an internal committee to assist in the gathering of materials and to make suggestions on implementing the external committee's recommendations. The external committee's most important recommendations addressed the need for more research by both students and faculty and the hiring of new faculty who had no previous ties to the department.[24]

Ralph Boatman stepped down as head of public health education in 1968 to direct the school's continuing education program. Dean Mayes appointed a search committee, and the committee selected Dr. Guy W. Steuart, a native South African then teaching at the School of Public Health at the University of California at Los Angeles. Mayes approved the appointment over the objections of the public health education faculty. Given Steuart's mandate to implement many of the recommendations of the review committee, particularly to upgrade the research capabilities of the department, the situation was ripe for misunderstanding and disagreement. In 1971 doctors Betty Mathews, Hiawatha Walker, Elizabeth McMahan, and Elta Mae Mast resigned.[25]

Staying afloat in the 1960s required constant adaptation to new trends in research and education. The Department of Public Health Administration, for instance, had to adjust very quickly to the enormous changes in the health care delivery system that took place in the 1960s. Robert Coker headed the department from 1960 until his death in 1966. With a small permanent faculty supplemented by part-time visiting instructors, the department taught students throughout the Division of Health Affairs. The complexities of modern health care management, however, posed problems. Bill Herzog, who became a member of the department in 1964, remembered, "The Department of Health Administration at the time didn't have much depth. Most of the principal faculty were physicians. It wasn't until the late sixties that they began pulling in faculty who were trained in public administration, sociology, health care finance, health care administration."[26]

The impetus for change came from the heightened demand for trained health administrators created by the medical care legislation of the mid-1960s. Preparations for that change started shortly before Coker's death in 1966, when the department undertook a review of its overall program. The review was put on hold, but the department did revamp its curriculum and develop new programs, thanks to grants from the Public Health Service. Arnold Kaluzny, Sagar Jain, Moye Freymann, and John Gentry were among the new faculty who joined the department in 1966. In 1967 Morris Schaefer was appointed head of the department. The next year the department changed its name to Health Administration.[27]

The Department of Parasitology also revamped part of its program to accommodate the demands for health professionals. In the late 1950s, representatives from the Centers for Disease Control (CDC) and the laboratory section of the American Public Health Association contacted the school about providing a training center for laboratory directors. "A large number of lab directors in state health departments were approaching retirement age, and there were no training sites," Hilton Goulson remembered. John Larsh and Ed McGavran expressed interest in the project but worried about how the students would fit into the existing degree program. The school and the CDC decided the appropriate degree would be the doctorate of public health. Although a Dr.P.H. had been in existence for many years, it was generally a degree earned in a year by M.D.'s. "That's not what we were interested in," Goulson remembered. "This program for laboratory directors was similar in most respects to the Ph.D., but rather than emphasizing basic research this was to emphasize applied research, things that could be carried back to the laboratories and implemented immediately. It was funded by the National Institutes of Health with the agreement that students would come to do their academic training here and their scientific research would be done at the CDC in Atlanta. We have provided a lot of much-needed manpower in the public health laboratory, not only the people who have obtained the training, but others who worked side by side with them." The program was so successful that in 1969 the department changed its name to Parasitology and Laboratory Practice.[28]

Relations between the School of Public Health and other schools in the Division of Health Affairs were either cooperative or competitive, depending on the people and the issues involved. The Department of Public Health Nursing and the School of Nursing sometimes worked together and at other times agreed to disagree. Soon after the creation of the School of Nursing in 1950, there was pressure to eliminate the baccalaureate degree in public health nursing. This pressure came from the dean of the School of Nursing, from the National League for Nurses, and from some people within the School of Public Health. Some of the conflict was no doubt territorial, but the major issue was whether or not specialized training (public health nursing as opposed to a more general course in nursing) was appropriate at the undergraduate level. Certain to lose accreditation for their program, the department finally stopped accepting undergraduates in 1962. Despite the uneasy relationship between the Department of Public Health Nursing and the School of Nursing, the two groups did successfully develop a program to prepare teachers of public health nursing, beginning in 1963. Margaret Shetland was the first director, followed by Marie McIntyre in 1967.[29]

Since the undergraduate and certificate programs had been the Department of Public Health Nursing's mainstays since the early days, their loss posed a threat to the department's survival. Nevertheless, the department was able to hang on and grow during the 1960s, thanks in part to the influence of Margaret Dolan. Dolan brought great distinction to the department and the school as president of the American Nurses Association (1963–65) and the National Health Council (1968–69). She also served as an advocate for improved health services on numerous state and local boards. Elizabeth Holley and Virginia Nelson had joined the department to fill positions opened by the retirement of Ruth Hay and Margaret Blee, and together with Margaret Dolan they formed the

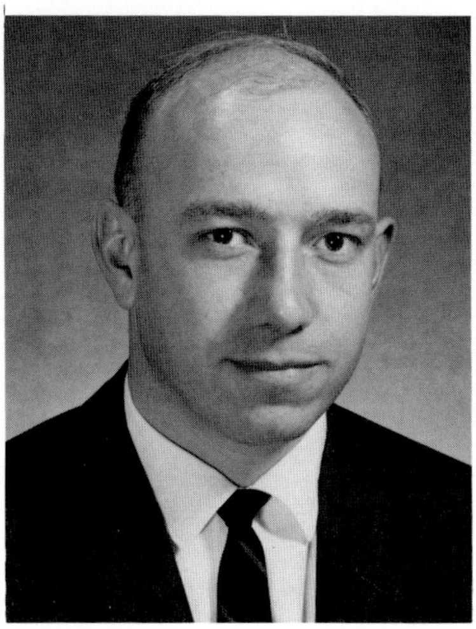
William Herzog

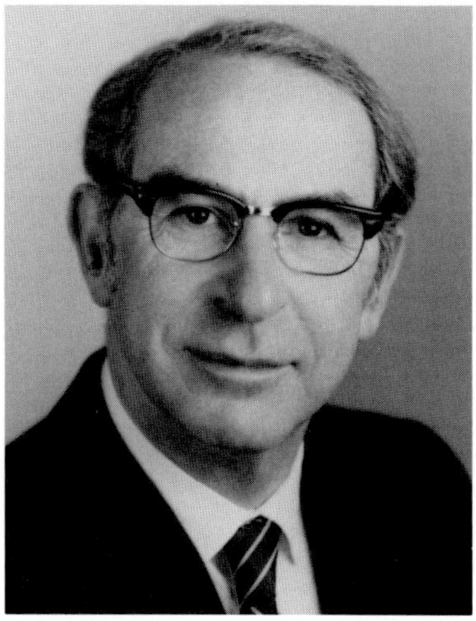
Harry Phillips

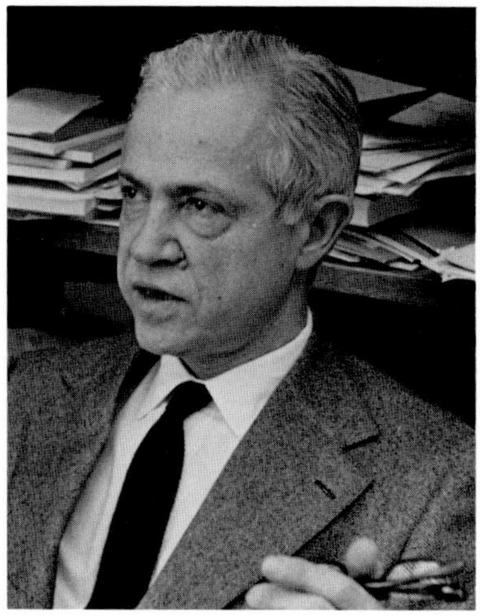
Leonard Rosenfeld

nucleus of the department. Grants from the Public Health Service and increases in state appropriations allowed the department to hire additional faculty.[30]

The department made two particularly important appointments in the late 1960s. In 1967 Elizabeth (Betty) Edmands came to the school with a joint appointment in public health nursing and maternal and child health and as a staff member of the Carolina Population Center. Margaret Dolan considered Edmands "the most knowledgeable public health nurse in the United States on family planning." Edmands used her expertise not only in training students but also as a consultant to numerous governments in Africa and Asia. Marion Highriter joined the department the next year to improve the research dimension of the program. Over the years Dr. Highriter supervised numerous research projects, many of which investigated the effectiveness of public health nurses in a variety of settings.[31]

The school's involvement with international health issues increased dramatically in the 1960s. The school had had a strong international orientation since the 1940s. A steady flow of students from Latin America, India, and the Middle East added a cosmopolitan flavor to MacNider and Rosenau Halls. Faculty passports bore stamps from all parts of the world. H. G. Baity's move to Geneva, Switzerland, to work for WHO; Lucy Morgan's travels to India, Burma, Ceylon, and Egypt the year she stepped down as head of the Department of Public Health Education; Ed McGavran's five-year stint in India for the Ford Foundation after he retired as Dean—all were indications of the faculty's deep involvement in the world scene.

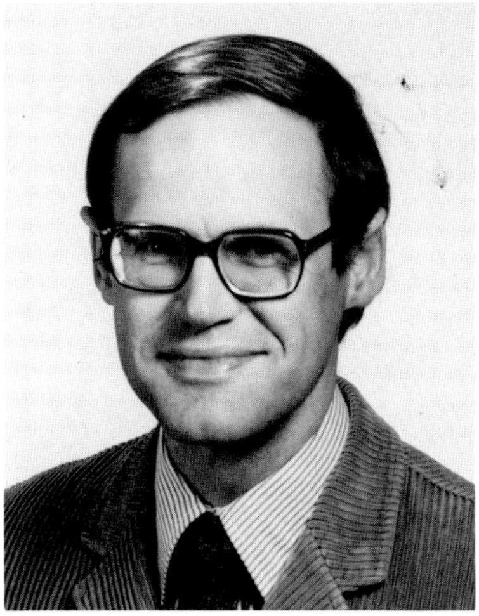
Arnold Kaluzny

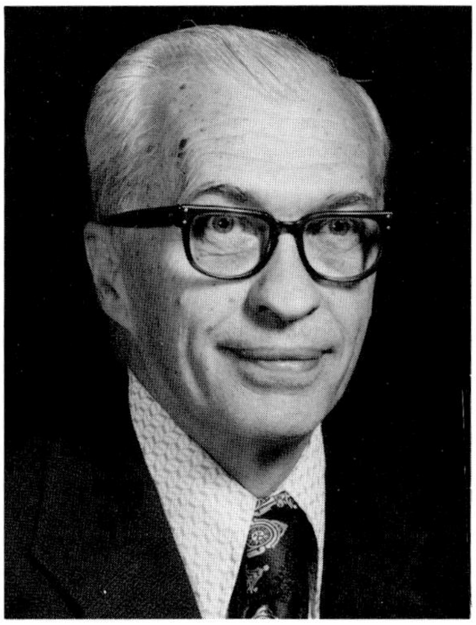
John Hughes

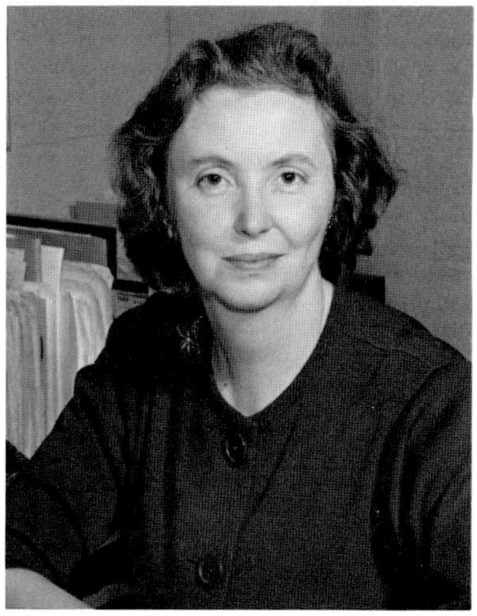
Frances McConnell

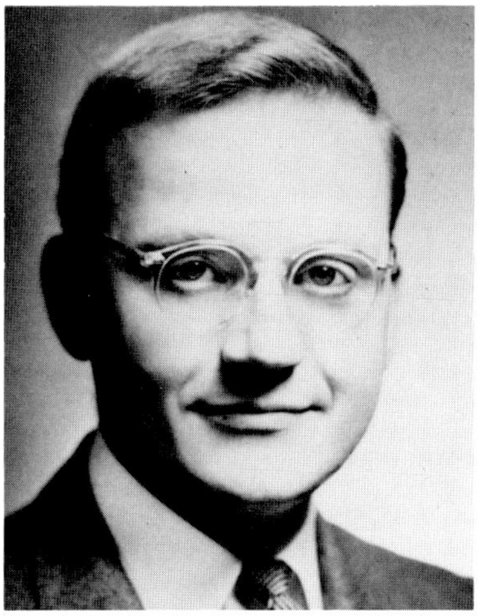
Moye Freymann

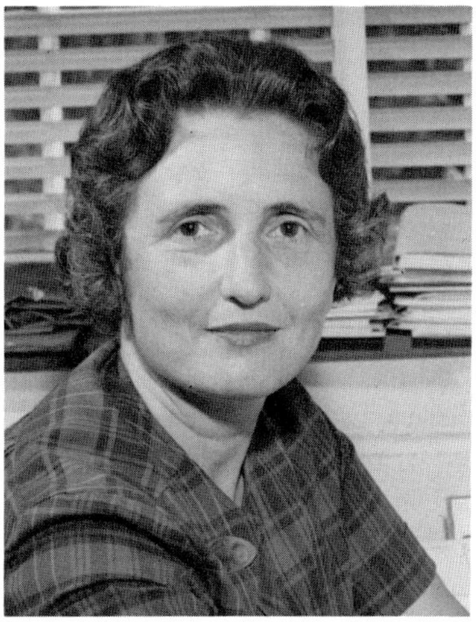
Janice Westaby

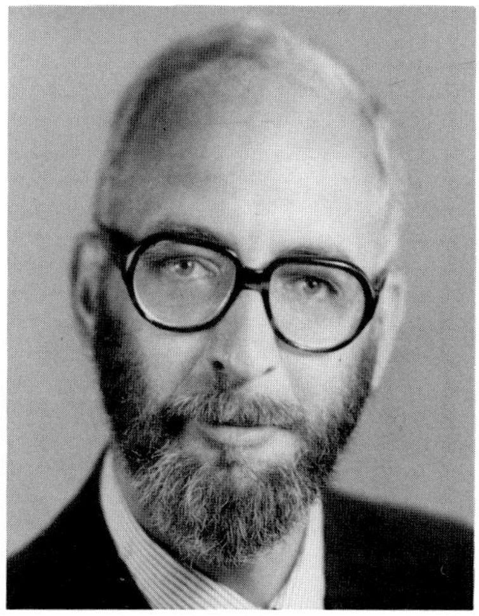
Dan Beauchamp

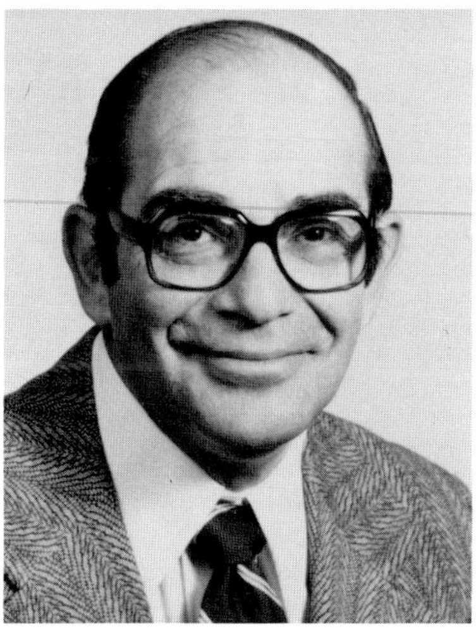
Morris Schaefer

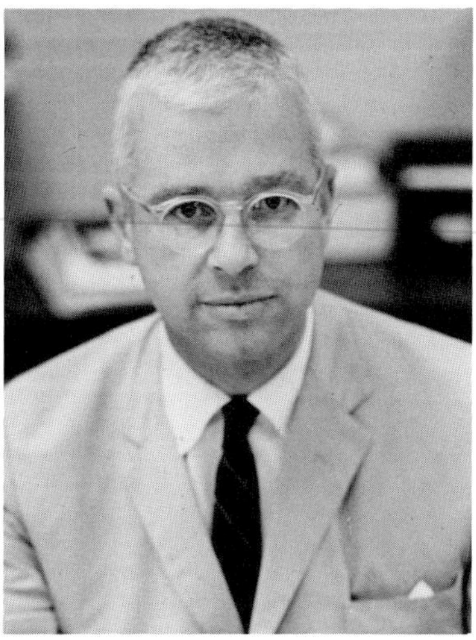
William Flash

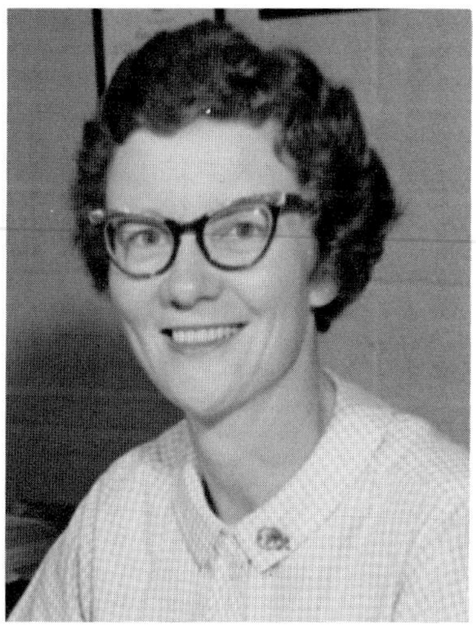
Lydia Holley

Some of the faculty who joined the Department of Public Health Administration in the late 1960s and early 1970s.

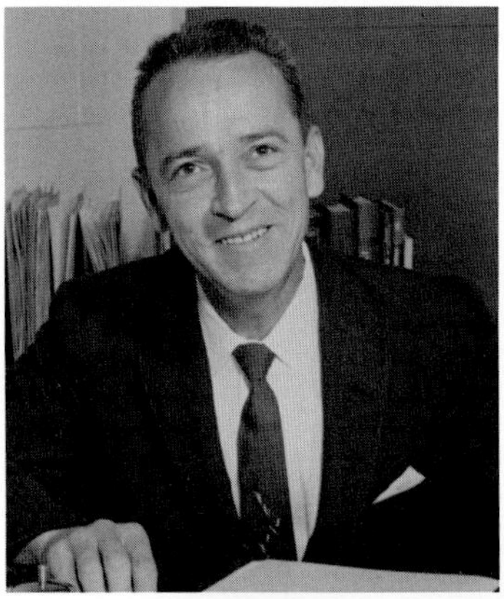
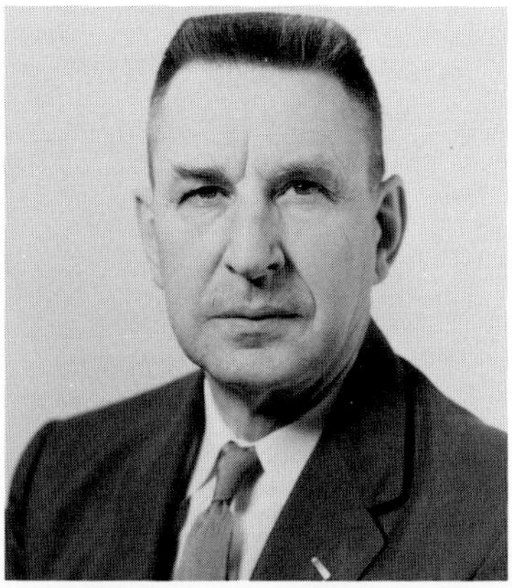
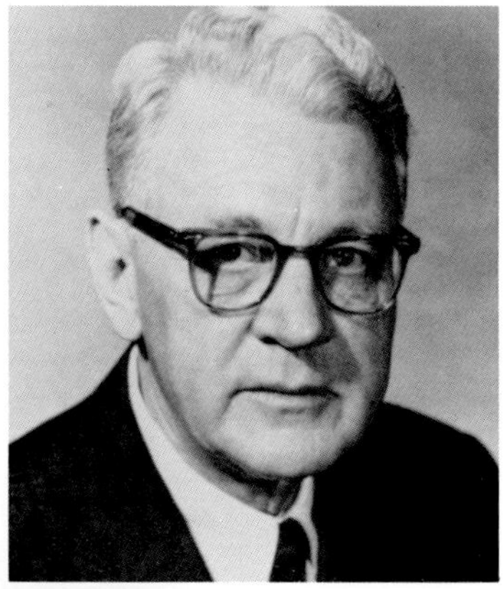
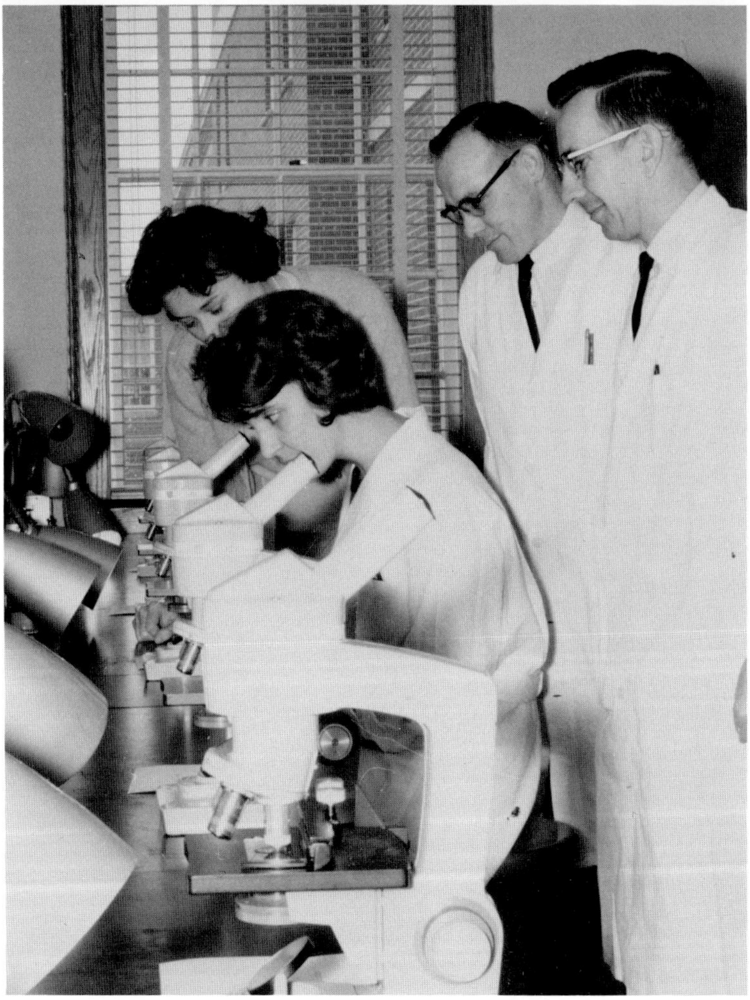

Norman Weatherly and Hilton Goulson observe students in parasitology lab. *Above, left to right:* James Hendricks, Elmer Chaffee, and Robert Watson.

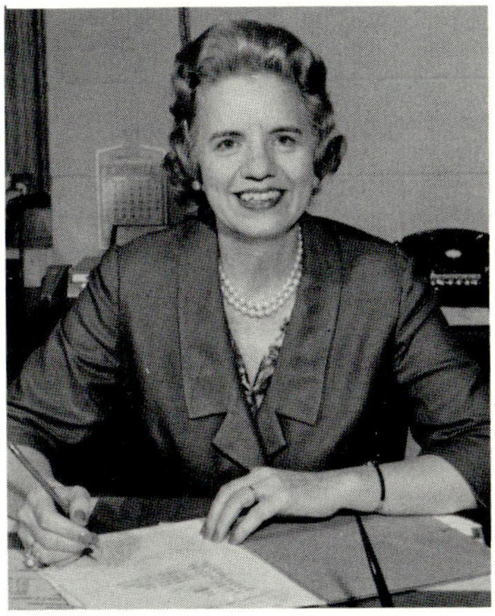

Margaret Dolan

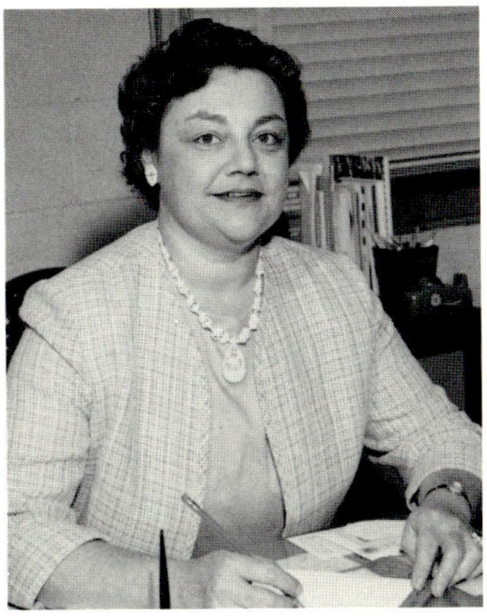

Elizabeth Holley

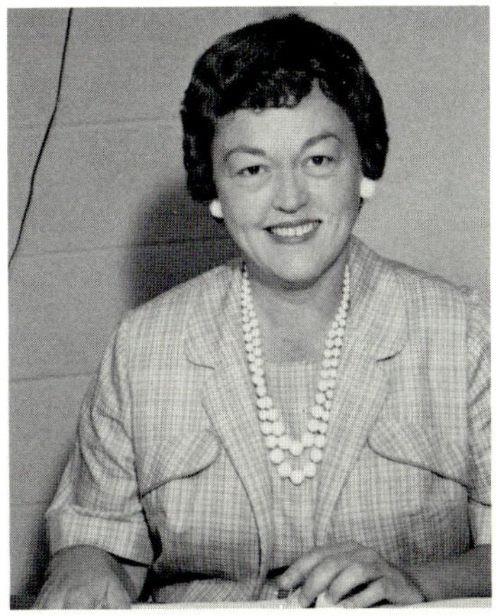

Virginia Nelson

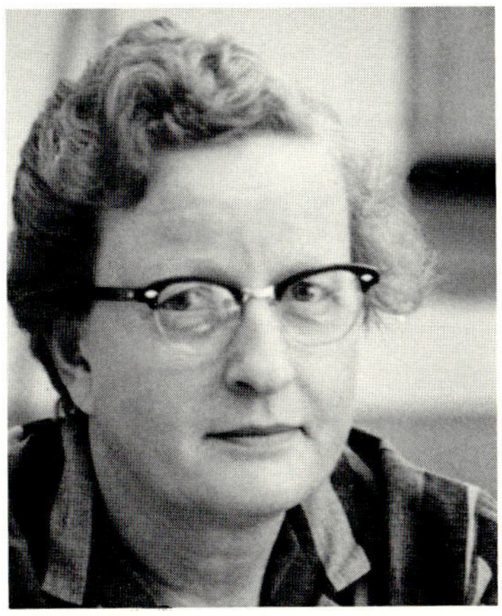

Marie Lowe

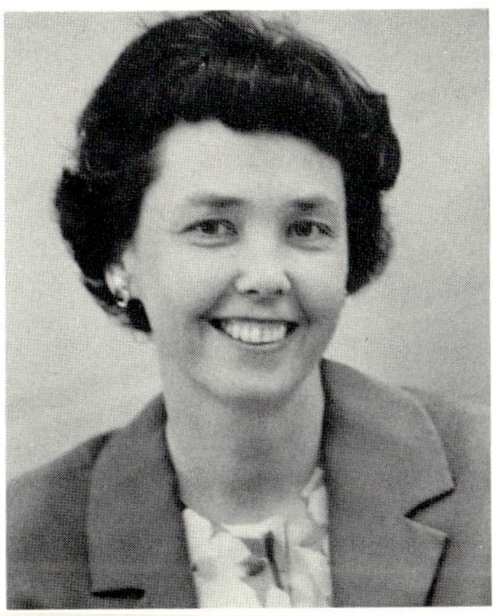

Doris Lister

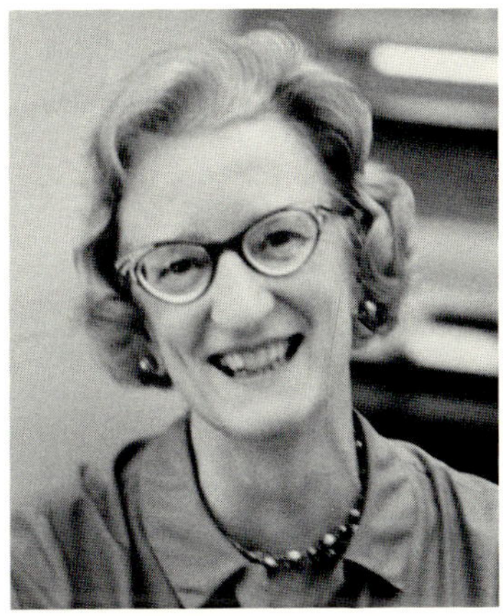

Margaret Shetland

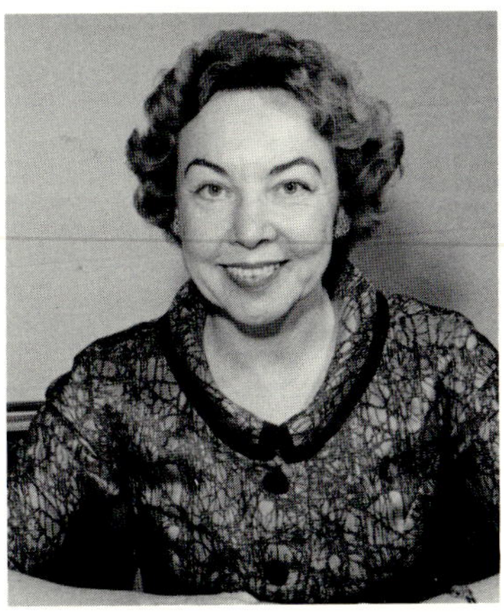

Nora Cline

Some members of the Department of Public Health Nursing during the 1960s and 1970s.

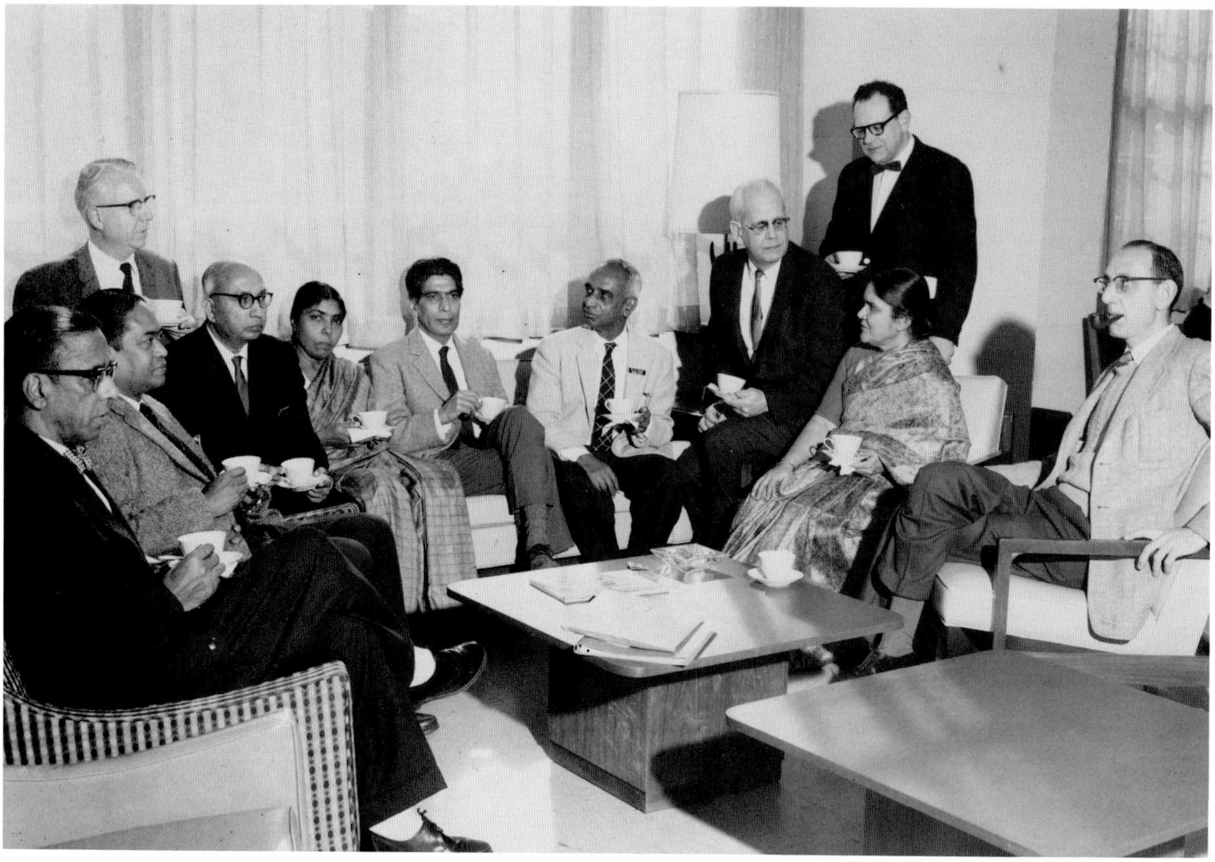

Dean Mayes, John Wright, Harry Spense, and John Cassel meet with a delegation of health administrators from India in 1964.

International efforts consisted of teaching, research, and service, the threefold mission of the school. The Department of Environmental Sciences and Engineering, for instance, established a nondegree training program for graduate sanitary engineers from developing countries in 1962, with grants from the Agency for International Development. The program eventually drew students from all over the world. The school also trained health workers for duty in foreign countries. In the summer of 1965, the public health faculty cooperated with the medical schools at UNC and Duke in a training program for Peace Corps doctors.[32]

A more ambitious training and service project was "The Malawi Public Health Program," a Peace Corps project supervised by the Department of Epidemiology. The program took Peace Corps volunteers with no professional health training, brought them to Chapel Hill for four months of instruction and then sent them to Malawi in south central Africa to work on the prevention and cure of tuberculosis. The program's objectives were twofold: implementation of an integrated health program using nonprofessionally trained personnel and the training of national counterparts so that health activities could continue following the Peace

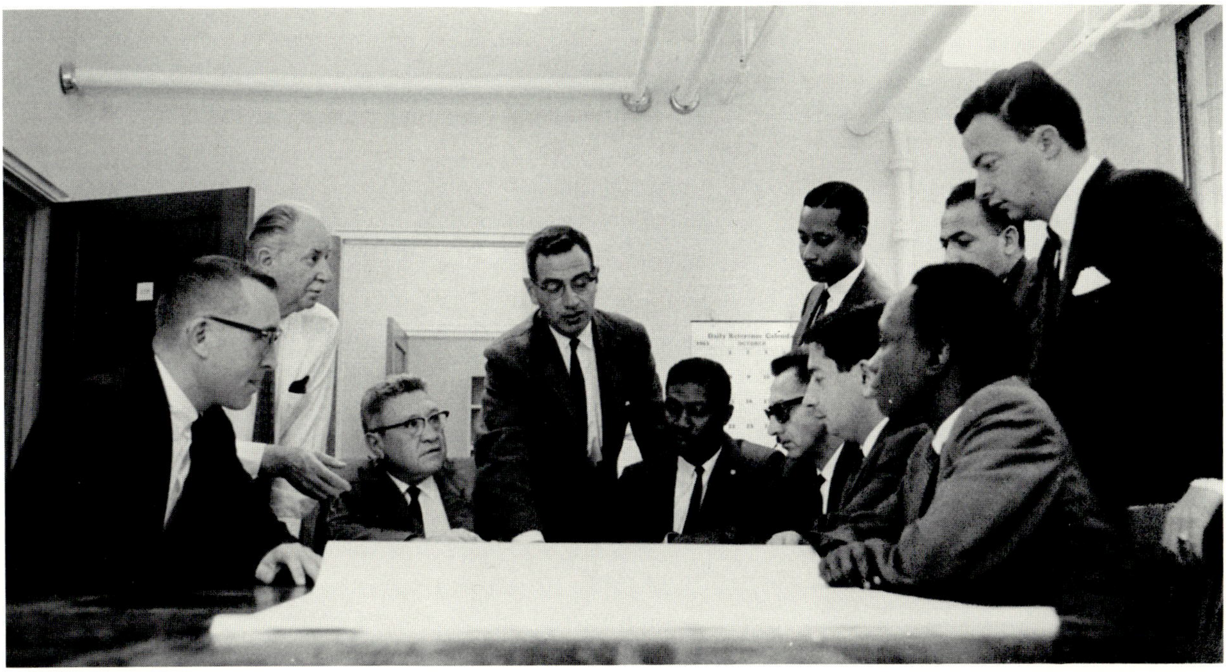

The International Program in Sanitary Engineering and Design, supported by the United States Agency for International Development, brought engineers to Chapel Hill for advanced study. *Seated, left to right:* James Brown (UNC), Jeff Flanagan (American technician from Burma), Vincent Hemming (Jamaica), Pedro Parada (Bolivia), Salman El-Rawi (Iraq), Emmanuel Ojo (Nigeria). *Standing, left to right:* George Barnes (UNC), Daniel Okun (UNC), Horace Beckford (Jamaica), Ali Shubber (Iraq), Walter Fabian (Costa Rica).

Corps's withdrawal. John Cassel beamed with pride as he inspected the troops. "I have just completed a tour of Malawi with Bill Peck looking at our Peace Corps project. I must say that even though I realize that it's still in its early stages, I was absolutely delighted with the way it had progressed. . . . I am really proud of the training they got in Chapel Hill. . . as they are probably the best-prepared bunch that have ever been sent out to Malawi."[33]

In the late 1950s and early 1960s, a pattern of social life oriented toward departments rather than the entire school had developed. The rapid growth of the school while Fred Mayes was dean reinforced this pattern. The Departments of Public Health Nursing and Public Health Education, with their large classes made up mostly of women, set the pace. Ruth Hay and Margaret Blee served Hogan stew to students at their home, Dun Roaming; while Lucy Morgan and Eunice (Pickie) Tyler's home, Lichenwood, served as the scene of numerous social events. As more faculty joined the Department of Environmental Sciences and Engineering and the student body increased in size, Dan Okun inaugurated annual parties for faculty and spouses, informal gatherings for students and faculty, and an annual banquet.

The Department of Maternal and Child Health exemplified this spirit of intradepartmental camaraderie and cooperation. Maternal and child health programs received special attention from the Johnson administration, particularly efforts to reduce infant mortality rates. The department benefited greatly from the increases in federal funds. Ann Peters, Naomi Morris, Jaroslav Hulka, Richard Udry, Earl Siegel, and Karl Bauman all joined the faculty in the mid-1960s. "One of the things that I look back on with great pleasure," Geraldine Gourley remembered, "was that the department was really close knit, it was like a family. The Chipmans, the Baumans, the Udrys, the Siegels, the Morrises, and I were really a very close-knit group, and the students felt that. The students were made to feel by everybody on the faculty that they were professional people to be respected and treated as coworkers in the health field. It was a wonderful time during those years."[34]

There were attempts to combat this increasing focus on department-centered activities, to try to maintain an "esprit de corps" that embraced the whole school. Dean Mayes and his wife Dorothy ('Mrs. Dean') played an important role in this effort. Mayes explained:

> In an effort to become personally acquainted with more students, Dorothy Mayes prepared food and hosted several groups of students each year for dinners and receptions in our home. Starting with a fall reception for international students, the entertaining proceeded at intervals through the year with home-prepared and served dinners for the officers, committee chairmen, and spouses of the student government; for officers and spouses of the Student Wives Club; for new faculty members and their spouses, and for other special groups. The year would end up with a final all-day Sunday open house for all students and their families during commencement week, opening with a 7:30 breakfast, going to a 10:00 coffee. . . , a 12:30 luncheon aimed at students who were leaving and in the throes of packing up, a 4:00 tea, and ending with a 6:30 Sunday night supper—thus breaking up the guest list into previously arranged manageable groups.[35]

Faculty, staff, and students at the school could not be unaffected by the upheavals of the 1960s. In many small ways, school programs and faculty had been catalysts for social change. The school, for instance, had confronted racial inequality through its cooperation with North Carolina College. The presence of foreign students, many of whom were dark skinned, challenged the racial myopia of the region. The civil rights sit-ins, which started in nearby Greensboro, spread to Chapel Hill in 1963, and members of the faculty were among the most vociferous

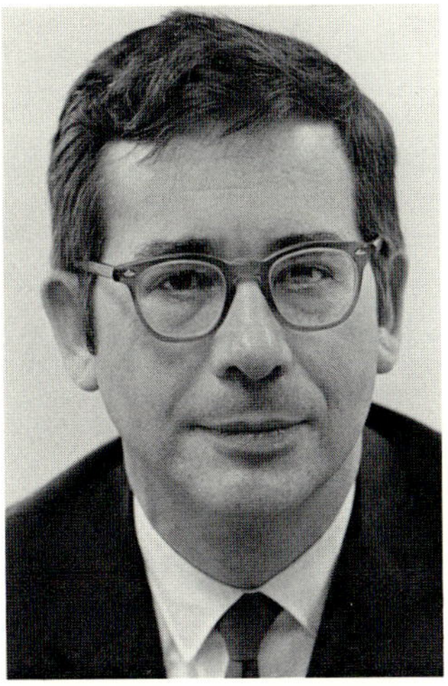

Earl Schaefer

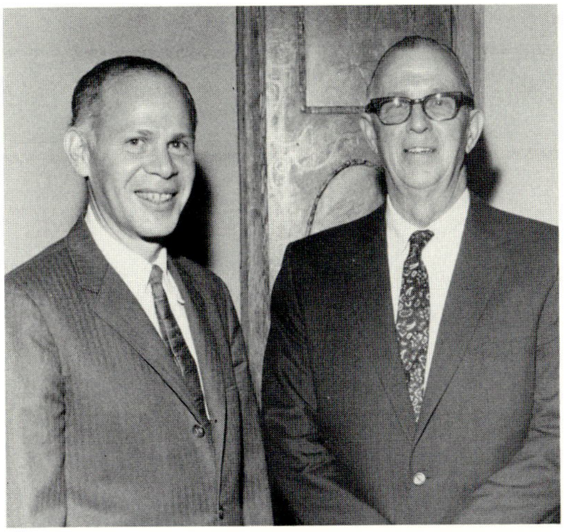

Earl Siegel Sidney Chipman

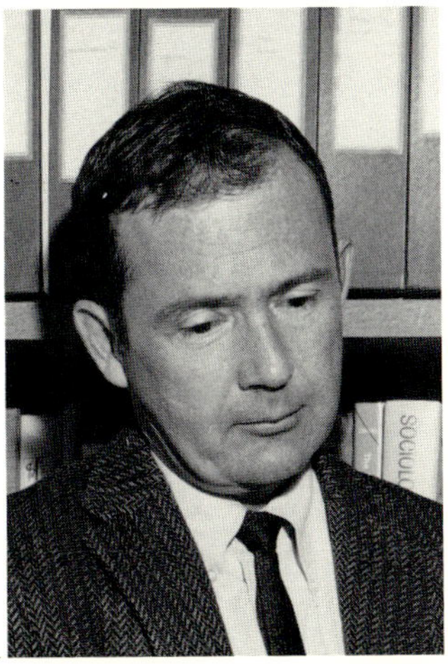

Richard Udry

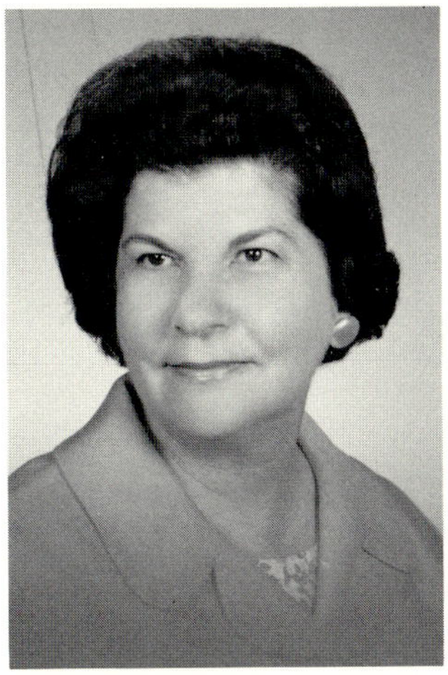

Barbara Stocking

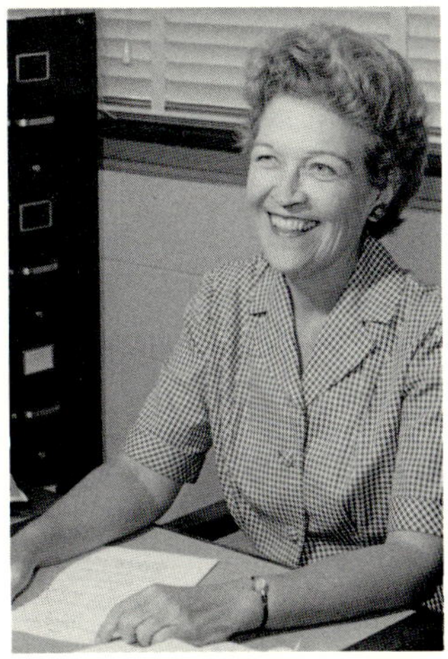

Geraldine Gourley

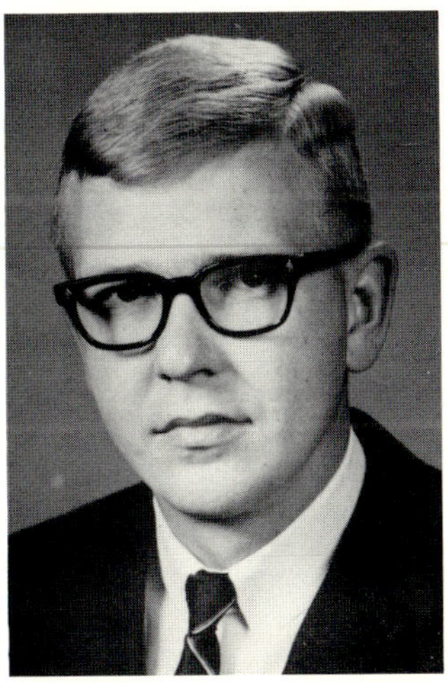

Karl Bauman

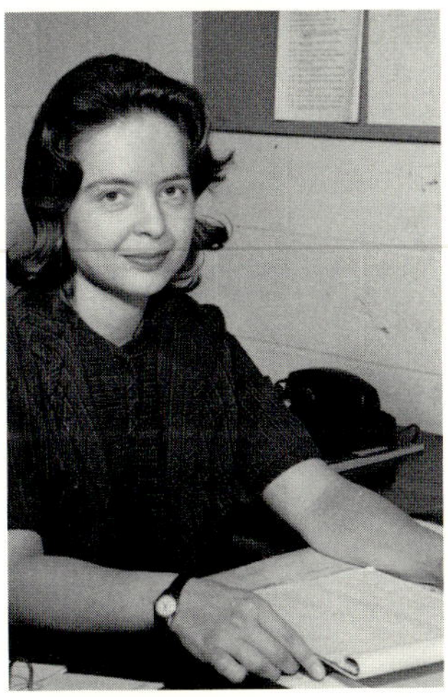

Naomi Morris

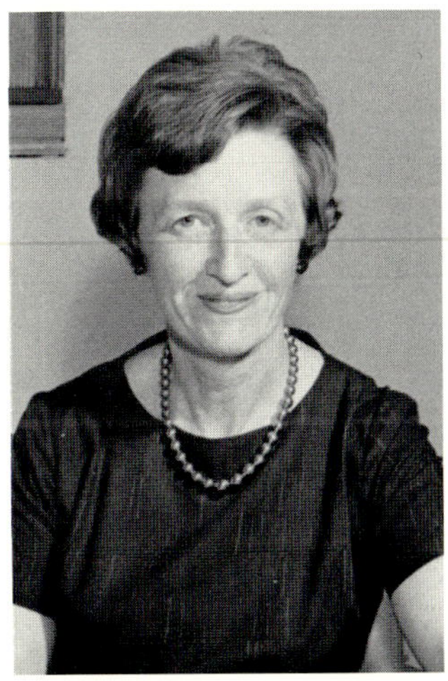

Ann Peters

Some members of the Department of Maternal and Child Health during the 1960s.

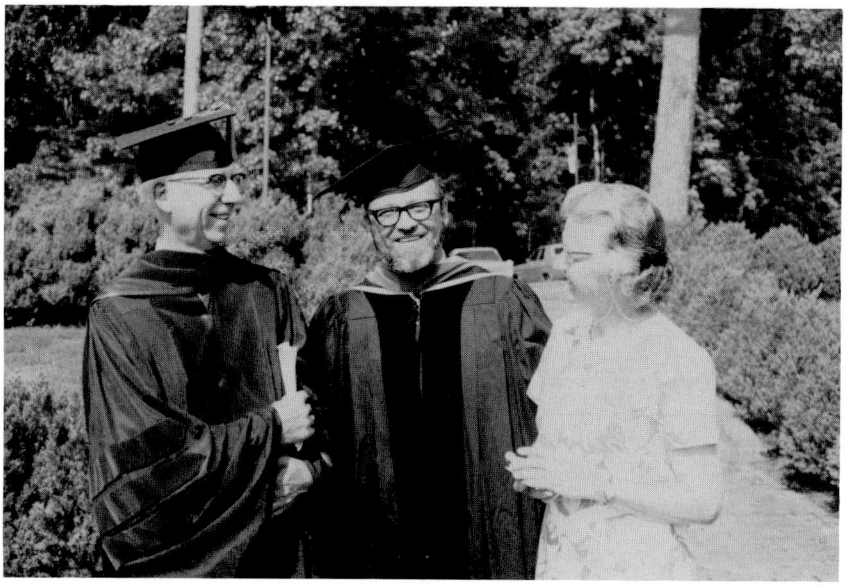

Dean Mayes and Dorothy Mayes congratulate School of Public Health graduate Robert Verhalen.

supporters of efforts to end segregation in Chapel Hill. Many of the same people lent a hand when food service workers at the university tried to organize a union in 1968 and 1969.[36]

Geraldine Gourley served on the school's speakers committee, and she remembered bringing in "some black activists to speak on the civil rights issue." "I always felt complete support if I wanted to take part in a demonstration. A lot of people on the faculty did that. I remember the strike of the cafeteria workers, and in those meetings it seemed like half of the faculty of the School of Public Health would be represented." Many faculty members signed a resolution supporting the recommendations of the Faculty Council for increased educational opportunities for minority students at UNC.[37]

Like most Americans, people at the school had been relatively apolitical during the 1950s. The protest movements of the sixties, however, widened the playing field and allowed a more direct challenge to the status quo. In the late 1960s the School of Public Health attracted advocacy-oriented students who saw adequate access to health care as a centerpiece of social change. Many of these students found a home in the Department of Public Health Education. A group of activists also centered around the Department of Environmental Sciences and Engineering. Here, they had professors who were outspoken critics of many environmental policies. In the classroom and in the field, students absorbed a passion for change, as well as a scientific understanding of the issues.[38]

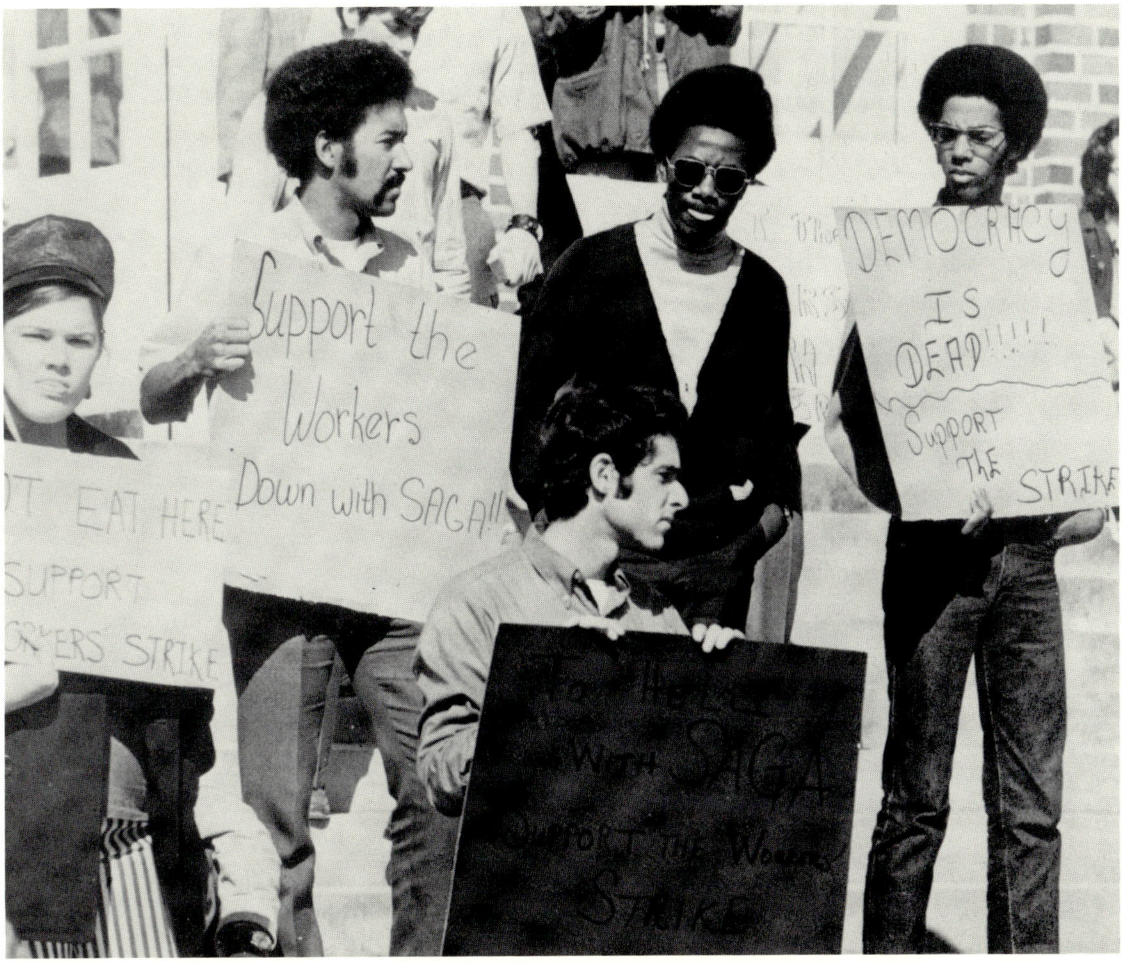
Support the
Workers
Down with SAGA!!
DEMOCRACY
IS
DEAD!!!!!
Support
THE
EAT HERE
SUPPORT
Students supporting the strike by food service workers at the university in 1969. Many faculty and students at the School of Public Health participated in the movements for social change in the 1960s.

Student activists were not content merely to challenge the larger political and economic structure, they also questioned some administrative and educational procedures in the school. Student organization dated back to 1947, when that year's class formed a Program and Steering Committee. The committee's primary purpose was to organize social activities that brought students and faculty together. An annual dinner-dance at the Chapel Hill Country Club and a picnic at Hogan's Lake highlighted the calendar. This committee functioned for many years, with Emil Chanlett as adviser.[39]

In 1968 students organized a student council, and in 1969 the Dean's Cabinet invited two students to attend the meetings as nonvoting members. A convocation address by the student council president in the Fall of 1970 was indicative of the new attitude.

> I welcome each of you . . . not in separate categories of 'students' and 'faculty', but as colleagues—co-participants in a mutual education

> process where all parties have an opportunity to define where they stand, to share whatever knowledges and experiences they may have, and to express openly what they expect from one another.
>
> Last year at convocation I alerted those present that emphasis would be placed upon the use of the student council as an action-oriented advocate of student educational interests with the desired outcome that of an improved and more creative learning environment. That was, and still *is*, based upon the following premises, the first of which I've already stated: (1) that students and faculty are *co*-participants in a mutual educational process; (2) that students enter this school, not as completely empty vessels into which a whole new set of concepts, attitudes, and values will be funneled by faculty, but with a rich variety of past experiences which can be tapped and built upon into a variety of new contexts and associations; and (3) that because students, as well as faculty, *do* have these sets of experience resources and special abilities, they have not only a right but a *responsibility* to be co-participants in the decisional processes which help determine the quality of their educational environment.[40]

Students were particularly critical of the core course, The Ecology of Health. There were too many lectures, a group of students wrote to Dean Mayes, and too much focus on research data. "Opportunities for full exploration of material and interchange of ideas were practically nil. [Faculty members] need to be aware of the desire of today's students for dynamic presentations of relevant course material on the ecology of health."[41]

By the end of the decade the school also began receiving criticism for its neglect of public health issues in North Carolina. A 1975 self-study characterized the period this way:

> Relationships with local communities and the state had deteriorated as departments were concerned with the federal dollar and were worshiping the idols in Washington and Bethesda. The image of the school in the state was not a pleasant one to contemplate because many local health department staffs as well as the state health department personnel felt the school's faculty were not interested in their problems. This was also evident by the relative lack of participation by the faculty in the operations and functions of the North Carolina Public Health Association.[42]

There were many reasons for this lagging interest in homegrown issues. First and foremost, was the lack of financial support from the state. The school's growth during the 1960s resulted from an infusion of soft money from the federal government, and many faculty members had no particular obligation to health agencies at the state or county level. Their careers centered on research and service to the agencies that gave them funding. Bill Herzog offered an example of the problems that situation created. One of Herzog's first jobs as assistant director of the Continued Education Service was running a six-week short course for sanitarians. "At that point," he remembered, "the Department of Environmental Sciences wouldn't run it, but they would participate. So I ran the course for two or three years and worked with them to convert it into an independent study course when it became more and more difficult to get participation of the faculty in teaching the course. The department had a person by the name of Gilbert Kelso. He kept a very good relationship with the health people. When Gilbert left, a significant point of contact was lost between the sanitarians in the local health departments and the school." Justified or not, the retreat from service to the state did little to help the school, particularly when it came time to ask for more money for buildings.[43]

Still, there were some notable exceptions. In the early 1960s, Charles Cameron helped secure a grant from the Public Health Service for a program in continuing education. John Wright served as director of the Continued Education Service (reorganized into Continuing Education and Field Service in 1969), and in 1964 Bill Herzog returned to the school after working at the Research Triangle Institute (RTI). Herzog spent much of his time at RTI scouting for federal money, experience that came in very handy in his new job. "At that time continuing education was federally financed and every time we wanted to do a short course we would write up a short grant proposal. Writing grant proposals had become a real art at that point, so we really took off with more and more short courses."[44]

The decline in service to the state was one of the issues university Chancellor J. Carlyle Sitterson asked a study commission to examine in 1970. Bernie Greenberg chaired the commission, which included representatives from the school's faculty and other areas of the university. The commission recognized the enormous changes that had taken place in the world since the end of World War II. Science and technology had advanced at a rapid pace, and people were putting increased pressure on government to distribute the benefits of those advances more equitably. Public health, the commission feared, had not kept up with these changes and, worse still, was not providing leadership in planning for future health needs.[45]

Unlike most self-study groups, the chancellor's committee made some far-reaching recommendations. The commission called, among other things, for the school to "institute baccalaureate programs to serve as a prototype for other universities and community colleges," to develop a model community health center, and to recruit minority faculty. The commission also suggested that the school's name should be changed to School of Community and Public Health, to reflect the broadened constituency it would serve in the 1970s.[46]

The most controversial recommendation centered on an administrative restructuring that would eventually combine the Departments of Health Administration, Health Education, Maternal and Child Health, Mental Health, Public Health Nursing, and Public Health Nutrition into a Department of Community Health Practices and Administration. The reorganization of the school was necessary, the commission said, because the present structure reflected "rather rigidly a constituency that is no longer in the ascendency." To survive, the school had to adapt more rapidly to the "changing marketplace for its product." This meant the school needed to streamline its operations according to the wealth and status of the departments as they stood after a decade of federal support. Since the service-oriented departments had not fared well during the federal funding battles of the 1960s, they should be consolidated, thus reducing their disciplinary independence. Given the nature of the recommendations, controversy was sure to follow.[47]

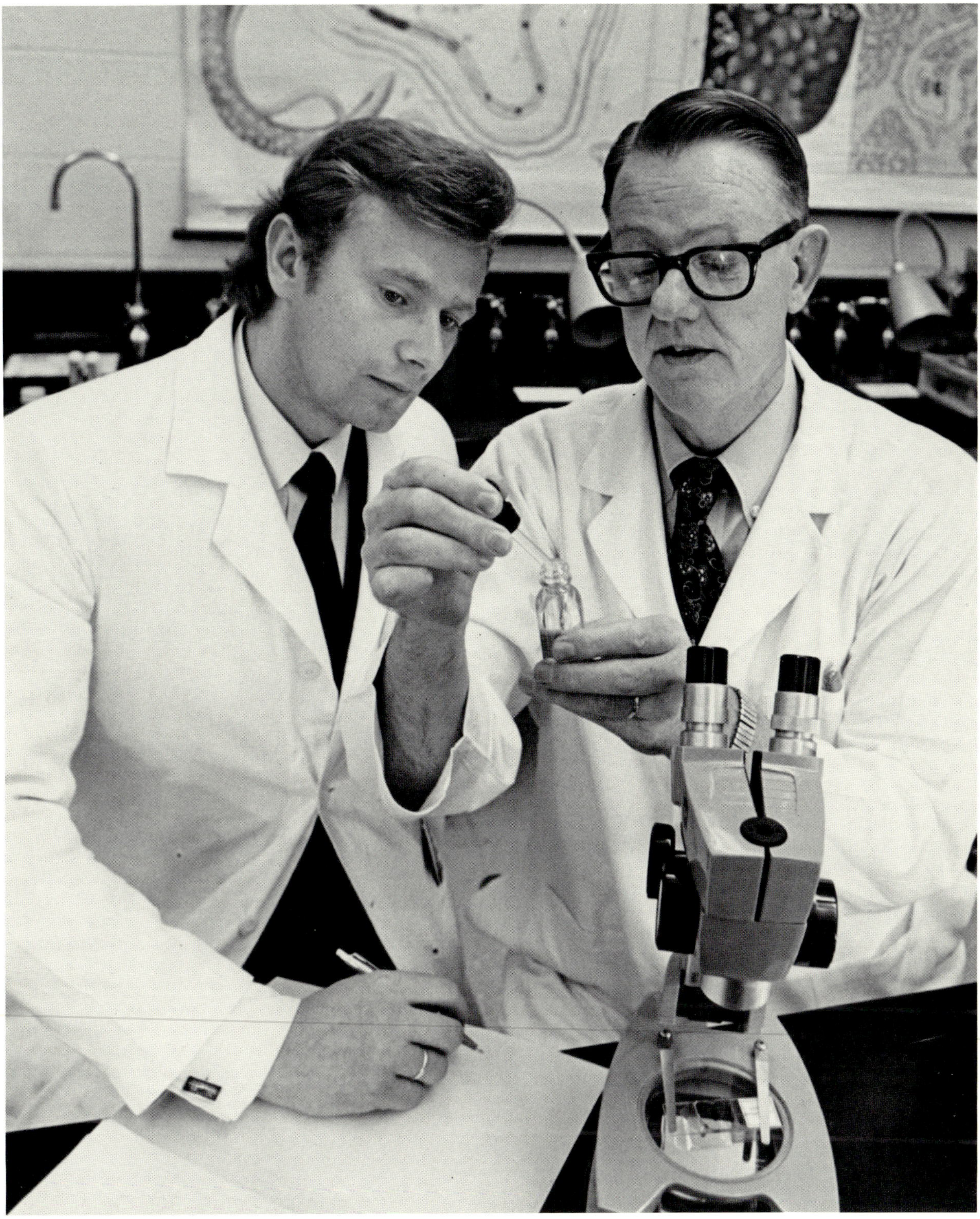

Dr. John Larsh (*right*), head of the Department of Parasitology and Laboratory Practice, confers with Polish scientist, Dr. M. Stankiewicz, about research on trichinosis.

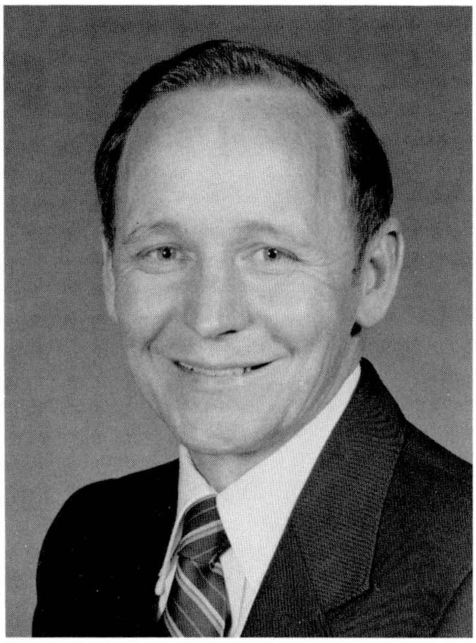

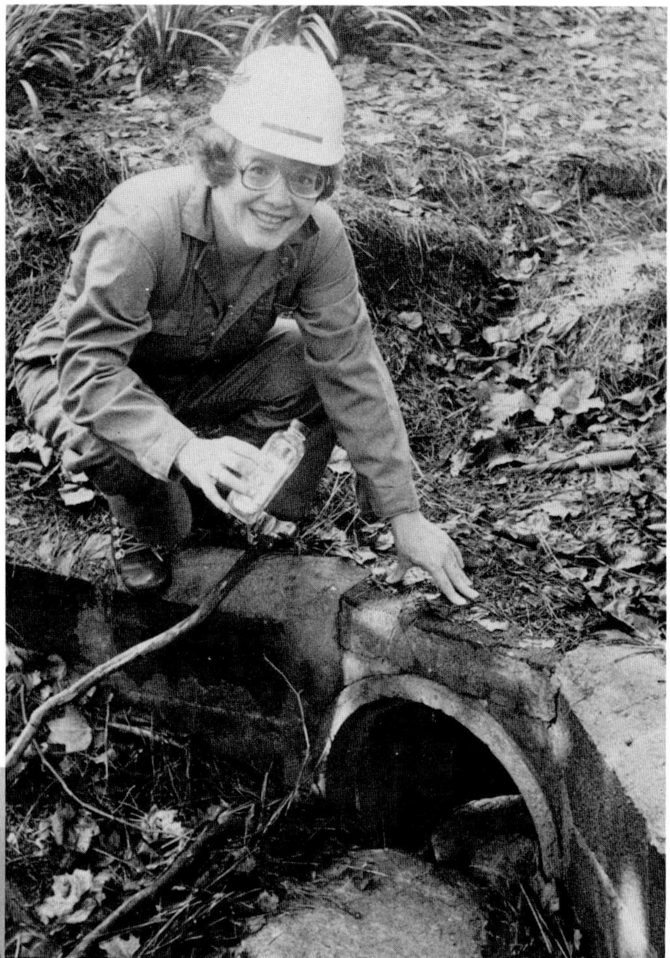

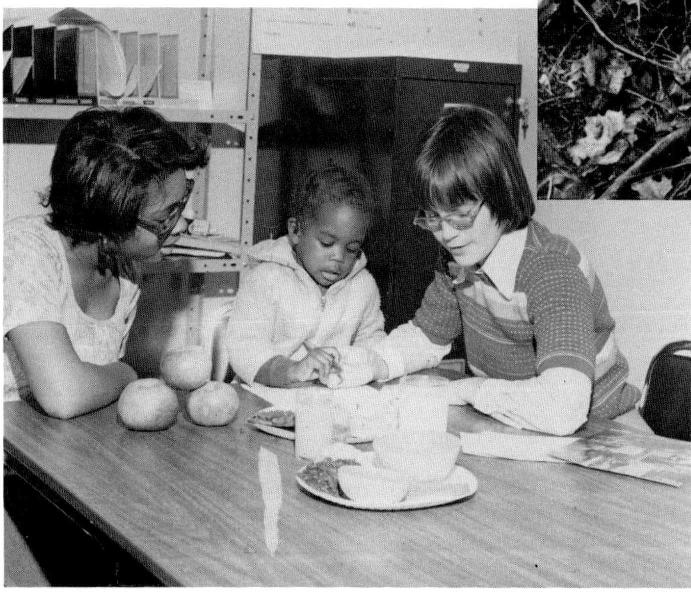

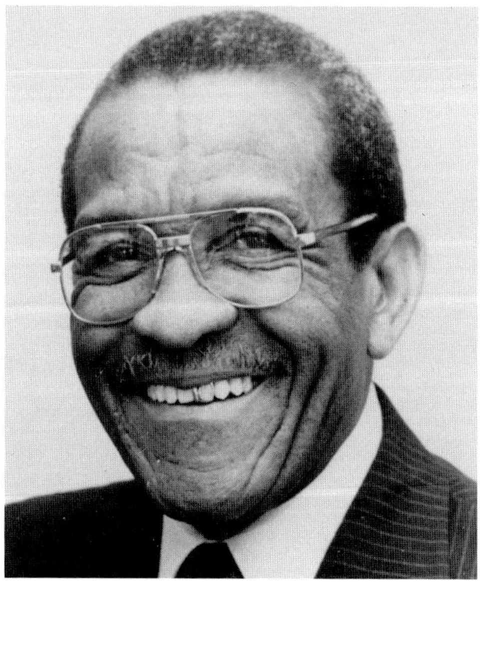

Dean Bernard Greenberg created the Division of Community Health Service in 1972 so that the school could better serve the needs of the state. Richard House (*upper left*) headed the continuing education program from 1976–1984 and became director of the division in 1984. Environmental consultant Linda Little (*upper right*) served as an adjunct professor in the Department of Environmental Sciences and Engineering. Howard Barnhill (*lower right*) coordinated the Area Health Education Centers in the western part of the state. A nutrition student (*lower left*) counsels a mother on the proper diet for her child as part of her field work.

Chapter 6

PRACTICE WHAT YOU TEACH

The 1970s was a period of remarkable contrasts. The decade opened with popular resistance to the war in Southeast Asia and protest movements among blacks, women, and students. Ten years later, the nation elected one of its most conservative presidents, Ronald Reagan. In between, Watergate, the oil embargo, runaway inflation, and the Iran hostage crisis seemed to mark the end of postwar confidence and prosperity.

Health care experienced similar ups and downs. The reformist impulses of the 1960s carried over until mid-decade as consumers demanded stricter regulation, advocates for the poor and minority groups pushed for more entitlement programs, and the environmental movement called for tougher laws to ensure clean air, clean water, and workplace safety. But stagflation put a break on further growth and experimentation, and by 1980 the political mood of the country turned against the Great Society programs that had spurred the expansion of public health programs since the 1960s.[1]

The School of Public Health did much soul-searching during the 1970s. A self-study committee seemed always to be in session. The volatility of national social and political life contributed to this reflective mood, but the school had its own problems. It had continued to grow, even after the mid-decade financial crisis. The operating budget for 1969–70 was almost $7 million; by 1979–80 it had jumped to over $20 million. Student enrollment rose from 391 to 702 during the same period. Faculty appointments (full- and part-time) increased from 158 to 317. But consolidation rather than innovation was the watchword of the decade. Dean Mayes had allowed departments to expand (or not to expand) on their own. The result was a great imbalance in the strength and resources of the departments. The 1970s demanded a more concerted effort at overall planning for the school.[2]

The school's mission also seemed unclear. Some faculty thought that the school was governed too often by a nose for financial support rather than a comprehensive plan for attacking the world's health problems. The status of women and minorities also caused concern. In earlier days women had played a major role, and the school had directed much effort toward the educational needs of blacks and American Indians. But by the 1970s, the recruitment of women and minorities had become a major problem.

The first problem addressed by the school was the issue of minority recruitment. The school had long been committed to public health training for minority groups. Until the 1960s, this commitment entailed support for graduate programs in public health nursing and public health education at North Carolina College in Durham. In 1960 those programs were disbanded, and black students enrolled at the school, albeit in relatively small numbers.

In 1970 the slow pace of integration and a general upsurge of black activism prompted black students to issue "A Statement of Concerns Regarding the Relevance & Responsiveness of the School of Public Health to the Needs of Black Americans." "The situation of Blacks in the South," the statement read, "is not unlike that of residents of developing countries. We have become increasingly cognizant of the magnitude and severity of the health problems and needs of our fellow Blacks and view this decade as a critical period for ourselves, the nation, and institutions that wish to be a part of the solution." The students requested increases in the number of black students and faculty, more courses geared to the needs of students planning to work in the black community, the appointment of a minority recruitment officer, and greater black involvement in projects relating to the black community.[3]

Dean Mayes appointed a committee to consider the students' demands. The committee recommended hiring a full-time minority recruiter, and William Small eventually took the job. A student had approached him about applying for the position. "He said 'We need someone who knows something about public health, who has been through the school, and who knows what it takes to get through,'" Small remembered.[4]

William Small knew the school quite well. A native of Wilmington, North Carolina, Small majored in chemistry at North Carolina College

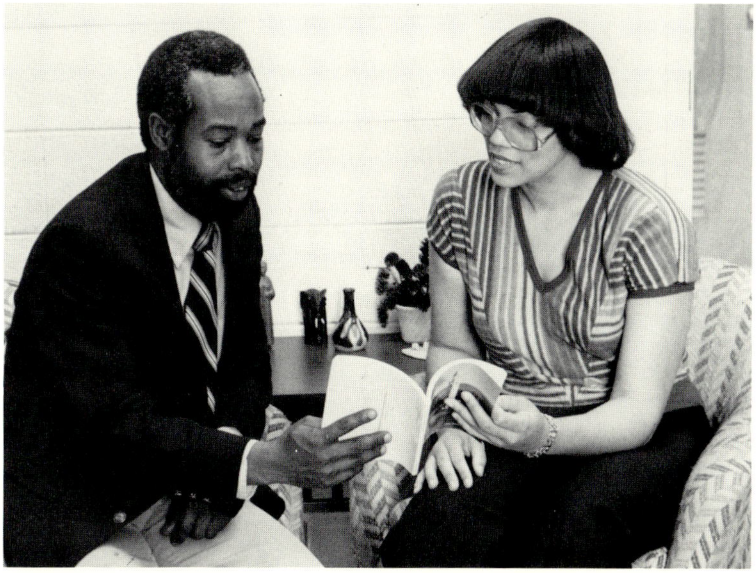

William Small advising Rebera Foston.

and then spent a few years with the American Tobacco Company. He returned to graduate school and received his M.S.P.H. from the Air and Industrial Hygiene program in the Department of Environmental Sciences and Engineering in 1969. Small was working as a chemist for the State Board of Health when he decided to apply for the recruitment position.[5]

"The School of Public Health was really in the forefront of efforts to recruit minority students at the graduate level," Small remarked. "We were the first school to hire someone full-time and go at it in a systematic manner. We involved faculty, students, staff and used all kinds of techniques to reach out into the community to attract students, and it paid off." In the fall of 1972, less than a year after Small accepted the job, the number of minority students increased from twenty to forty-nine. The next year the school began to concentrate on black faculty.[6]

A stronger minority presence in the school highlighted the need to make the curriculum more relevant to the needs of the black community. Concerns included white instructors' insensitivity to black students and a lack of understanding of the complexities of black community life. A minority health conference, initiated in 1977, helped "create a feeling of pride and understanding among the students," Small recalled. "We felt that minority students who were training here would be the leaders of tomorrow in the health field. They needed to know how to get organized and put on programs. The conference was planned and run by the students. It was learning outside the classroom."[7]

Increased minority recruitment was one of the many recommendations made by the Chancellor's Study Commission in 1971, and it boded well for the future that the school moved quickly on this issue. By contrast, a number of factors conspired to prevent the implementation of the commission's plan for far-reaching changes in the school's administrative structure. Little could be done until after Dean Mayes's retirement, scheduled for 1973. Nevertheless, Dr. Dorothea C. Leighton of the Department of Mental Health chaired a committee that began to canvass faculty opinion on the report. Virtually no one supported changing the school's name to the School of Community and Public Health. "The school is community-oriented by definition," Robert Watson of the Department of Parasitology and Laboratory Practice wrote, "why gild the lily by stating this in the name of the school." Strong opposition to departmental reorganization also surfaced. "Consolidation of the nutrition department with five unrelated 'service' units is a retrograde step," wrote Department of Nutrition Chair Joseph Edozien. "Nutrition is as much a science in its own right as are parasitology, biostatistics and epidemiology."[8]

When Dean Mayes elected to step down early at the end of the 1971–72 academic year, the chancellor appointed a search committee. But there was little question who the next dean would be. When the committee polled the faculty, the name of Dr. Bernard Greenberg came up time after time. "By any standard—professional competence, administrative skill, innovative practice, regard for staff well-being," Roy Kuebler wrote, "[Bernard Greenberg] merits and receives the respect and loyalty of all who work with him. . . . His devotion to the university and his long intimate knowledge of its ins and outs combined with his professional and personal characteristics lead me to see him as a top ranking nominee for our new dean."[9]

As a faculty member since 1949, the only chairman of the Department of Biostatistics, and chairman of the Chancellor's Study Commission, Greenberg knew the strengths and weaknesses of the school as well as anyone. He, John Cassel, and Dan Okun had talked for years about how they would do things if they got the chance. Now Greenberg had the opportunity. In brief, he envisioned a more rigorous academic institution, dedicated to research and teaching. Greenberg was also determined to secure a new building and to improve the school's standing in the state. In the end, the effort to acquire a building and the rededication to North Carolina, more than academic restructuring, guided his tenure as dean.

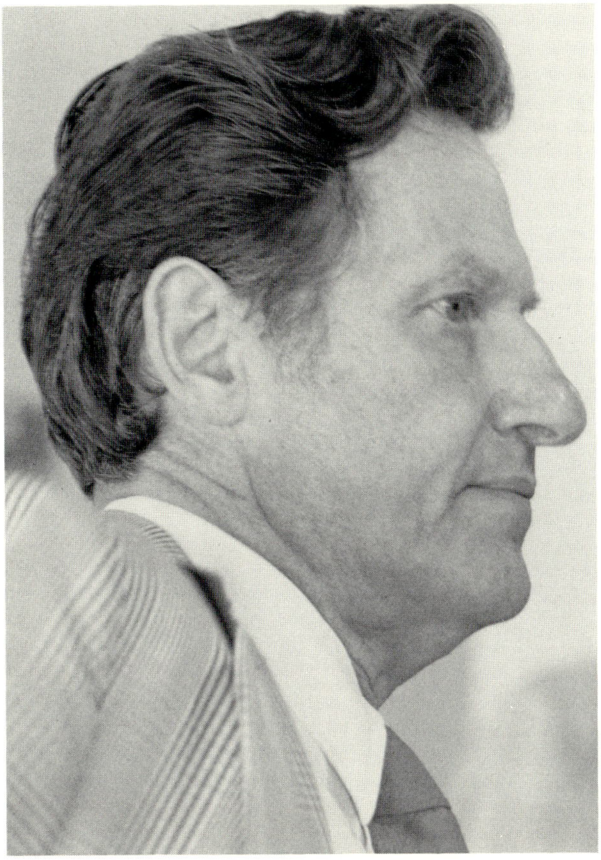

Dean Bernard Greenberg

If Washington and Bethesda had been the center of the school's attention in the 1960s, Raleigh became the focus of the 1970s. Greenberg surveyed the school's problems and concluded that poor relationships with state and local health agencies constituted the school's most serious failing. Determined to mend fences, he moved ahead on a number of fronts.[10]

Greenberg's first move was to reactivate the Alumni Association and resume publication of *The Body Politic.* He believed that a strong alumni association would keep the school in better touch with public health practitioners, whose involvement would then increase the effectiveness of the school's programs. Harriet Barr became director of public relations for the school, with responsibility for the Alumni Association. Barr received her M.P.H. in public health education in 1948 and returned to the school in 1965 as a research associate in that department. She was an assistant professor at the time she undertook her work in public relations.[11]

The school held its first annual Alumni Day in 1973, at which time the association was formally established. A steering committee worked out the fine points of organization over the next year, and in

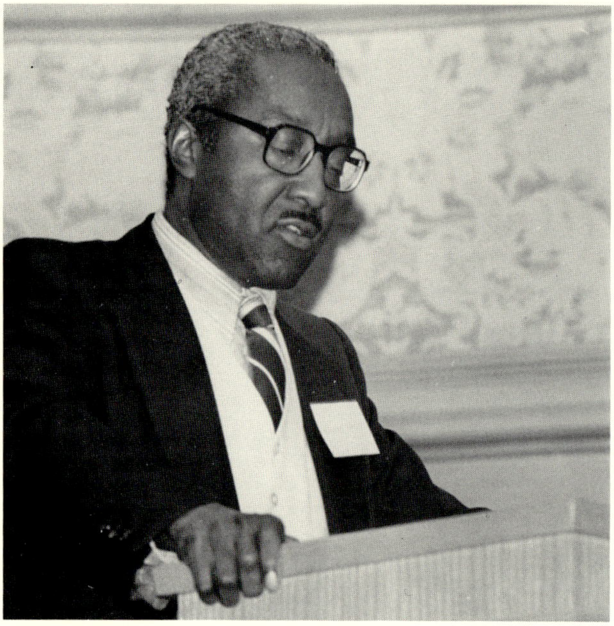

William A. Darity

April, 1974, Dr. William A. Darity, dean of the School of Health Sciences at the University of Massachusetts, became the first president. Within a few years the Alumni Association had become a highly visible arm of the school. *The Body Politic* began appearing three times a year in 1975. Social hours at the American Public Health Association and North Carolina Public Health Association meetings provided opportunities for alumni to keep in touch with one another and with the faculty. The Fred T. Foard Memorial Lecture, delivered by a distinguished public health person, anchored the annual Alumni Day, and the association established numerous awards to recognize the contributions of former students of the School of Public Health.[12]

Dean Greenberg moved to improve the school's standing among the state's health officials by creating the Division of Community Health Service in 1973. The division included Continuing Education, the Off-Campus Master's Degree Program, the Area Health Education Centers, the Technical Assistance Unit, and Field Relations. Dr. Charles Harper directed the division and was very clear about its purpose. "Originally, the school had a strong North Carolina focus, beginning as it did with a continuing education program in 1936," he said. "As the school grew in size and prestige, we responded to strong pressures from national and international sources for training programs in public health. As a result, the school, over time, developed an international and national focus that overshadowed its original commitment to North Carolina. The division's role has been to right that balance."[13]

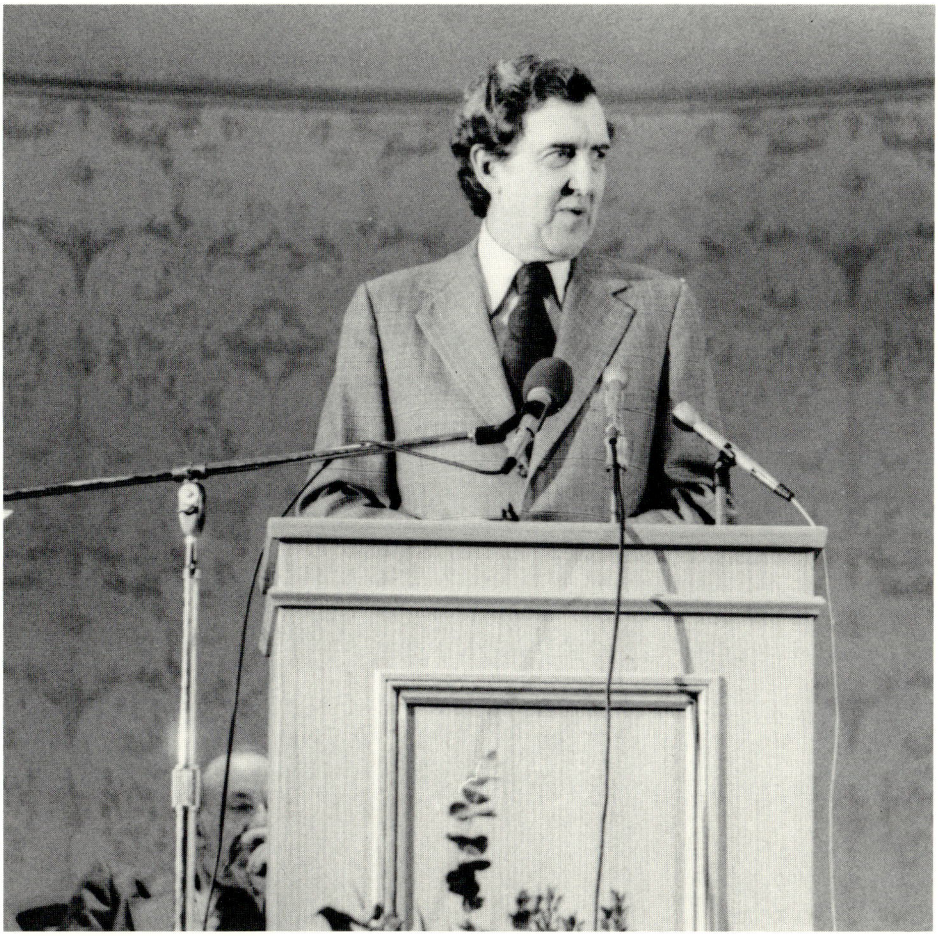

Senator Edmund S. Muskie delivers the 1976 Fred T. Foard Memorial Lecture.

Dr. John Hughes assumed direction of Continuing Education. Hughes had extensive contacts with public health officials in the state because of his work with the Dental Health Division of the State Board of Health. He joined the Department of Health Administration in 1966, heading the Dental Public Health Program. Under his leadership, Continuing Education attempted to bring the latest public health knowledge to professionals in the field. Through noncredit short courses and training sessions, the unit upgraded skills that were learned in earlier years and introduced new techniques.[14]

Under Dr. Morris Schaefer's leadership, the school initiated the Off-Campus Master's Degree Program in 1969 to allow employees of state and local health departments to complete degree requirements on a part-time basis while they continued to work. Students received an M.P.H. in health administration at the end of three years. The first program was held in Raleigh, followed by programs in Asheville in 1974

Lydia Holley and Howard Fitts attend the School of Public Health reception at the annual North Carolina Public Health Association meeting. School faculty and alumni became more involved in the association in the 1970s.

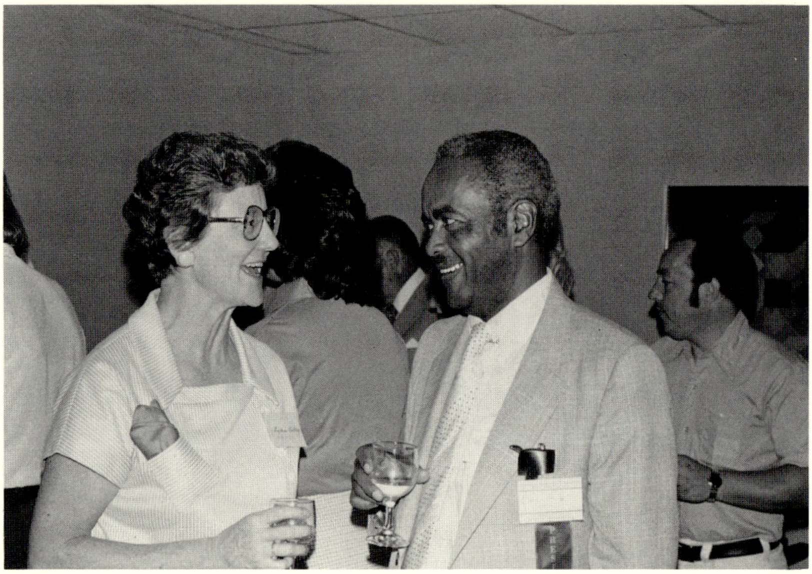

and in Fayetteville in 1977. The school added a degree in public health nursing in Greenville (1977) and Hickory (1980).[15]

The Technical Assistance Unit of the division represented Greenberg's efforts to strengthen the school's contact with state and local health agencies. In its pure form, technical assistance involved members of the faculty in a direct consulting role; for example, they would help to devise a health survey for a county. But assistance also took the form of serving on the boards of agencies, such as the North Carolina Affiliate American Heart Association.

Another development geared to the public health needs of the state was the bachelor of science in public health program. The training of undergraduate public health nurses had ceased in 1962. But the need for entry-level community health workers put pressure on the school to resume the program. Frances Gust and Ed McGavran tried to build a resource for the training of local public health workers by cooperating with the newly established community college system, but to no avail. Responding to recommendations by the Chancellor's Study Commission and the 1972 Legislative Study Commission on Public Health in North Carolina, the school moved to reinstitute the baccalaureate degree in public health. A grant from the federal government helped establish undergraduate concentrations in biostatistics, health administration, health education, nutrition, and environmental protection. Students entered at the beginning of their junior year.[16]

The Area Health Education Center (AHEC) was a bold initiative of national importance. Operated as a cooperative program of the Schools

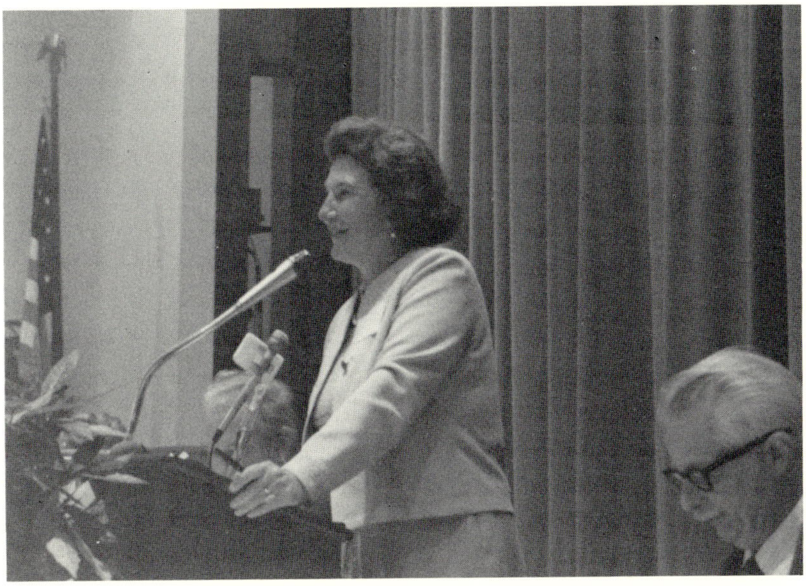

Sarah Morrow, a School of Public Health alumna and secretary of Human Resources during the administration of Governor James B. Hunt, delivers an address during public health week. At right is Jacob Koomen, Jr., another school alumnus who served as State Health Officer from 1966–1972.

of Medicine, Dentistry, Nursing, Pharmacy, and Public Health, AHEC established educational programs in areas that lacked easy access to major health centers. A gross imbalance in health personnel existed in North Carolina, as in other states, and one way to right that was to decentralize health and medical education. The regional centers provided training for practicing professionals, course development for technical and community colleges, and student trainees. The School of Public Health assigned some students whose programs required field training to the centers.[17]

No sooner had Dean Greenberg embarked on these various efforts to improve the teaching and service components of the school, than President Richard Nixon delivered a budget message that sent shock waves through the public health community. As part of his administration's "New Federalism," Nixon recommended termination of federal support for schools of public health and for research training grants as of June 30, 1973. Greenberg declared the proposed cuts would "cripple schools of public health across the country. Some of the nation's 18 schools will almost certainly have to close if they do not receive emergency funds."[18]

The school took a number of steps to meet the threatened fiscal crisis. University officials lobbied congressmen and senators in an effort to restore the cuts. The dean appealed to the North Carolina General Assembly for emergency funds and to private foundations for additional scholarships. The school also instituted some minor restructuring in an effort to economize.

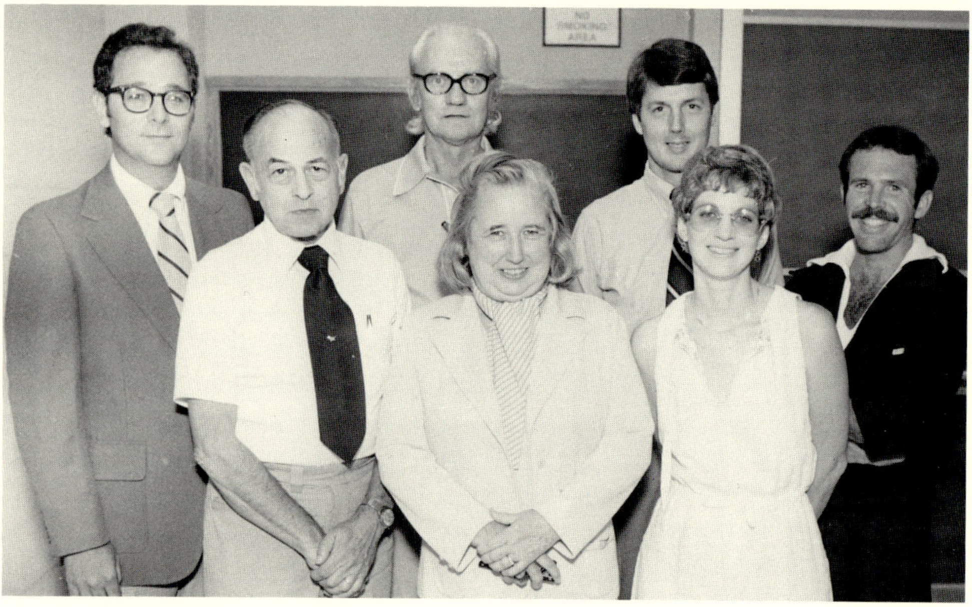

The School of Public Health reinstated an undergraduate degree program in 1976, as part of Dean Greenberg's efforts to train more North Carolinians. *Above,* members of the Bachelor of Science in Public Health Advisory Committee. *Left to right:* Craig Turnbull, Godfrey Hochbaum, Ralph Patrick, Elizabeth Coulter, Fred Stevens, Laurel Files, and Terry Bazzarre.

Fortunately, the lobbying effort proved successful, and Congress extended the Hill-Rhodes Act for another year. But with the financial future anything but stable, Greenberg tried to overcome the resistance to the reorganization recommended by the Chancellor's Study Commission. "He had a honeymoon period," Dan Okun recalled. "I said, 'do it now. Get rid of some of those departments.' [But] he felt he couldn't do it." Pressure from alumni and faculty in the affected departments, Okun concluded, held Greenberg back. Others felt that the political and personal costs of making major changes in the face of strong opposition had simply been too great. In the end, the school eliminated the Department of Mental Health and left everything else intact.[19]

The strain on schools of public health brought about by the legacy of social and technological upheaval and the threatened funding cutbacks was highlighted by a much-discussed report, "Higher Education for Public Health," compiled for the Association of Schools of Public Health by the Milbank Memorial Fund. Dr. Cecil Sheps, a former member of the school's faculty and vice chancellor for health sciences at the university, chaired the Milbank Commission. The commission's thirty-four recommendations called for the "reorganization and systematization" of the educational system. "What exists now is chaotic, wasteful, and dysfunctional," Sheps wrote. "What is needed is greater clarity of purpose to serve urgent public needs."[20]

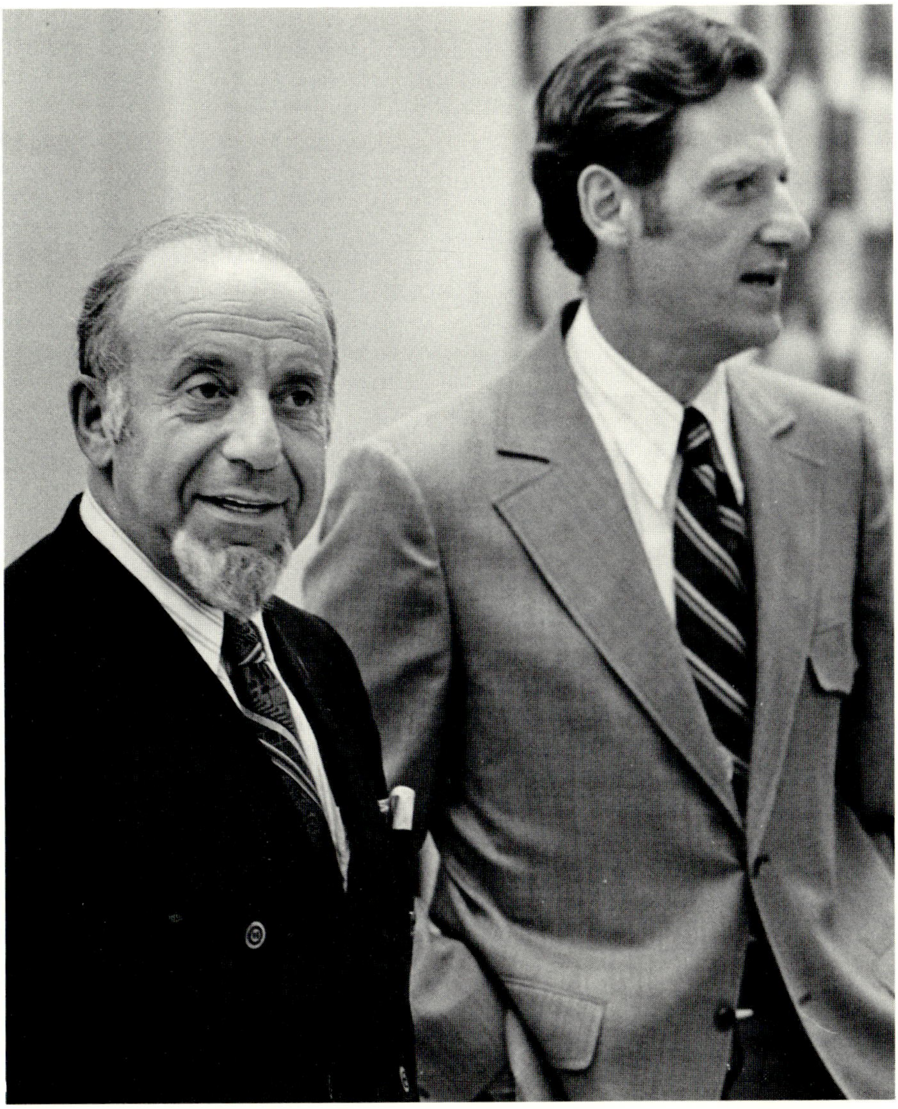

Vice Chancellor for Health Affairs Cecil Sheps and Dean Bernard Greenberg.

The commission also stressed the need for improved leadership in public health and urged the schools to focus their energies in that direction. The commission encouraged public health faculty to become advocates "for effective health policies, programs, and practices." Although such actions would often "entangle them in political or otherwise controversial efforts," the commission felt that the problems of the environment and in the delivery of health services required that those who knew the most about the issues speak up.[21]

Dean Greenberg and Dr. Sheps discussed some of the Milbank Commission's early assessments in *The Body Politic.* Greenberg pointed to a number of areas where the school had already moved to implement the commission's recommendations: undergraduate training and greater

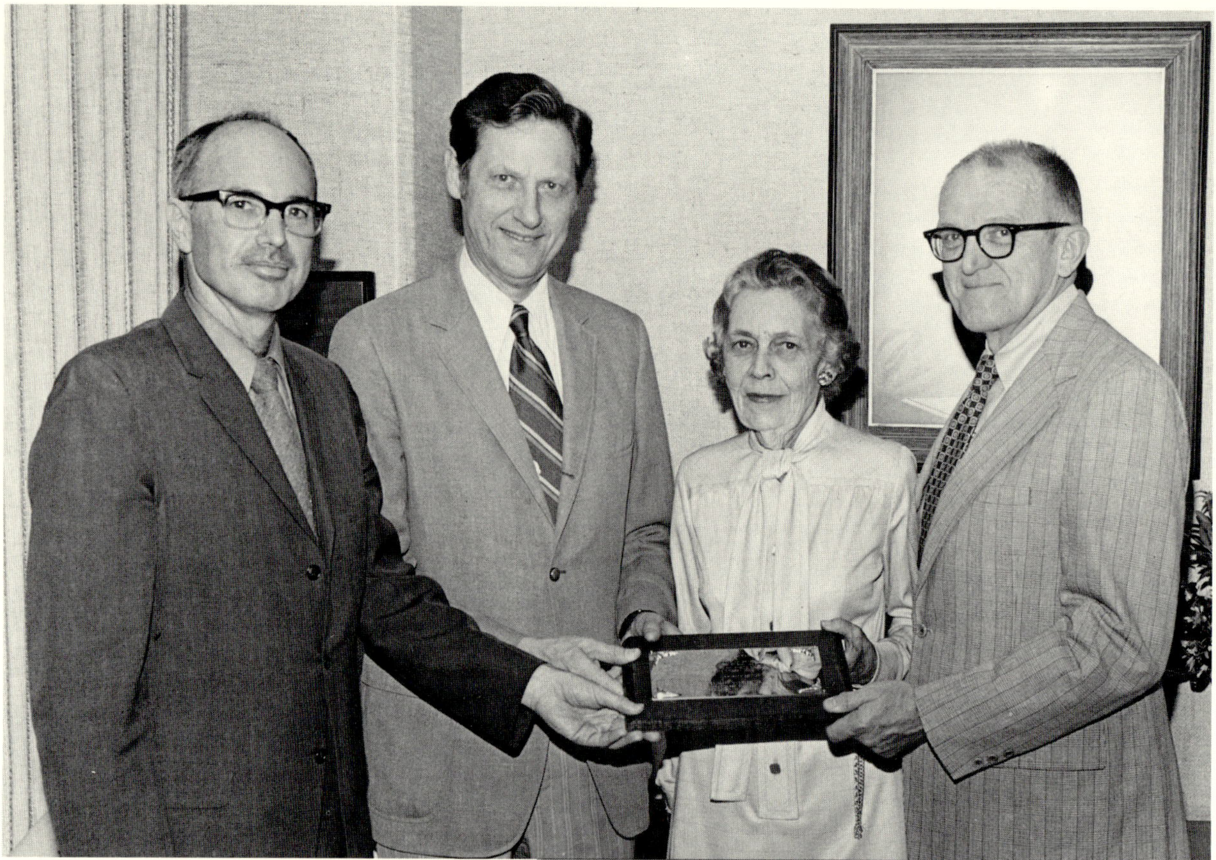

Roy R. Kuebler, Jr., of the Department of Biostatistics, receives the school's first Edward G. McGavran Award for excellence in teaching. *Left to right:* Bert Kaplan, chairman of the selection committee, Dean Greenberg, Mary McGavran, and Kuebler.

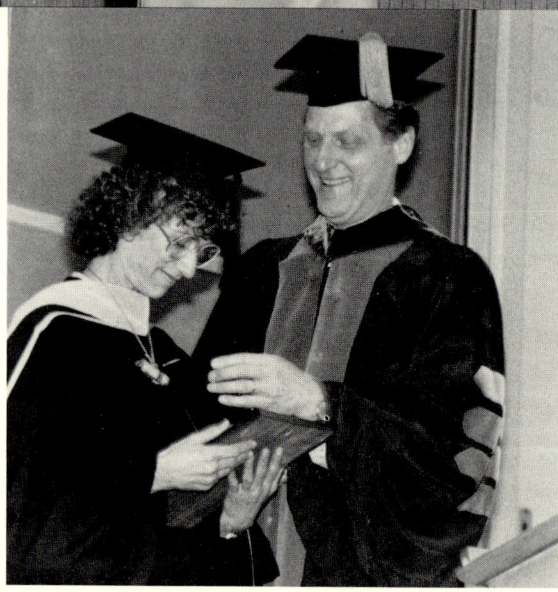

Dean Greenberg presents the McGavran Award in 1981 to Patricia Z. Barry of the Department of Health Policy and Administration for her innovative use of small groups in classroom teaching.

service to the state, for instance. But Greenberg admitted "it is a difficult process to change organizational structures within the school." Since collapsing practice-oriented departments seemed an impossibility, whether desirable or not, Greenberg's only choice was to strengthen the weaker departments. In doing so, Greenberg had the help of a new group of young department chairs who worked hard to improve the standing of their faculty and of the school.[22]

Each of the practice-oriented departments—health education, public health nursing, health administration, nutrition, and maternal and child health—took a different route and developed in unique ways over the next few years. Health administration and maternal and child health experienced the greatest successes, although in different ways.

Thanks to increased federal support for local health agencies in the sixties and early seventies and the rapid growth in the field of health care, the demand for qualified health administrators far outran the available supply. Unfortunately, the Department of Health Administration lacked the ability to train large numbers of capable administrators when Dr. Sagar Jain assumed the chair in 1971, and the Schools of Medicine, Business, and Public Administration competed for interested students. Instruction suffered from the lack of faculty trained in the

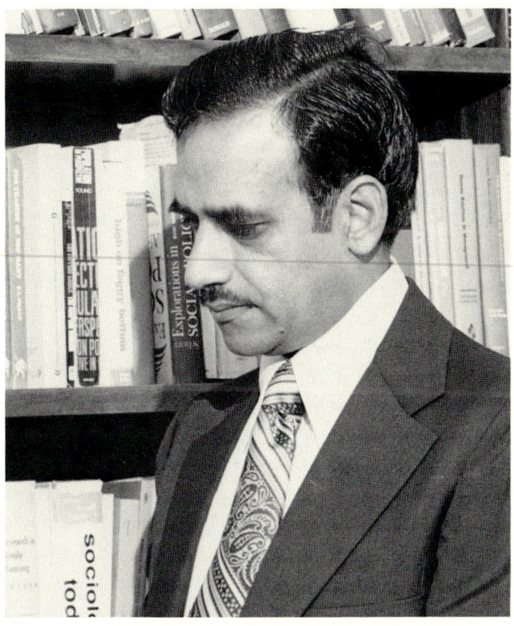

Sagar Jain

social and administrative sciences. The department, at the time, was made up of health clinicians—physicians, nurses, therapists. "They could describe the health care system very well," Jain recalled. "Often they could identify the issues on the basis of their personal observation. The only question was how to solve them." Experience and "wisdom" substituted for methodology, Jain believed. He went to work to change that, with the support of both Dean Mayes and Dean Greenberg.[23]

Jain's own degree was in public administration, and he began hiring people with training in operations research, finance, and economics. Research continued to suffer, however, because of the teaching loads and service responsibilities of these new faculty members and because the department lacked a "critical mass" in the various disciplines. Prodded by criticism of the department's teaching capabilities and its limited contact with former health administrators, the school increased the faculty in these key areas. By 1981 Jain's strategy paid off and the department changed its name to Health Policy and Administration and began offering a Ph.D. degree.[24]

The women's movement and changing attitudes toward sexuality heightened the public's awareness of maternal and child health issues and increased the demand for public programs. The Department of Maternal and Child Health benefited from this increased exposure and grew dramatically during the seventies. The department experienced two changes of leadership during the decade. When Earl Siegel stepped

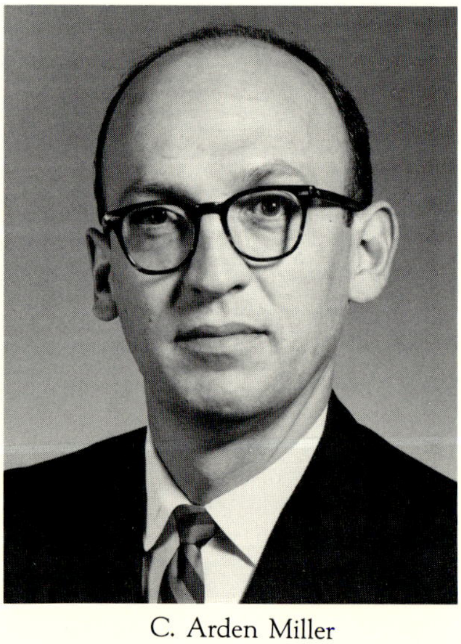

C. Arden Miller

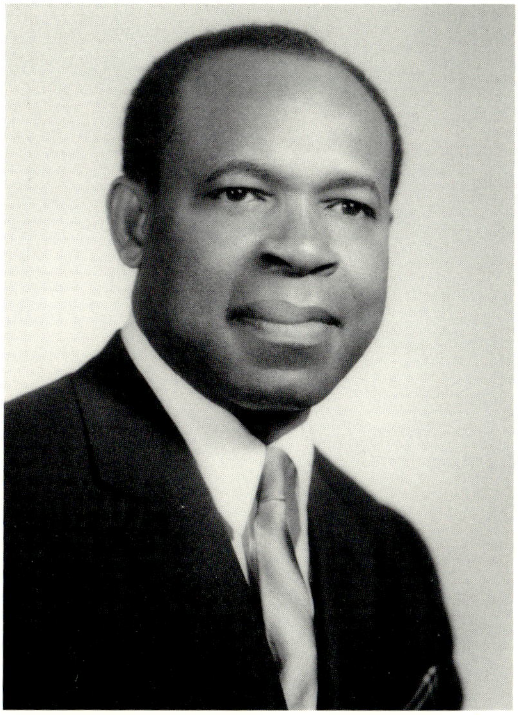

Joseph Edozien

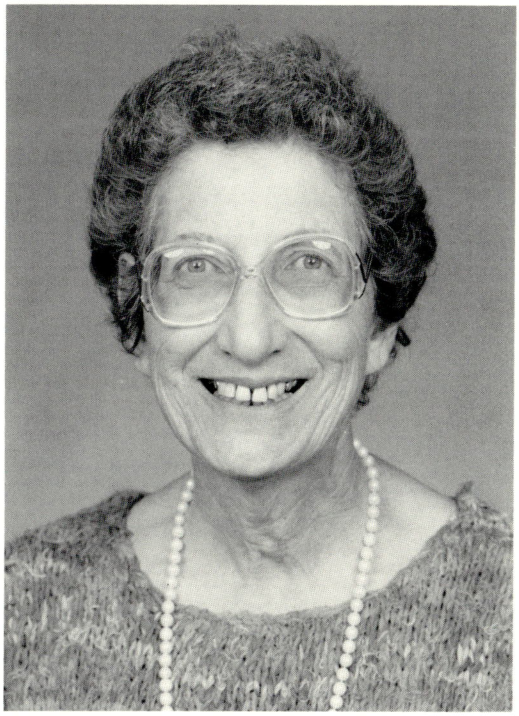

Mildred Kaufman

down as chair in 1975, Dean Greenberg named Dr. Naomi Morris as Siegel's replacement. As a pediatrician and public health physician, Morris had combined clinical experience with a successful career as a teacher and researcher. For Morris, the department's primary purpose was to train the physicians, nurses, and social workers needed by local, state, and national programs. But the department also had an active research component aimed at providing a better understanding of the problems mothers and children faced. Teenage pregnancies, delayed child bearing, and day care were some of the issues that interested faculty.[25]

In 1977 Dr. Morris moved to Chicago, and Dr. C. Arden Miller took charge of the department. Miller brought extensive administrative experience to the job, having served as dean of the University of Kansas School of Medicine before coming to the University of North Carolina as vice chancellor for health sciences (1966–1971).[26]

Nutrition became an important national and international concern in the 1970s, and the Department of Nutrition attracted increasing numbers of students, faculty, and research grants. Dr. Joseph Edozien's appointment as chair in 1971 allowed Rebecca Bryan to return to full-time teaching and consulting. Dr. Edozien also reclaimed the department's laboratory space and began to attract students interested in biochemical

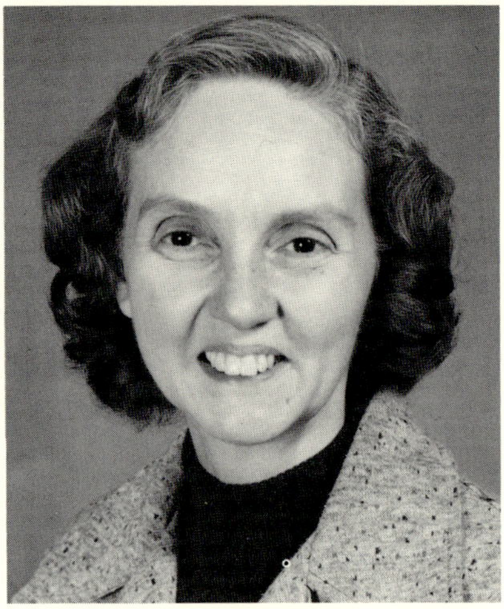
Marion Highriter

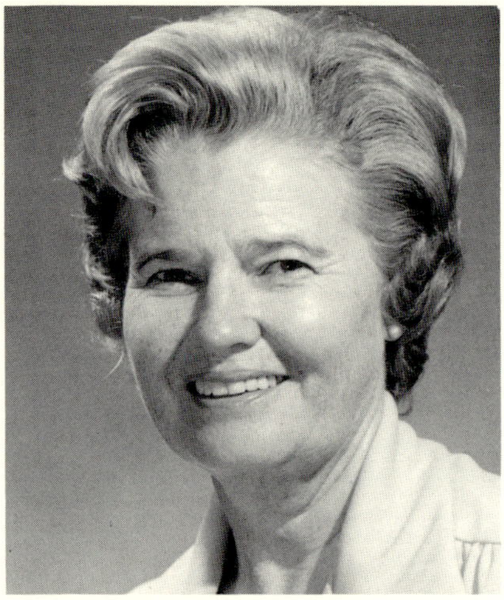
Dorothy Talbot

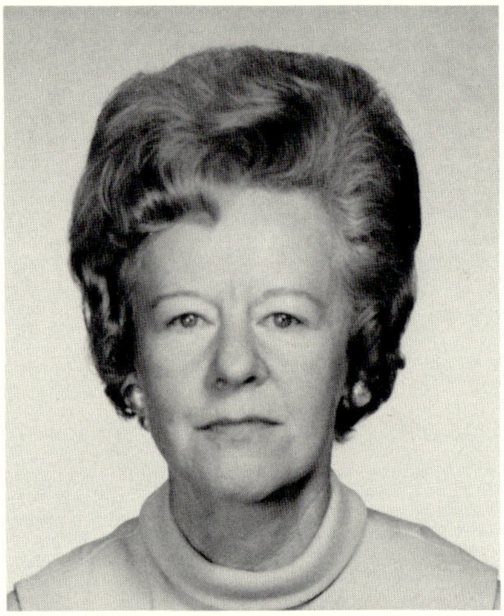
Elizabeth Edmands

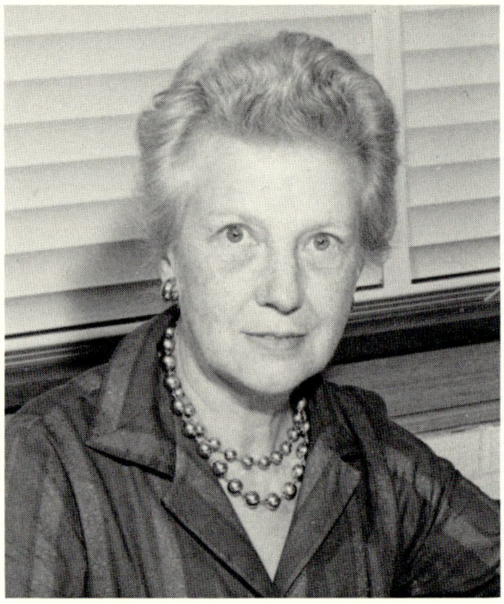
Ann Hansen

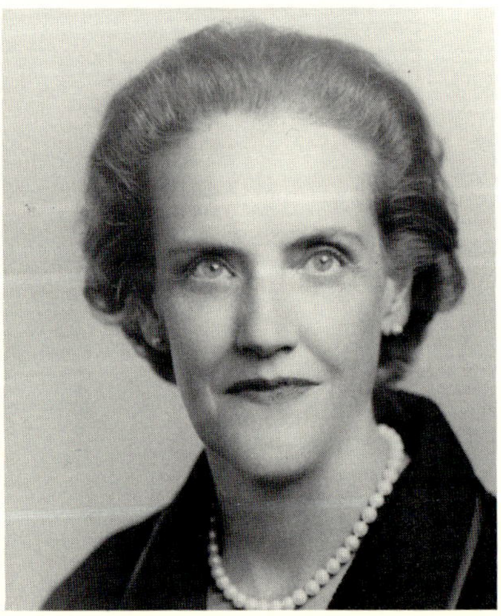
Marie McIntyre

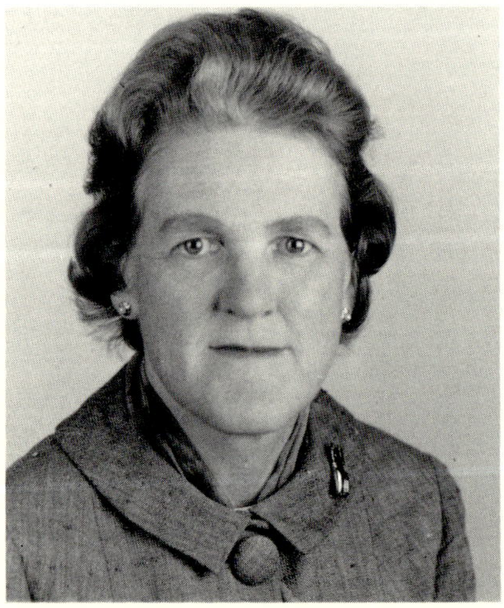
Julia Watkins

Some faculty members in public health nursing in the 1970s.

research. In fact, there was some concern by the mid-1970s that the department had become too research oriented.[27]

The department's projects, however, often had policy implications. The school's nutritionists, for instance, found themselves caught up in political battles in Washington as part of their evaluation of the Special Supplemental Food Program for Women, Infants, and Children (WIC). The department's three-year study concluded that the supplements increased the weight and the health of the infants and children in the program and reduced anemia among mothers. "The WIC program is one of the most important and successful of the food assistance programs," Dr. Edozien remarked. The Department of Agriculture and President Gerald Ford were less enthusiastic, and it took a congressional override of a presidential veto to sustain the program.[28]

By the early 1980s, education was being proposed to replace such entitlement programs as solutions to the problem of poverty. A 1982 project headed by Mildred Kaufman of the Department of Nutrition, with Jonathan Kotch of the Maternal and Child Health Department and Robert Cefalo from the School of Medicine, was a case in point. The project, funded by the March of Dimes Birth Defects Project, sought to improve the health and nutrition of pregnant women by training health professionals who would counsel them. Behavior modification and diet counseling were certainly helpful in reducing infant mortality, but as the WIC program had shown, low-income women needed more than education to sustain a healthy diet.[29]

The Departments of Health Education and Public Health Nursing expanded their research bases in the seventies, but preparation of front-line practitioners and service to health agencies continued to be their strong suit. The Department of Health Education maintained its direct involvement with local groups through the Rural Community Environmental Education Project. The environmental movement had largely bypassed poor rural residents, Dr. John Hatch noted, and problems such as substandard housing, improper waste disposal, poor water quality, and fire hazards abounded. John Hatch, Ethel Jackson, and graduate students in the department worked with residents of a rural black community in Chatham County to reduce environmental health and safety risks.[30]

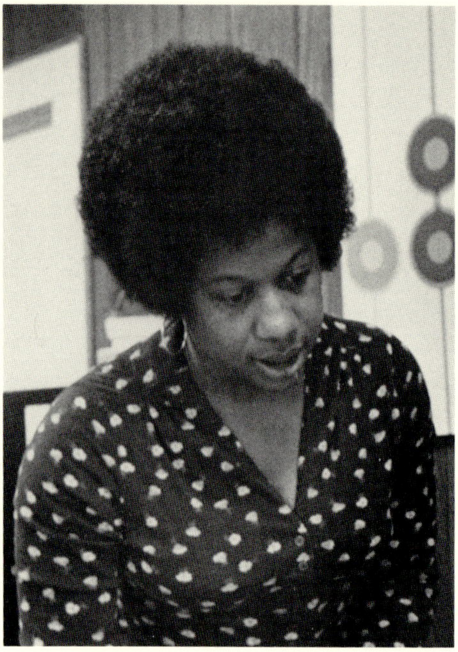

Ethel Jackson

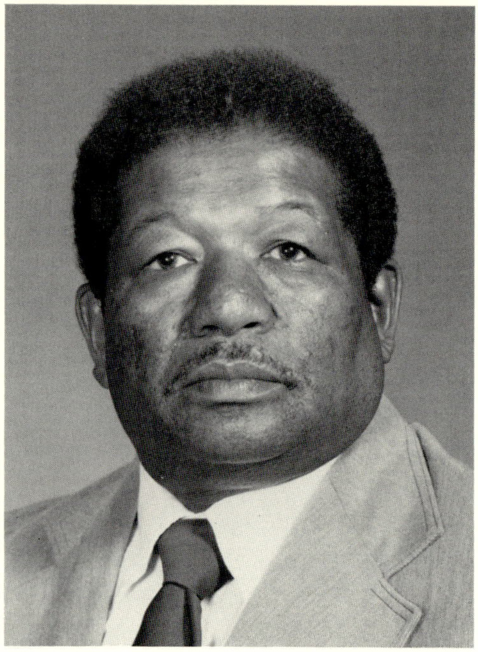

John Hatch

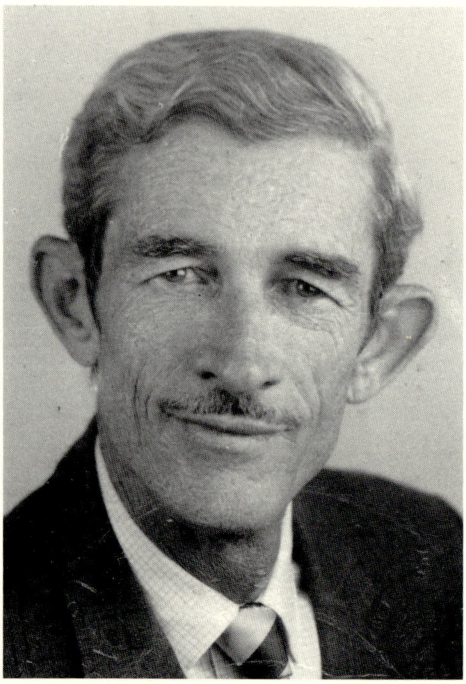

Guy Steuart chaired the Department of Health Education from 1969 to 1985. During that time the department led the school in the recruitment of minority faculty and students. Dr. Steuart later served as director of the Office of International Public Health Programs.

John Hatch oversaw a more ambitious education project in the Republic of Cameroon in western Africa. Funded by a $1.9 million grant from the U.S. Agency for International Development, the project emphasized education and self-help as means of preventing disease and lowering mortality. It encouraged the Cameroon government to undertake a modernization campaign aimed at changing traditional health beliefs and habits. The team of consultants from various departments in the school worked with health officials to improve their understanding of health issues and suggest ways of communicating this knowledge to their countrymen.[31]

Although the practice-oriented departments improved during the 1970s, the research-oriented departments—epidemiology, environmental sciences and engineering, biostatistics, and parasitology and laboratory practice—remained the key to the school's national standing. A centerpiece of the Department of Biostatistics's research program in the 1970s was the Lipid Research Clinics Program. Begun in June, 1971, with a grant from the National Heart, Lung and Blood Institute, the program

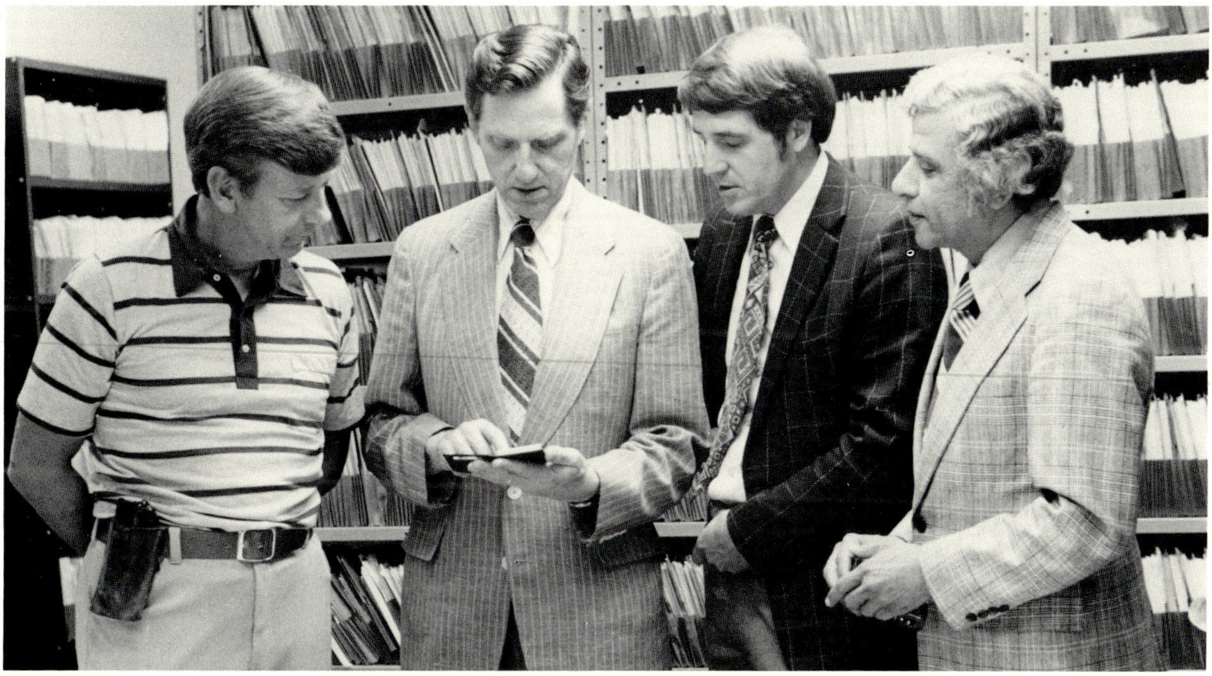

Left to right: James Grizzle, Bernard Greenberg, Dale Williams, and Michel Ibrahim work on the renewal contract for the Lipids project.

measured blood fat levels in subjects at selected hospitals in the United States, as well as in Canada, Israel, and the Soviet Union. The program sought to determine the relationship between lipids and heart disease and in particular to discover whether lowering cholesterol levels reduced the risk of heart attacks and strokes. The grant established the Central Patient Registry and Coordinating Center (CPR) at the School of Public Health. From its offices in the NCNB building in downtown Chapel Hill, the CPR established standard procedures for patient testing and collected and analyzed data.[32]

One of the more intriguing aspects of the program was the participation of two clinics in the Soviet Union. In 1973 James Grizzle of the Biostatistics Department and Herman Tyroler of the Epidemiology Department visited the Soviet Union to work out plans for a cooperative United States-Soviet Union lipids research project. A few years later, Soviet specialists began visiting Chapel Hill. "Flowering in the climate of detente," an observer noted, "the historic collaboration has seen visiting teams of scientists and physicians traveling back and forth . . . between the two countries working toward the mutual goals of cutting the high number of deaths from heart disease in both countries."[33]

In 1973 Daniel Okun stepped down as chair of the Department of Environmental Sciences and Engineering. He was replaced by Russell F. Christman, who came to Chapel Hill from the University of Washington. A chemist by training, Christman, like Okun, was interested in water quality control. Christman did not see the department as having a direct role to play in solving environmental problems. "Our principal goal," he explained, "is to seek through research more accurate descriptions of basic environmental problems which would be useful for public decision making."[34]

By the mid-1970s, those environmental problems were immense. During the energy crisis brought on by the oil embargo, the nation turned to coal, nuclear power, and wood as alternative fuel sources, all of which posed potential, but little understood, dangers to the atmosphere. The pesticides and other chemicals that helped make the United States the leading producer of food in the world also caused cancer in farm workers and consumers alike.

The environmental movement spurred a major expansion of health-related activities in the private sector. The federal government, through the Environmental Protection Agency and the Occupational Health

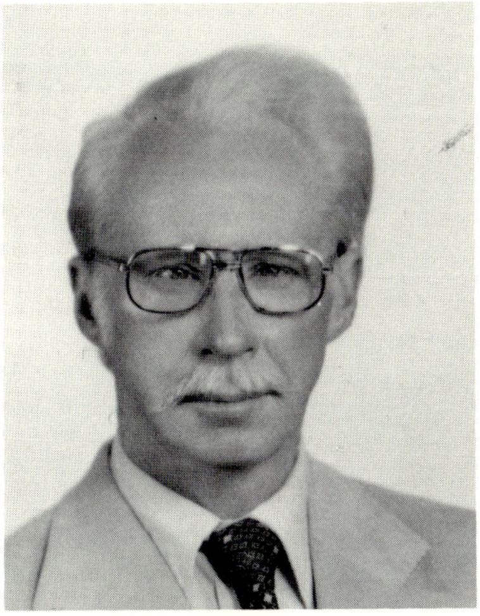

James Abernathy

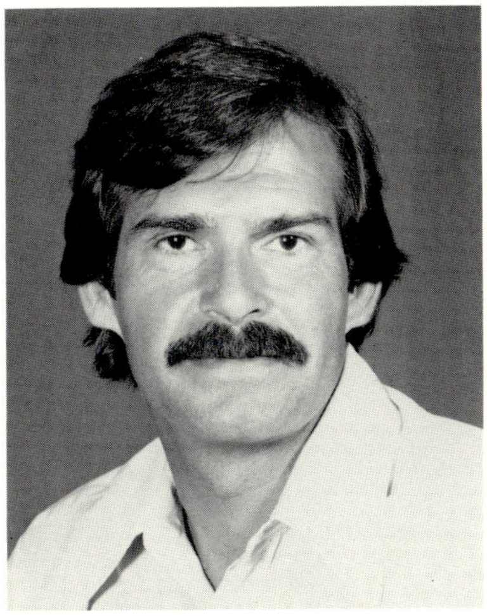

Michael Symons

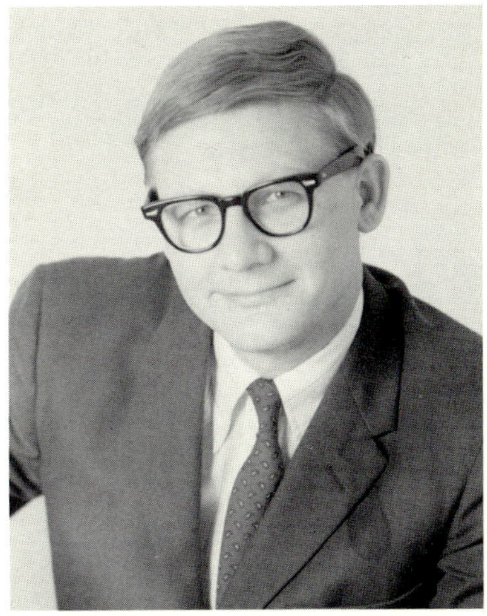

Ronald Helms

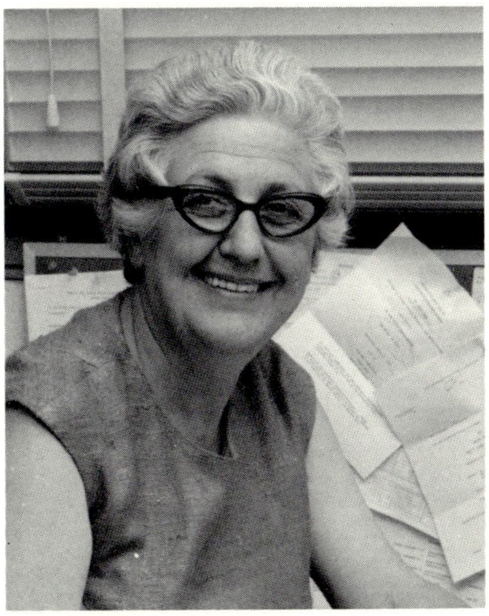

Mindel Sheps

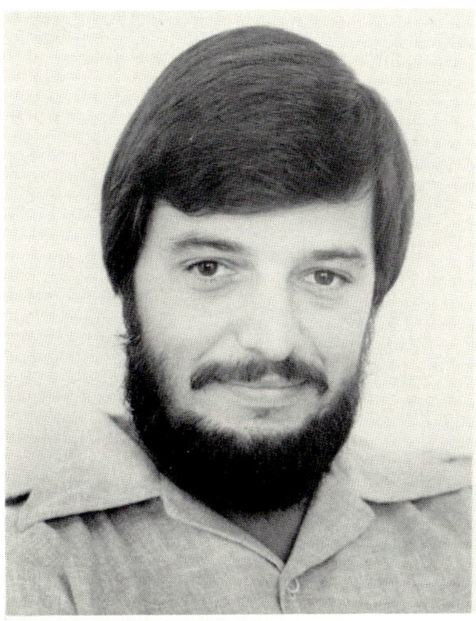

Richard Shachtman

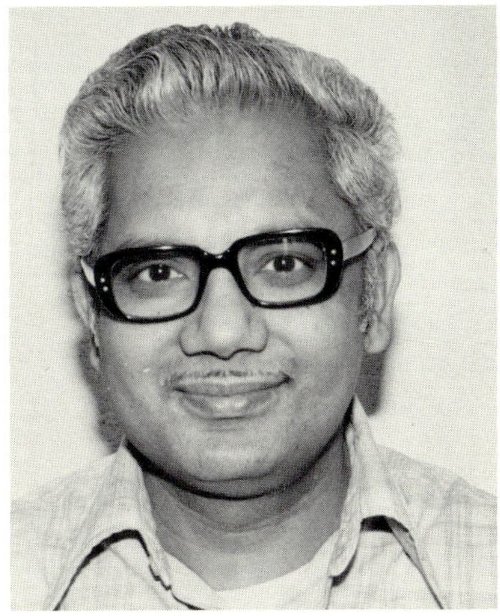

Pranab Sen

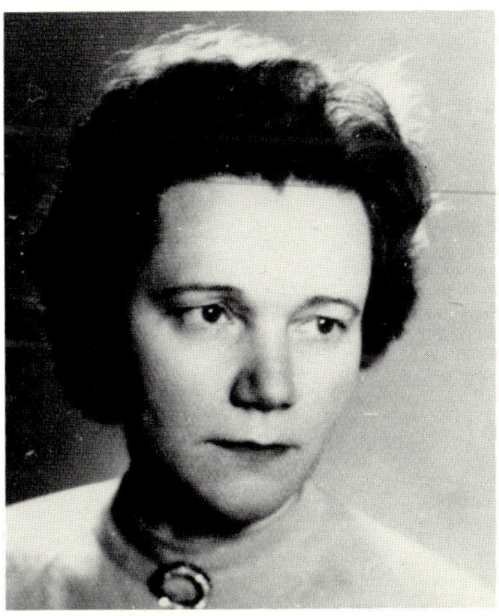

Regina Elandt-Johnson

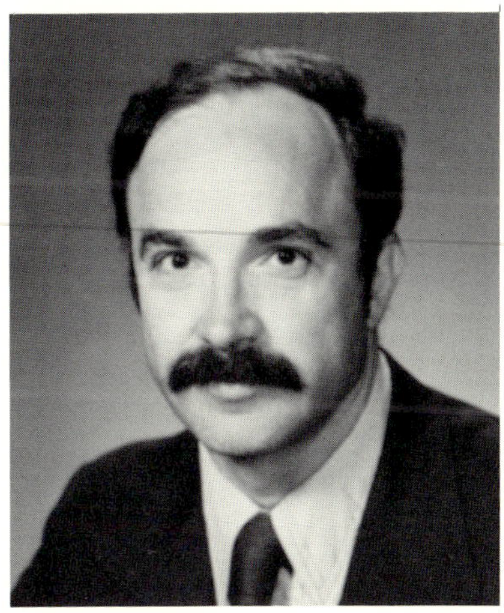

Gary G. Koch

Some faculty members in biostatistics in the 1970s.

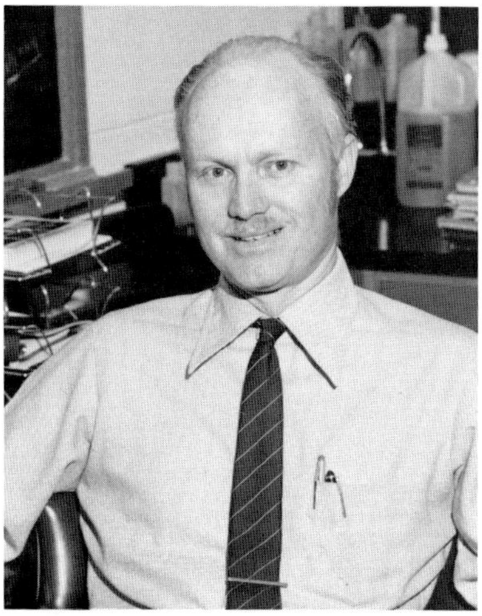

Edward Kuenzler

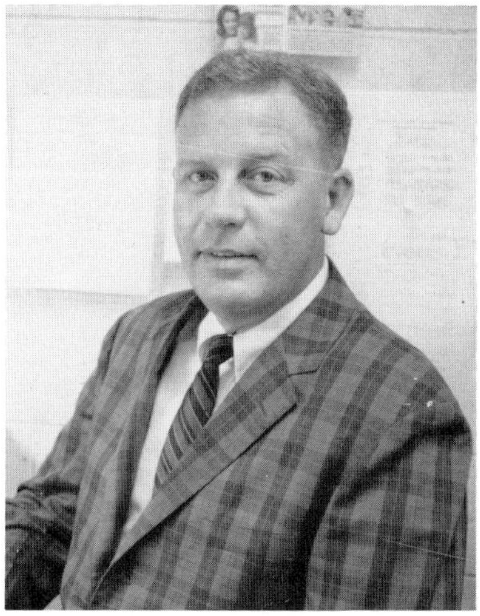

Alvis Turner, Jr.

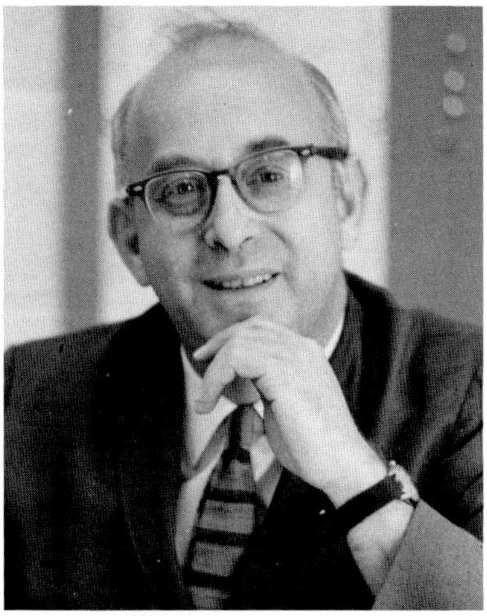

Morris Shiffman

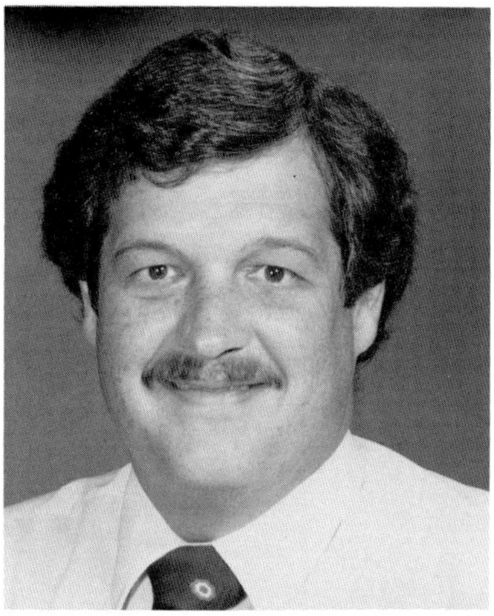

Frederic Pfaender

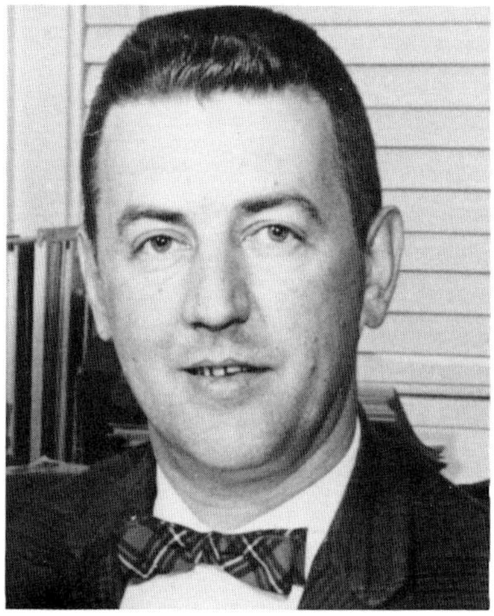

James Lamb III

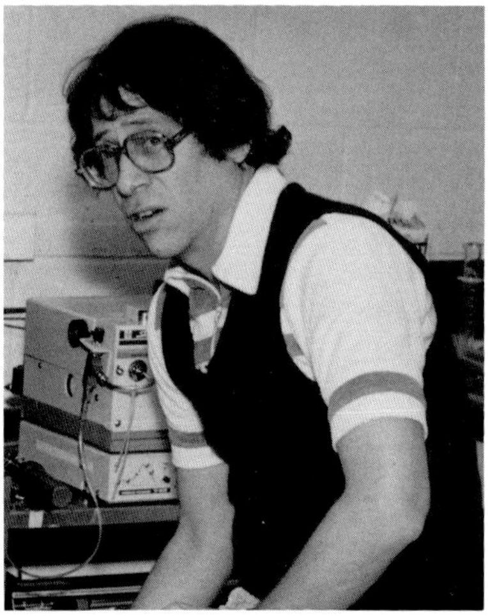

Richard Kamens

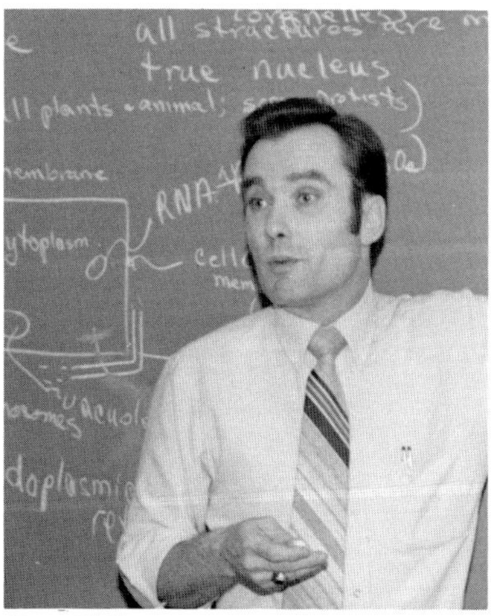

Donald Francisco

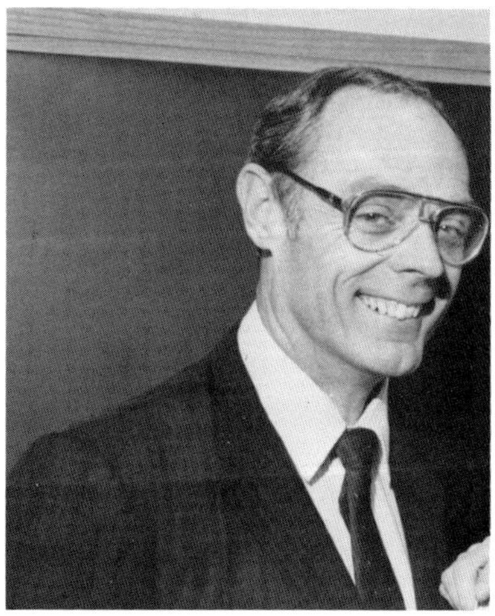

Donald Johnson

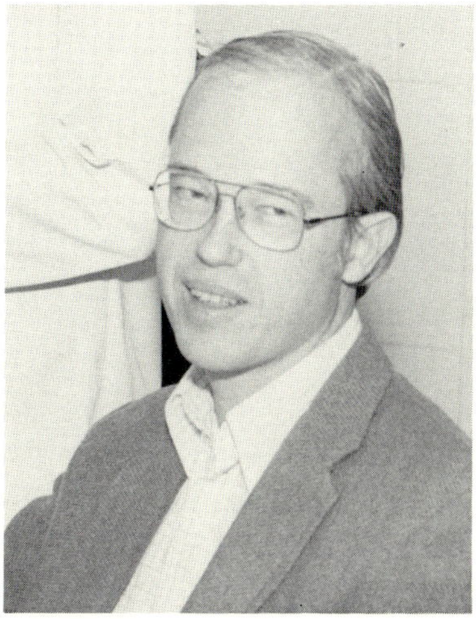

Mark Shuman

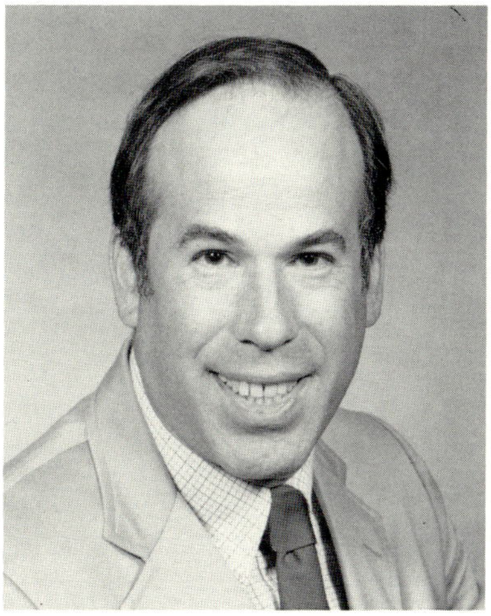

Philip Singer

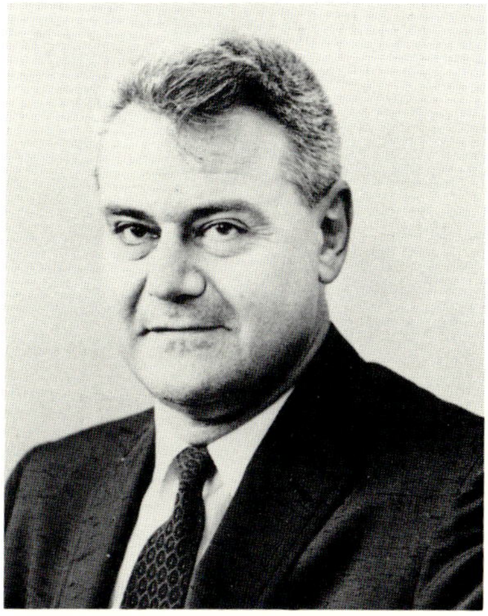

Arthur Stern

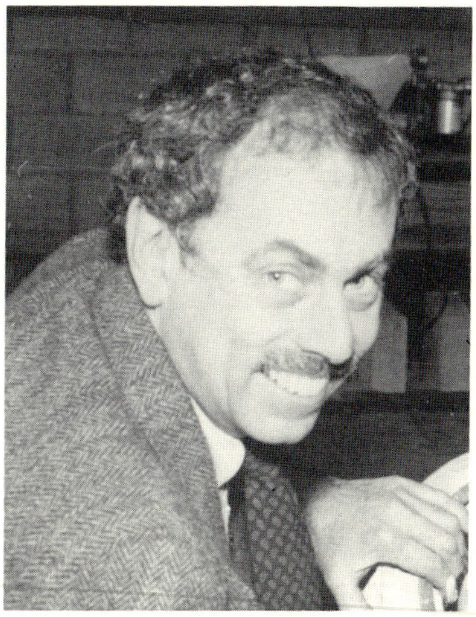

Parker Reist

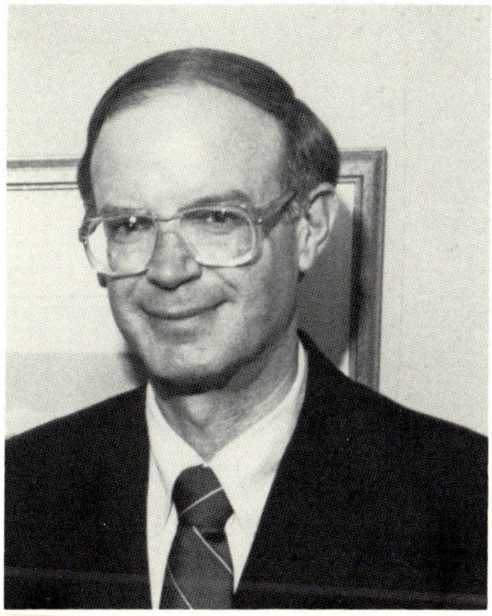

James Watson, Jr.

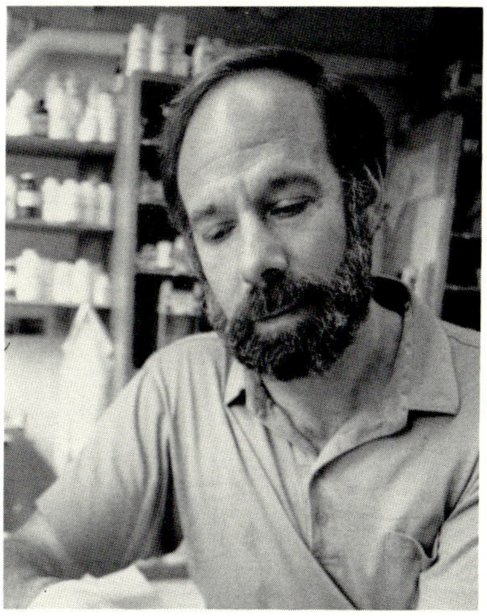

Mark Sobsey

Some members of the Department of Environmental Sciences and Engineering in the 1970s.

and Safety Act, required tougher health and safety standards in the workplace, reductions in pollution levels, and safer consumer products. To comply with these new requirements and improve public relations, corporations began efforts to address some of their problems. This corporate campaign had two effects on the school. First, departments such as epidemiology, environmental sciences and engineering, and biostatistics contracted with firms to conduct health studies and run training programs. Second, a larger proportion of the school's graduates found employment in industry and nonprofit organizations.

One of the more interesting consulting projects involved the school in a cooperative venture with the United Rubber Workers Union and major tire companies. In 1970 the discovery of a respiratory illness associated with a chemical process in tire manufacturing spurred the creation of the Joint Occupational Health Program involving both the union and the tire manufacturers. The program contracted with the school to study health problems among rubber workers. Led by Dr. David Fraser, the Occupational Health Studies Group first conducted mortality studies and then began investigating environmental problems in the workplace. The long-term goal was to establish a system to monitor employees' health and to evaluate the health risks of new manufacturing processes.[35]

The Department of Epidemiology also addressed itself to more local concerns. In cooperation with the North Carolina Affiliate American Heart Association and the Tarboro Clinic, Dr. Michel Ibrahim and Dr. Lawrence Cutchin directed a hypertension control program in Edgecombe County. High blood pressure was a major health problem in North Carolina, particularly among blacks and other rural people. The program sought to identify patients suffering from hypertension who could then be treated with different methods to determine levels of effectiveness. The program also taught physicians new ways of encouraging patients to maintain their treatment regimen.[36]

Under the circumstances, the school navigated the uncertainties of the seventies well. It continued to be ranked as one of the best schools of public health in the country, and many of its faculty members won individual honors, highlighted by the election first of Margaret Dolan and then of C. Arden Miller to the presidency of the American Public Health Association. Dean Greenberg's admonition to the faculty "to practice what you teach" proved moderately successful, and relations

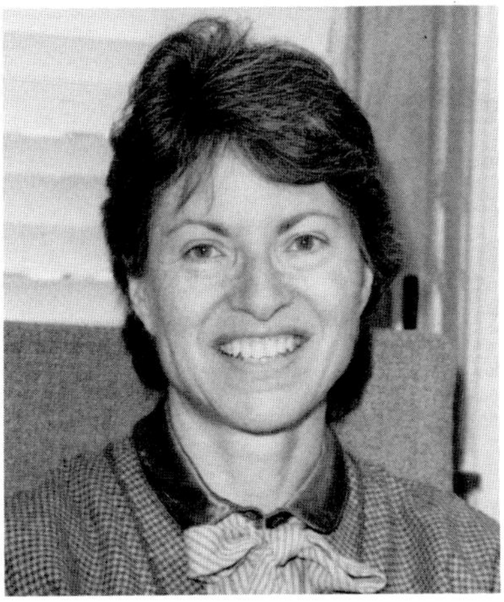

Barbara Hulka

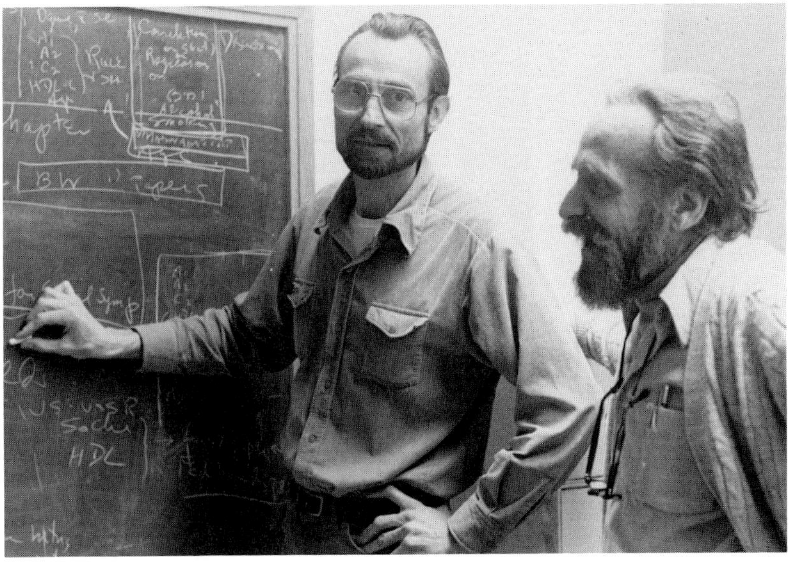

Gerardo Heiss and Herman Tyroler

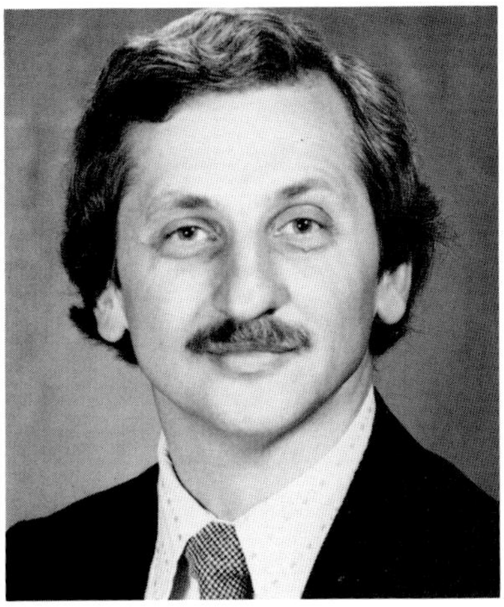

Carl Shy

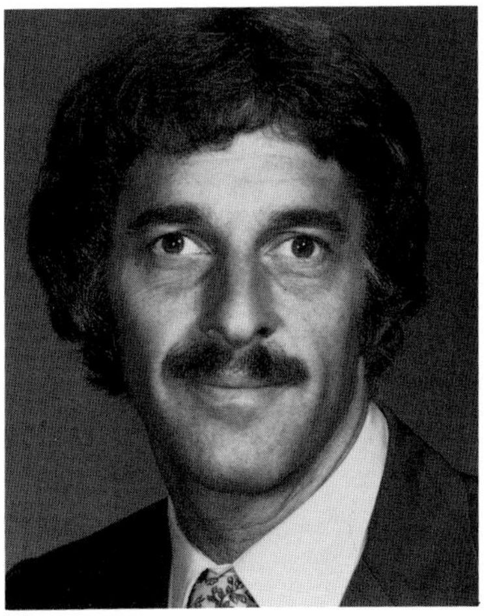

David Kleinbaum

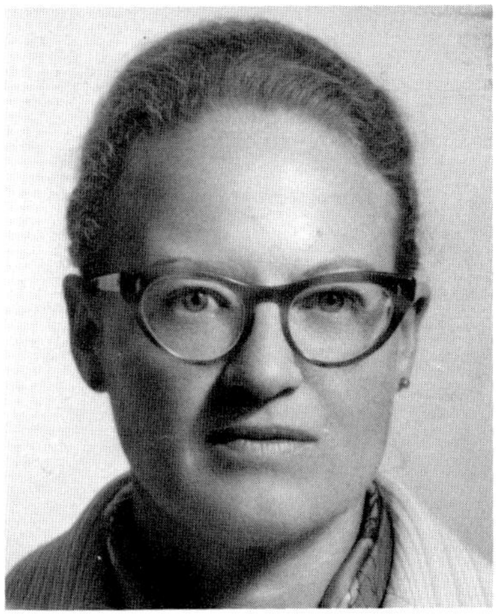

Caroline Becker

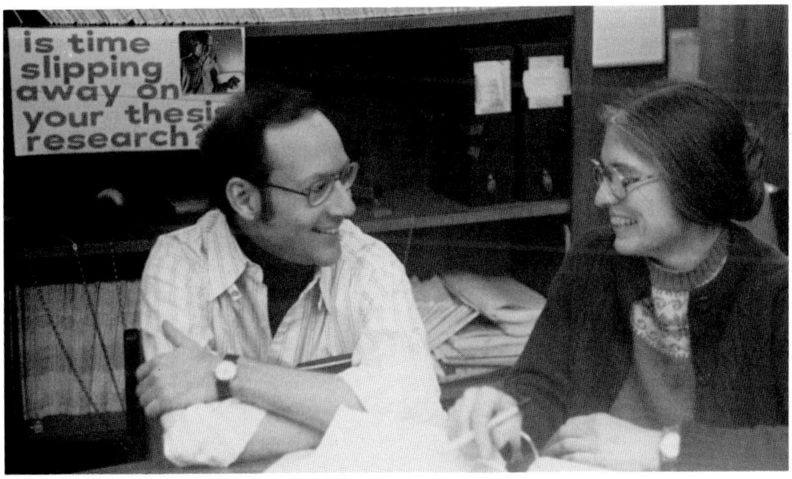

Victor Schoenbach and Joyce Allen

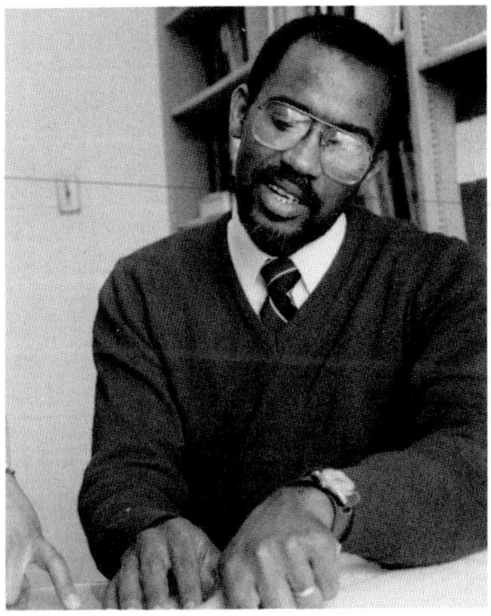

Sherman James

Some members of the Department of Epidemiology during the 1970s.

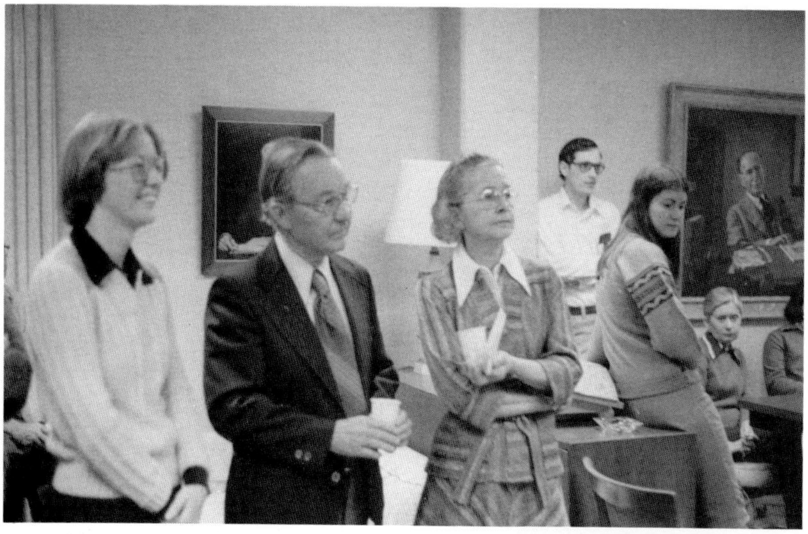

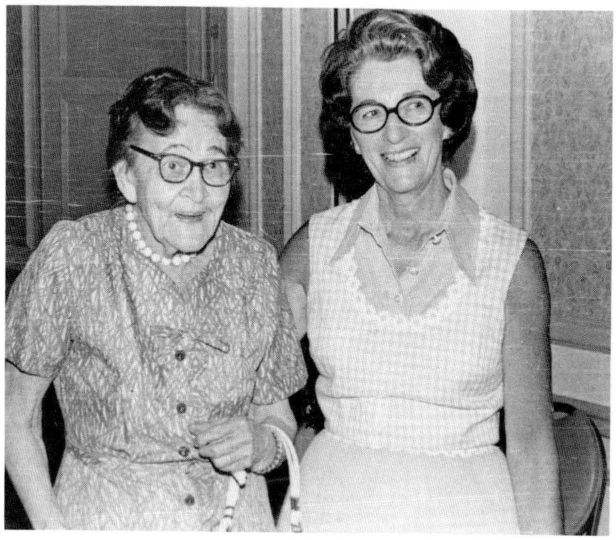

Top: The retirement party for Gil Clarke *(center).* Mrs. Clarke is at right and Kay Cox Wijnberg on the left.

Right: Registrar Emmy Lou Palladino escorts Madeline Harbin at her retirement party. Through an administrative oversight, Mrs. Harbin worked at the school until she was 80 years old.

with state and local health agencies improved. The Division of Community Health Services oversaw an array of services that benefited the delivery of health programs in the state, and the faculty served North Carolina in many capacities in numerous organizations.

Still, problems remained. The inflationary crisis of the 1970s put a severe strain on the university's budget. Some feared the School of Public Health was losing ground to other institutions. "Increases in faculty salaries have not matched inflation during the last four or five years," the 1976 annual report declared. "Special perquisites, such as free parking and preference in tickets to sports events, have been reduced or eliminated. This erosion will reach a breaking point soon and when the dam bursts, small patchwork efforts will not suffice." The lack of a sabbatical program also made it difficult to attract and keep good faculty and detracted from their research and instructional efforts.[37]

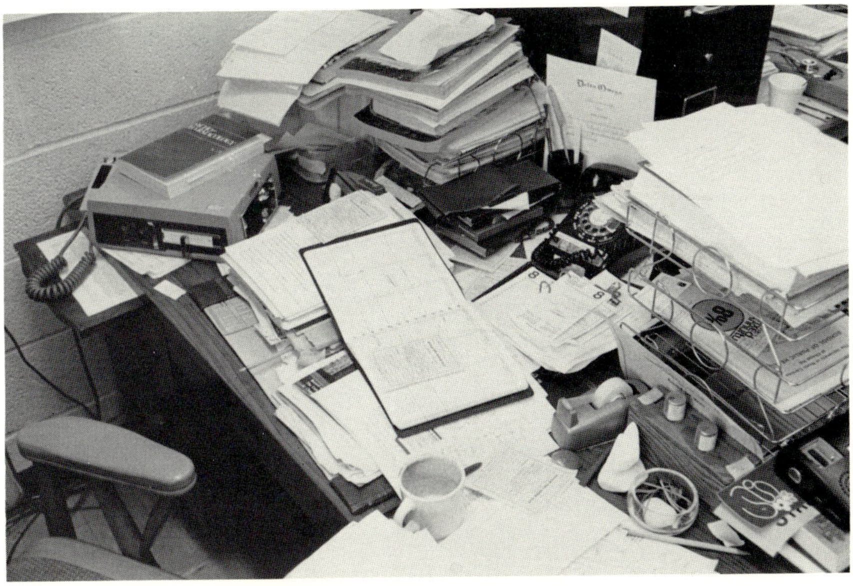

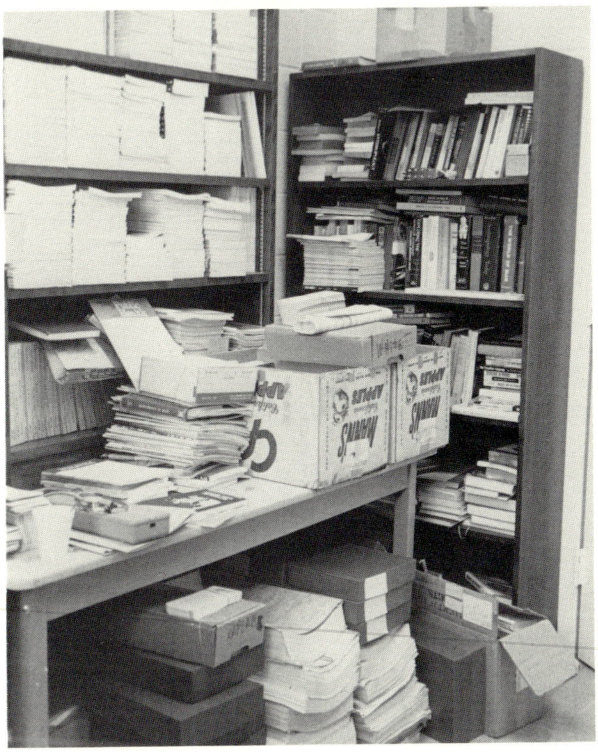

Typical office scenes in Rosenau Hall. Overcrowding was an extreme problem at the school during the 1980s.

The school's record in regard to women and minorities also needed improvement. Despite early success in recruiting, the black presence in the student body leveled off at 12 percent by the end of the decade. Medical and dental schools competed more effectively for blacks in the post-civil rights era. Moreover, the pool of qualified students increasingly came from northern cities, and some potential students from outside the region, black and white, hesitated to attend school in the South.

Efforts to recruit Native American students were even less successful. In response, the school hired Ronald Oxendine, a Lumbee Indian from Maxton, as director of American Indian Recruitment Services.[38]

Recruiting minority faculty proved even more difficult. The pool of qualified candidates for most jobs was quite small, and in some fields nonexistent. Furthermore, pressures on minority faculty once they were at the school made it difficult to retain them. The demand for minority members to serve on departmental, school, and university committees, as well as minority students' need for counseling and advice, made it difficult for them to find time for research.[39]

The relatively small percentage of women on the faculty stemmed from structural factors, as well as from decisions by the school. In 1960, twenty years after the school began granting graduate degrees, women occupied roughly one-third of the faculty positions. By 1980 the proportion had slipped to less than 20 percent. The Departments of Public Health Nursing and Public Health Education accounted for the majority of the 1960 positions. The presence of these programs was notable because few schools of public health had either one. The federal gov-

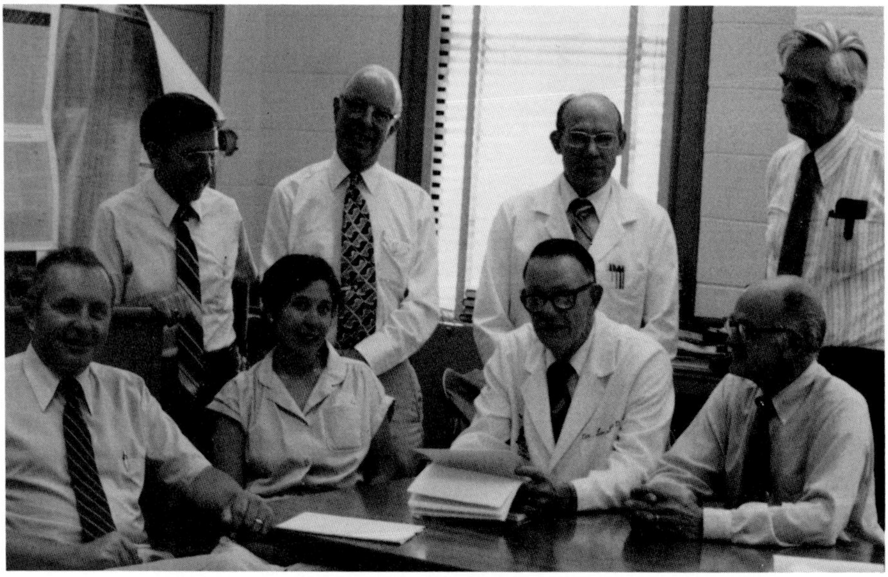

Committee for the 99th doctoral examination presided over by John Larsh. *Standing, left to right:* Hilton Goulson, William Fleming, Norman Weatherly, John Reed. *Seated, left to right:* John Feeley, doctoral candidate Sally Liska, John Larsh, and Charles Okey.

ernment's romance with health issues in the 1960s, however, benefited medical and scientific endeavors—disciplines that were dominated by men—rather than the helping professions, which were dominated by women. Nursing, education, nutrition, and maternal and child health lost ground to hard sciences such as epidemiology and biostatistics. The result was an erosion of the number of women at the school.

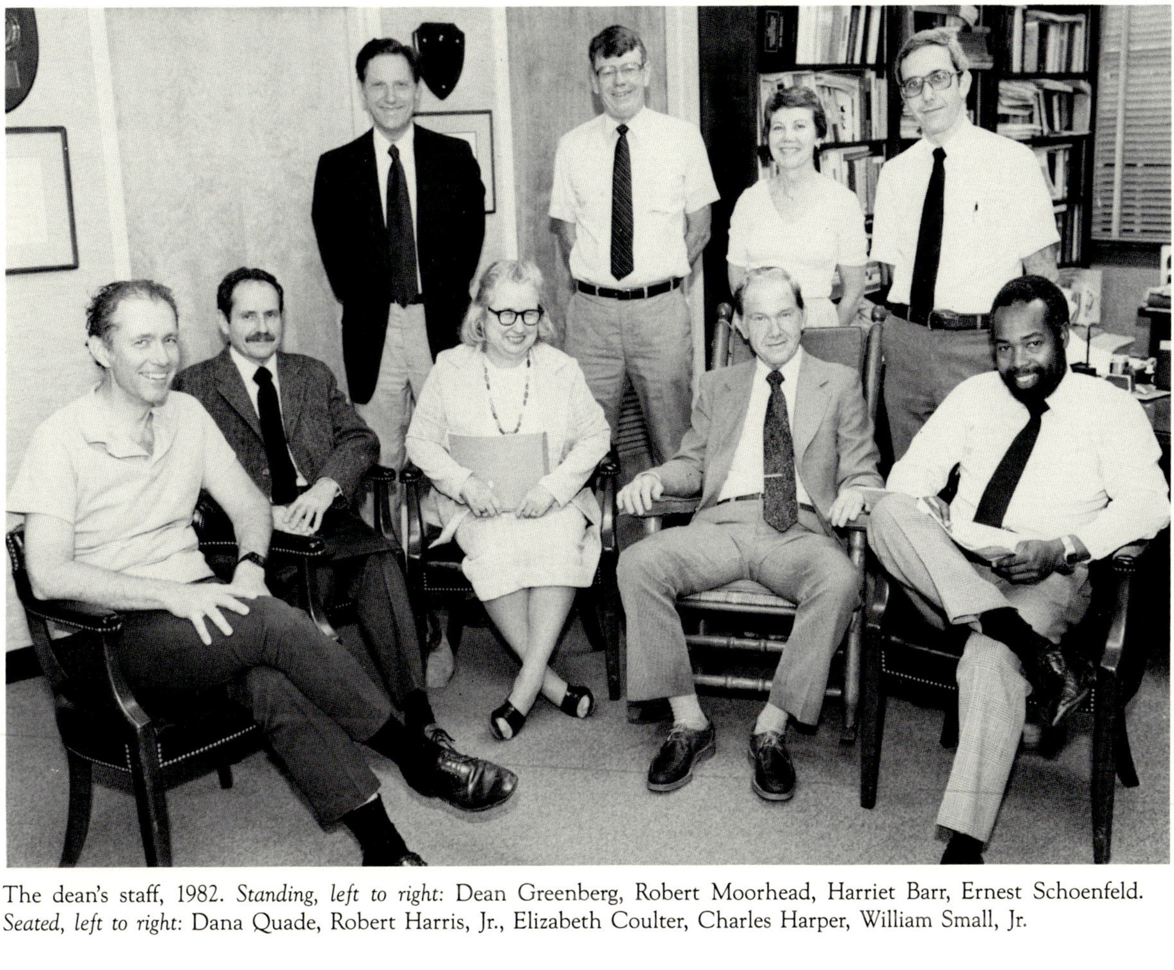

The dean's staff, 1982. *Standing, left to right:* Dean Greenberg, Robert Moorhead, Harriet Barr, Ernest Schoenfeld. *Seated, left to right:* Dana Quade, Robert Harris, Jr., Elizabeth Coulter, Charles Harper, William Small, Jr.

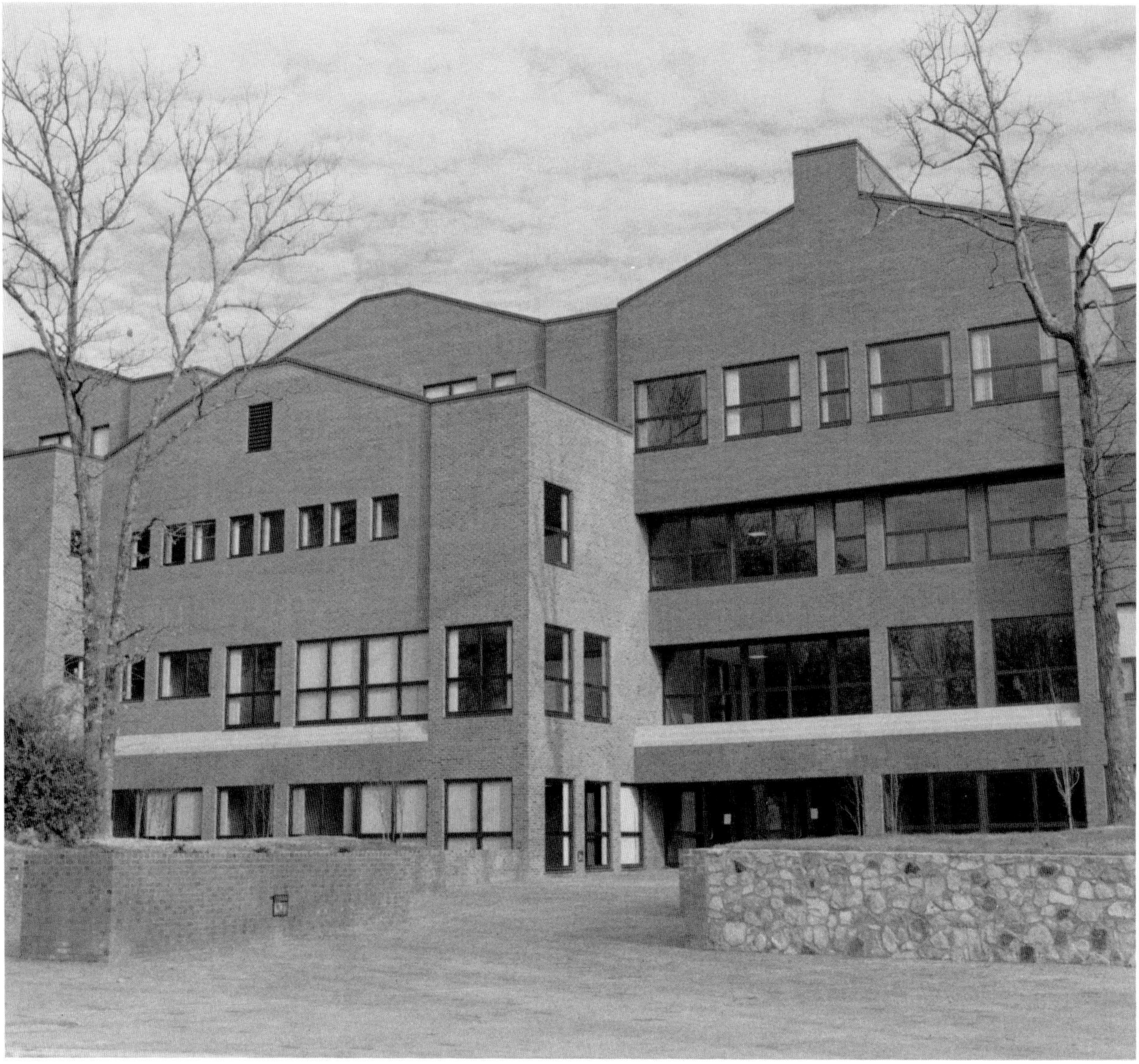

McGavran-Greenberg Hall

Epilogue

The 1980s brought extensive cutbacks in federal funding for health-related programs. At the same time the rising cost of medical care and the growing number of uninsured families put added pressures on the public health system in the United States. By the end of the decade an Institute of Medicine report concluded that the United States had "allowed the system of public health activities to fall into disarray." As in the past, many health problems were related to poverty, but many others cut across class and racial lines. Toxic wastes that contaminated the water, air, soil, and food affected everyone. Drug and alcohol abuse, AIDS, accidents, Alzheimer's disease, unwanted pregnancies, and the aging of the population constituted the decade's most pressing health problems.[1]

The School of Public Health weathered the attack on federal spending for social services, as the state increased its contribution to the school and the private sector invested more dollars in university-based research. Between 1979 and 1989, the school's budget increased from $17 million to $30 million, student enrollment from 652 to 878, and the number of full-time faculty from 146 to 162. Growth, however, exacerbated a perennial problem: lack of space. By 1980 faculty offices and classrooms were scattered in eighteen separate locations across campus and in the town of Chapel Hill, and Rosenau Hall was bursting at the seams.[2]

As soon as he became dean in 1972, Bernie Greenberg began lobbying the Division of Health Affairs, the chancellor, and the General Administration to support his request for additional space. But there always seemed to be more urgent needs. The first good news came in January, 1980, when University of North Carolina President William Friday informed Dean Greenberg that the school would receive $100,000 for the planning of a new building. That same year the Board of Governors gave top priority to a Public Health and Environmental Sciences building. The architects prepared drawings and a scale model of the proposed building, but the General Assembly did not appropriate the necessary funds. When Dean Greenberg retired in 1982, his dreams of a major expansion of the school's physical facilities had not been realized.[3]

University officials chose Dr. Michel A. Ibrahim, professor and chair of the Department of Epidemiology, to succeed Greenberg. Ibrahim had been a member of the school's community since 1960, when he began study for an M.P.H. in biostatistics. He switched fields and took a Ph.D. in epidemiology in 1964 before leaving for Buffalo, New York, to serve on the faculty of the State University of New York at Buffalo Medical School. In conjunction with his faculty position, he later became first deputy commissioner in the Erie County Health Department. Ibrahim returned to Chapel Hill in 1971 as a professor in the Department of Epidemiology and succeeded John Cassel as chair of that department in 1976. This combination of academic excellence, administrative ability, and familiarity with the school made Dr. Ibrahim an outstanding choice for the deanship.

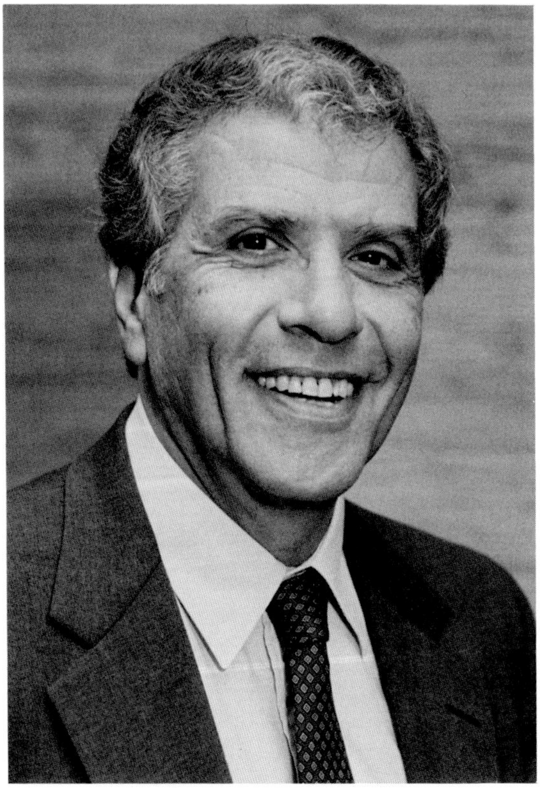

Dean Michael A. Ibrahim

"When I took over," Dr. Ibrahim remembered, "the school was well respected nationally. My job was to preserve that high standing and improve on it if I could. One of the first things I wanted to do was get the building for the school, because you can't achieve your mission without proper facilities. The facilities here were very inferior compared to other schools and other places on campus, especially the laboratories and classrooms."[4]

Dean Ibrahim, along with faculty, staff, and the school's supporters throughout the state, went to work to secure funding for a new building. "It was now or never," Ibrahim felt. The North Carolina General Assembly finally approved funds for a Public Health and Environmental Sciences building in June, 1985. Construction began in 1986, and the 125,000 square-foot building opened in the early part of 1990.[5]

In addition to helping secure McGavran-Greenberg Hall and the Herman G. Baity Environmental Engineering Laboratory, Dean Ibrahim instituted a number of important changes at the school. Between 1982 and 1989 he appointed a new chair in every department. In many cases the search committees and the dean selected people from outside the school. "The majority were people from the outside," Ibrahim observed, "[but] I went for the best person. Now we have a team of fresh, new chairs who will be looking ahead and pushing the departments and the school to greater and better horizons."[6]

Although the school maintained the tradition of strong, independent departments, complex health problems increasingly required that people from different disciplines work together. To encourage interdisciplinary teaching and research, which the school had deemphasized in the 1960s and 1970s, Ibrahim established three new programs: the Program on Health Promotion and Disease Prevention, the Office of International Public Health Programs, and the Program on Aging. These combined with the Institute for Environmental Studies and the Occupational Health Studies Program to give the school vital centers for addressing some of the most pressing health problems.

Improved teaching continued to be a primary concern for faculty and administrators. Students of the 1980s were younger than their counterparts of earlier years and brought less public health experience to the classroom. They required different teaching methods and more extensive contact with adjunct professors drawn from various health

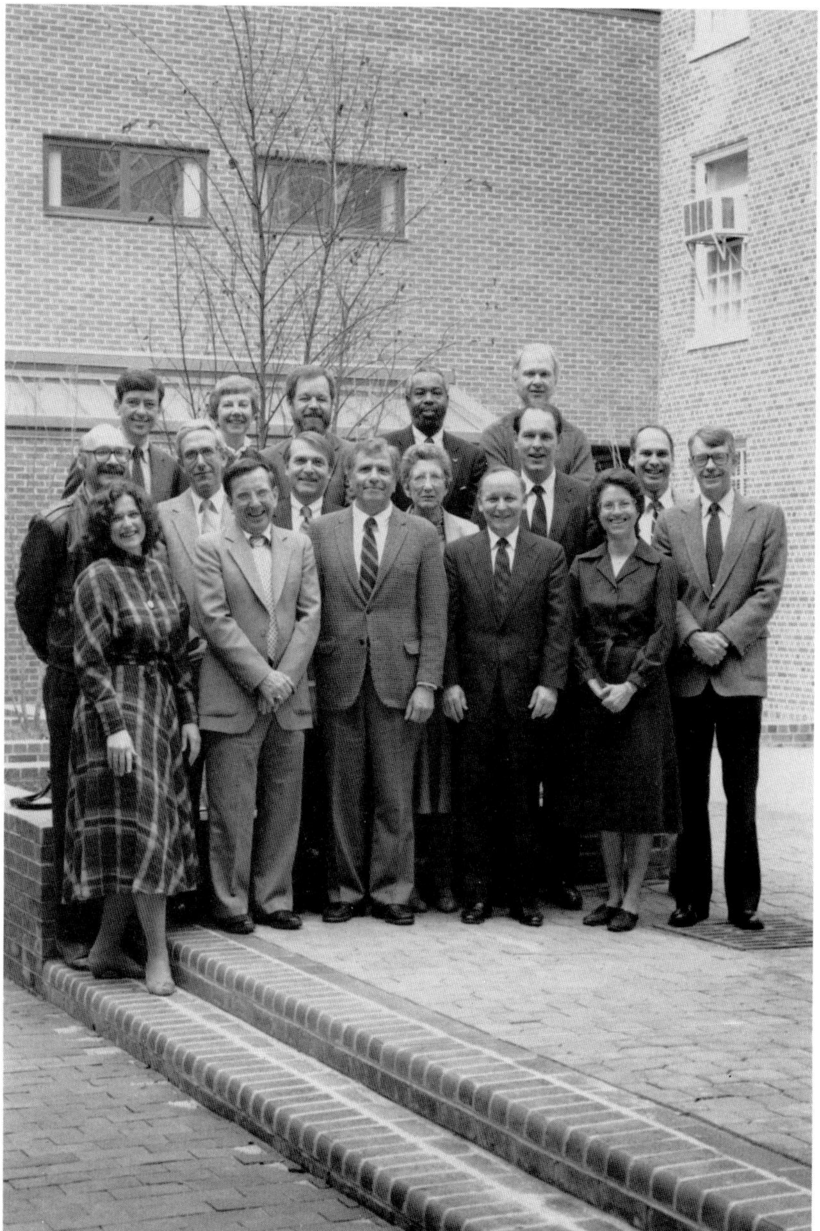

The Dean's Cabinet and Staff, 1990. *First row, left to right:* Marla Salmon, Hilton Goulson, Michel Ibrahim, Richard House, Barbara Hulka, Robert Moorhead. *Second row:* Milton Kotelchuck, Ernest Schoenfeld, James Sorenson, Mildred Kaufman, Charles Rasberry, Kerry Kilpatrick. *Third row:* Barry Margolin, Harriet Barr, Donald Fox, William Small, William Glaze.

agencies. The Learning Resources Center (established in 1986) represented an effort by the school to enhance teaching. The center produced a variety of media materials for classroom use, as well as for professional presentations and public information. It also provided faculty with consultation on new educational and communications technologies.

Although the school paid more attention to teaching, research continued to be the yardstick by which faculty were judged, and in that regard the school played a leading role among schools of public health. The scope of both basic and applied research conducted by faculty and staff during the 1980s would have startled yet pleased the school's pioneers. From laboratory research aimed at developing a vaccine for syphilis to field studies seeking to reduce smoking among teenagers, the school's research efforts covered virtually every serious public health problem. There was continuity in many of the projects. The Lipids Research Clinics Program continued its international collaborations on the relationship between lipids and cardiovascular disease. A follow-up of the Evans County, Georgia, study found a steady decline in deaths due to strokes and heart attacks over the previous two decades. A new study of the WIC nutritional program included faculty from a number of departments. But many new health problems, such as radon, AIDS, magnetic field exposure, and eating disorders, also received attention by researchers.

Smoking was probably the most sensitive public health issue in North Carolina during the 1980s, and the school took the lead in analyzing the effects of tobacco and in developing ways to help people quit smoking. In the school's early days tobacco was an accepted part of daily life: Rosenau kept a pipe at his side and Dean McGavran was rarely without a cigarette. But by 1989, the school no longer permitted smoking in any of its buildings. Spurred on by the antismoking campaign of Surgeon General C. Everett Koop, researchers associated with the school worked to develop new methods for breaking the tobacco habit. One such program focused on blacks, who, by the late 1980s, had smoking rates above the national average and as a result had higher incidences of heart disease and lung cancer. School researchers were not unmindful of the economic impact of reduced tobacco consumption on the state's farmers and also studied ways to ease farmers' dependence on the crop.

Public service remained an important component of the school's overall mission, and the school maintained the ties to state and local health agencies built during the 1970s. But in addition to the county health departments, in the 1980s the school gave assistance to voluntary health organizations, schools, local environmental agencies, and corporations. To adapt to this changing constituency and to improve the school's service efforts and to communicate them to the general public, Dean Ibrahim established the School of Public Health Board of Advisors in 1985. Members represented civic and advocacy groups, voluntary health organizations, professional associations, and various government agencies.[7]

As the school approached its golden anniversary, it began planning for the future. With the support of Dean Ibrahim, the school developed a strategic planning process. Begun as a loosely structured discussion among administrators and faculty in 1986, the process became more formalized the next year with the appointment of a Strategic Planning Committee headed by Arnold Kaluzny, professor of Health Policy and Administration. The size and diversity of the school required a more systematic approach to growth than had prevailed in the past. The faculty could no longer hash out ideas over lunch in the dean's office. Rapid technological changes and uncertain political developments also necessitated more careful forays into the future.

The committee defined strategic planning "as a continuous process conducted by the leadership of the school in order to identify important school-wide issues, analyze these issues from the perspective of existing and future environmental forces and organizational characteristics, and develop mechanisms for their resolution." Although similar to past patterns of dealing with critical issues, the new process structured planning into the everyday life of the school.[8]

As a start the committee solicited the opinions of the faculty and outside evaluators on the critical issues facing the school. Not unexpectedly, the faculty focused on improving the educational environment at the school—the need to attract high quality faculty and students, the need for improvements in the curriculum, the need for space and support services—while outsiders emphasized the need for the school to expand its involvement with state and local health agencies. All parties agreed that the school had to continue to find ways of addressing serious contemporary health problems.

In identifying the issues the planning process should address, the committee confronted a host of institutional and social issues. It was a

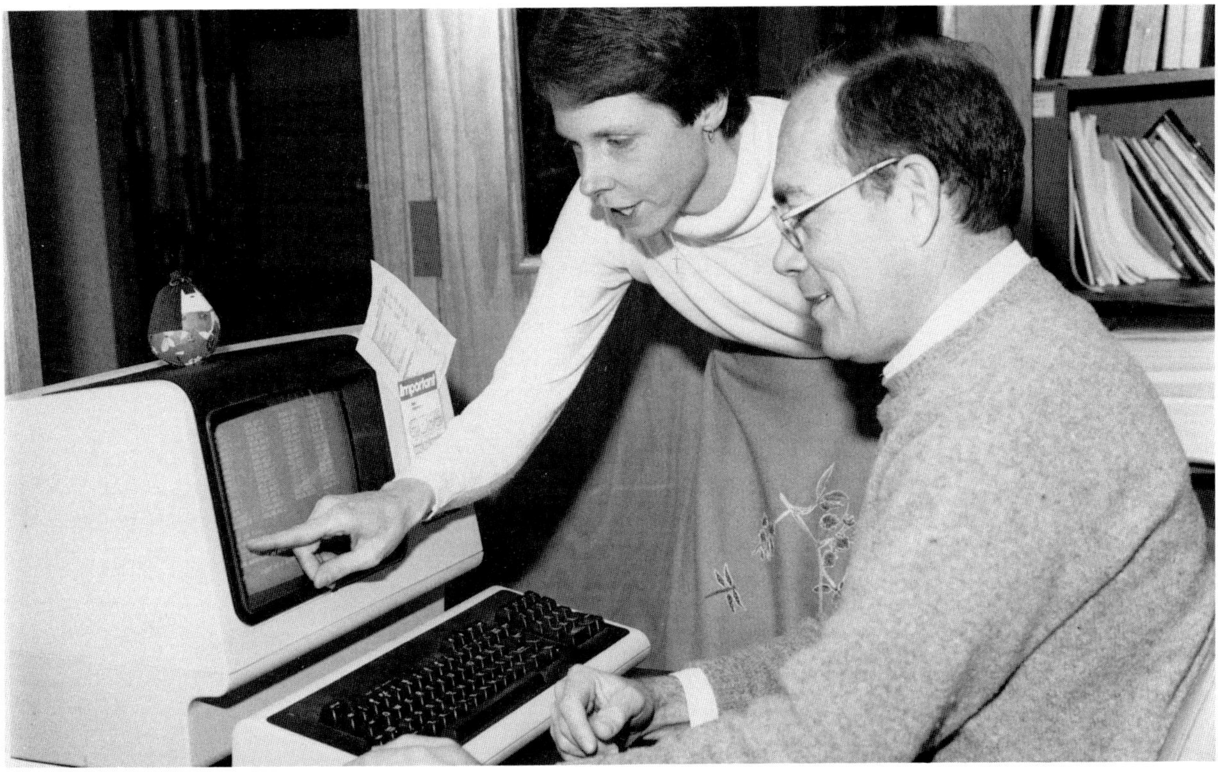

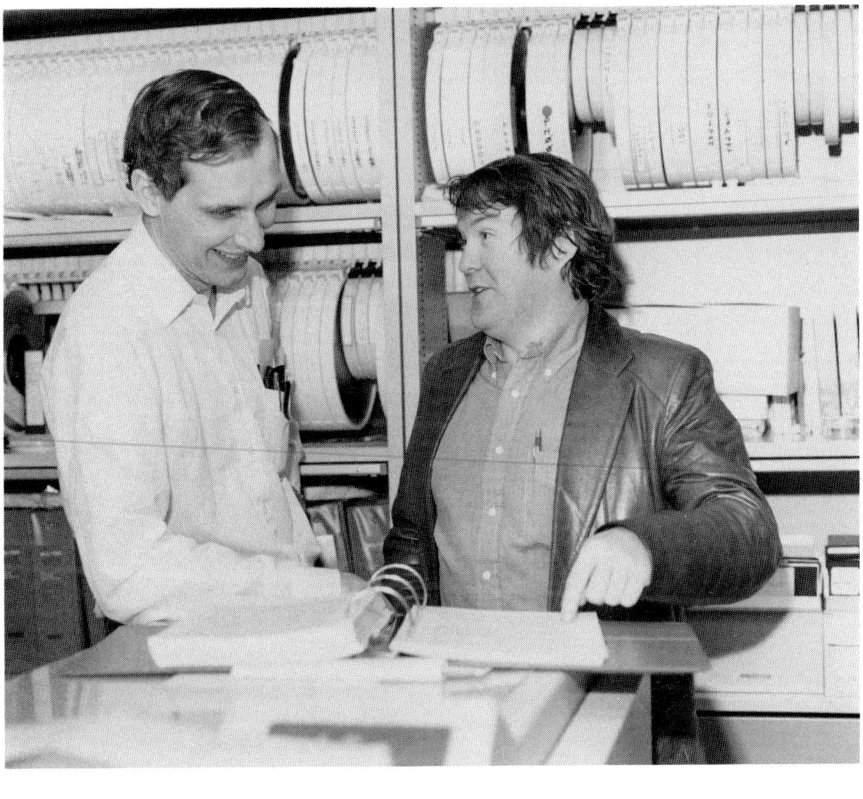

Long a leader in the use of computers for scientific work, in 1982 the school led the way into the office automation era by installing a mini-computer for word processing, electronic mail, and other office and administrative tasks. *Above,* Russell Christman receives instruction from his administrative assistant, Maggie Schimert, on the use of electronic mail. *Below,* Harvey Jeffries, who was instrumental in establishing the new system, confers with Operations Manager Robert Middour.

question of which problems were paramount and the manner in which the school could best organize itself to address and solve them. There were dozens of institutional issues that had no direct relation to the larger health concerns, but which were of critical importance if the school were to accomplish its mission. The committee decided to focus on problems facing the school and identified eight issues for the planning process to address: departmental versus school mission; the School of Public Health's administrative and financial structure; the appropriate balance between education, research, and service; public education about health; policy development and advocacy; research dissemination; student enrollment; and continuing education.

The highlight of the strategic planning process was an afternoon and evening retreat attended by 117 faculty members in March, 1989. For the first time in almost forty years, the faculty formally sat down to discuss the school's purpose and direction. The issues were not that different from the discussions instigated by Dean McGavran in the early 1950s, and as always the faculty expressed a wide range of opinions. There was general consensus that the committee had raised important questions, but there was also an understanding that there were no simple answers.

As it planned for the future, the School of Public Health could take pride in the many accomplishments of its first fifty years. From its beginnings in 1936 as a division of the Medical School, it had emerged as one of the outstanding schools of public health in the world. Thousands of students had left the school for jobs in private and public health agencies in every state and in numerous foreign countries. Their contributions, and those of the faculty, in basic and applied research and in the improvement of the health of people around the world were incalculable.

The school's success can be attributed in large part to the breadth of its scientific and educational undertakings and its flexible response to changes in the public health agenda. The school was blessed with outstanding leaders—administrators, educators, and scientists. These men and women came from numerous disciplines—engineering, education, biomedical research, administration, and statistical analysis—to build a school with a wide range of research and educational activities. Adherents of an administrative and social reform philosophy of the health movement worked side-by-side (though not always seeing eye-to-eye) with proponents of a more scientifically oriented model. The University of North

Carolina was the first school of public health to train all members of the public health team: public health nurses, health educators, biostatisticians, sanitary engineers, nutritionists, and epidemiologists.

This makeup insured a student body with diverse interests and expectations. The short courses of the late 1930s helped the employees of southeastern health departments better perform their duties as health officers, sanitarians, and engineers. The public health nurses and health educators who filled the classrooms during the 1940s and early 1950s staffed growing state and local health agencies. The training of front-line health practitioners declined over the years as more students prepared for administrative, research, and teaching positions. But off-campus and continuing education programs helped keep practitioners up to date.

As the school approaches its fiftieth anniversary, it can celebrate the realization of Dr. Rosenau's dream of developing a "real" school of public health. But Rosenau's other dream, "of a time when . . .every man shall possess sufficient for the needs of his body and the demands of health," has proved more illusive. Despite a century of extraordinary progress, serious public health problems—some old, some new—continue to plague the state, nation, and world. Infant mortality rates in North Carolina are the highest in the country; AIDS has reached epidemic proportions in parts of the United States; and millions of people around the globe suffer from malnutrition. In attempting to address the problems of the 1990s, health officials will be plagued by the same situation that led to the founding of the School of Public Health in the 1940s, the shortage of trained health workers. Even today the majority of public health practitioners lack formal training.

The School of Public Health cannot solve the state's (or the world's) problems by itself. Poverty, ignorance, and governmental neglect continue to impede the creation of a healthy society. Still, if progress is to be made, the school must remain dedicated to finding solutions to today's health problems, educating the public about means of disease prevention, and advocating increases in social expenditures for health. Dr. Rosenau's credo can provide a guidepost for the next half century. "When young men have vision, the dreams of old men come true."

NoteS

CHAPTER 1

1. Carl V. Reynolds to Rosemary M. Kent, July 30, 1962, School of Public Health Records, University of North Carolina Archives, University of North Carolina, Chapel Hill (hereafter cited as SPH).
2. C. S. Mangum to Milton J. Rosenau, September 26, 1935, SPH.
3. Milton J. Rosenau to A. S. Rose, September 29, 1939, SPH.
4. Milton J. Rosenau, Curriculum Vitae, SPH.
5. George Rosen, *A History of Public Health* (New York: MD Publications, 1958), 201.
6. Rosen, *A History of Public Health*, 278, 287–90; Paul Starr, *The Social Transformation of American Medicine* (New York: Basic Books, 1982), 181; Barbara Rosenkrantz, *Public Health and the State: Changing Views in Massachusetts, 1842–1936* (Cambridge: Harvard University Press, 1972), 97–127; Elizabeth Fee, *Disease and Discovery: A History of The Johns Hopkins School of Hygiene and Public Health, 1916–1939* (Baltimore: The Johns Hopkins University Press, 1987), 13.
7. Rosen, *A History of Public Health*, 294; Fee, *Disease and Discovery*, 22.
8. Fee, *Disease and Discovery*, 14–22.
9. Benjamin E. Washburn, *A History of the North Carolina State Board of Health, 1877–1925* (Raleigh, N. C.: North Carolina State Board of Health, 1966), 8–22.
10. Washburn, *History of N. C. Board of Health*, 38.
11. Washburn, *History of N. C. Board of Health*, 41–2; J. W. Roy Norton and Benjamin Drake, "History of Public Health in North Carolina," in *Essays in the History of Medical Science and Medical Service, 1524–1960*, vol. II, ed. Dorothy Long (Raleigh, N. C.: The North Carolina Medical Society, 1972), 593.
12. Quoted in Allen Tullos, "The Great Hookworm Crusade," *Southern Exposure* 6 (1978): 41; James Leloudis, "'A More Certain Means of Grace': Pedagogy, Self, and Society in North Carolina, 1880–1920" (Ph.D. diss., University of North Carolina at Chapel Hill, 1989), 293–300. Also see John Ettling, *The Germ of Laziness: Rockefeller Philanthropy and Public Health in the New South* (Cambridge: Harvard University Press, 1981) for an analysis of the hookworm campaign.
13. Washburn, *History of N. C. Board of Health*, 46–9.
14. Washburn, *History of N. C. Board of Health*, 48.
15. Fee, *Disease and Discovery*, 28.

16. Steven C. Wheatley, *The Politics of Philanthropy: Abraham Flexner and Medical Education* (Madison: The University of Wisconsin Press, 1988), 57–107; Fee, *Disease and Discovery*, 29–30.

17. Fee, *Disease and Discovery*, 37–40.

18. B. E. Washburn, *As I Recall: The Hookworm Campaigns Initiated by the Rockefeller Sanitary Commission and the Rockefeller Foundation in the Southern United States and Tropical America* (New York: The Rockefeller Foundation, 1960), 15, 111–181.

19. B. E. Washburn, "Report on Proposed Cooperation for Training Public Health Workers Between the State Board of Health and the University of North Carolina," [1919], North Carolina State Board of Health Records, Division of Archives and History, Raleigh, North Carolina (hereafter cited as NCSBH); "Tentative Report from the North Carolina Board of Health to the University of North Carolina Regarding the Establishment of a Post Graduate Course of Study for Health Officers and Public Health Nurses," March 17, 1919, University Papers, University of North Carolina Archives, University of North Carolina, Chapel Hill (hereafter cited as University Papers).

20. H. W. Chase to W. P. Jacocks, April 30, 1919, University Papers.

21. Washburn, *History of N. C. Board of Health*, 53; Washburn, "Report on Proposed Cooperation for Training Public Health Workers Between the State Board of Health and the University of North Carolina" and William deB. MacNider to H. W. Chase, November 7, 1919, University Papers.

22. Washburn, *History of N. C. Board of Health*, 72–3.

23. *Bulletin of the North Carolina State Board of Health* 37 (January 1922): 3–11.

24. *Biennial Report, North Carolina Board of Health (1936–38)* (Raleigh, N. C.: North Carolina Board of Health, 1938), 22–25.

25. *Report on a Survey of the Organization and Administration of the State Government of North Carolina* (Washington: The Brookings Institution, 1930), iv, 176–90.

26. *Biennial Report (1936–38)*, 25–29.

27. James M. Parrott to John A. Ferrell, July 16, 1931; John A Ferrell to James M. Parrott, July 20, 1931; James M. Parrott to John A. Ferrell, July 24, 1931; John A. Ferrell to James M. Parrott, July 28, 1931, Record Group 2, Series 236, Rockefeller Foundation Archives of the Rockefeller Archive Center, Pocantico Hills, North Tarrytown, New York (hereafter cited as RFA).

28. H. G. Baity to Frank P. Graham, February 1, 1932, Office of the President Records, Frank Porter Graham Series, University of North Carolina Archives, University of North Carolina, Chapel Hill (hereafter cited as Graham Series).

29. Memorandum by John A. Ferrell, March 24, 1932, RG 2, Ser. 236, RFA.

30. Daniel Singal, *The War Within: From Victorian to Modernist Thought in the South, 1919–1945* (Chapel Hill: University of North Carolina Press, 1982), 115–152, 265–301.

31. Albert Coates, *The Story of the Institute of Government: the University of North Carolina at Chapel Hill* (Chapel Hill: n.p., 1981), 27–8.

32. Howard W. Odum to Frank Graham, May 21, 1931; W. C. Jackson to Frank P. Graham, January 8, 1934, Graham Series.

33. Carl V. Reynolds to Charles S. Mangum, July 10, 1935, "Plan for Educational Unit in the Field of Public Health in the University of North Carolina, School of Medicine"; C. S. Mangum to M. V. Ziegler, March 18, 1935, NCSBH.
34. Committee on Economic Security, *Report to the President of the Committee on Economic Security* (Washington: United States Government Printing Office, 1935), 38–41.
35. Edwin E. Witte, *The Development of the Social Security Act* (Madison, Wisconsin: The University of Wisconsin Press, 1963), 171–2; Roy Lubove, "The New Deal and National Health," *Current History* 45 (July 1963): 83.
36. Memorandum by M. V. Ziegler, December 27, 1935, Office of the Chancellor: R. B. House Series, University of North Carolina Archives, University of North Carolina, Chapel Hill (hereafter cited as House Series).

CHAPTER 2

1. Frank P. Graham to Milton J. Rosenau, December 30, 1935, Graham Series; "State Is Slated to Get Regional Health School," *News and Observer*, January 7, 1936; Matthew S. Broun to Frank P. Graham, January 22, 1936, Graham Series. See also C. C. Hudson to Milton J. Rosenau, January 16, 1936, SPH.
2. C. S. Mangum to Frank P. Graham, February 5, 1936, Graham Series; "Rosenau on Epidemics," *The Chapel Hill Weekly*, February 14, 1936; "Rosenau Speaks on Epidemiology," *The Daily Tarheel*, February 6, 1936.
3. M. J. Rosenau to R. B. House, December 18, 1936, House Series.
4. Jean Alonzo Curran, *Founders of the Harvard School of Public Health, with Biographical Notes, 1909–1946* (New York: Josiah Macy, Jr. Foundation, 1970), 28; Fee, *Disease and Discovery*, 88–9.
5. M. J. Rosenau to C. S. Mangum, April 28, 1936, SPH.
6. Charles M. Weiss, "An Historical Outline of the Department of Environmental Sciences and Engineering," (Chapel Hill: School of Public Health, 1967, mimeographed), 1.
7. M. J. Rosenau to Frank P. Graham, June 6, 1936, Graham Series; Albert Coates, "A Portrait in Words," in *Presentation of the Herman G. Baity Portrait to the University of North Carolina* (Chapel Hill: School of Public Health, [1966]), 7–9.
8. A. Worth Petty, interview with author, Virginia Beach, Va., November 10, 1988.
9. Petty interview.
10. Petty interview; Minutes of Administrative Board of the Division of Public Health, November 13, 1936, SPH.
11. M. J. Rosenau to Charles S. Mangum, September 12, 1936, SPH; Frank P. Graham to Charles S. Mangum, June 18, 1936, SPH; Frank P. Graham to Charles S. Mangum, W. deB. MacNider, M. J. Rosenau, Herman G. Baity, and W. R. Berryhill, March 22, 1937, SPH.

12. "University of North Carolina Public Health and Medical School Project," March, 1937, SPH.

13. H. G. Baity to Raymond J. Rosenberger, June 12, 1937; H. G. Baity to Milton J. Rosenau, June 25, 1937, SPH.

14. M. J. Rosenau to R. B. House, March 3, 1938; R. B. House to M. J. Rosenau, March 7, 1938, SPH.

15. John Larsh, interview with author, Edenton, N. C., October 3, 1988; M. J. Rosenau to A. S. Rose, October 27, 1937, SPH.

16. M. J. Rosenau to My Friends, September 25, 1939, SPH; memorandum by William A. McIntosh, December 4, 1939, RG 2.1, RFA.

17. Emil Chanlett, interview with author, Chapel Hill, N. C., October 26, 1988; Thomas J. Brooks, Jr., "Reflections," *The Body Politic* 4 (Summer 1976): 3.

18. Fee, *Disease and Discovery*, 42; Record of Faculty Meeting, February 10, 1940, SPH; R. B. House to M. J. Rosenau, June 15, 1940, Graham Series.

19. Allan Brandt, *No Magic Bullet: A Social History of Venereal Disease in the United States Since 1880* (New York: Oxford University Press, 1985), 6.

20. Bryan Haislip, *A History of the Z. Smith Reynolds Foundation* (Winston-Salem, N. C.: John F. Blair, Publisher, 1967), n.p.; "Enormous Sum is Given State for Battle Against Syphilis," *News and Observer*, December 19, 1937.

21. M. J. Rosenau to R. B. House, October 3, 1939; J. E. Moore to Wm. deB. MacNider, June 19, 1939, SPH.

22. "A Study in the Epidemiology of Syphilis, Orange, Person, Chatham Counties, North Carolina," July 1, 1940, to December 31, 1940, n.d., 3; "Summary of the Activities of the Field Epidemiological Study of Syphilis in the Orange-Chatham-Person Health District and the City of Durham and Durham County During the Year 1942," n.d., SPH.

23. E. A. Kelley, Bessie Baker, Ruth Council, and Bessie M. Chapman to Frank P. Graham, August 23, 1937; M. J. Rosenau to R. B. House, December 6, 1937; Record of Faculty Meeting, December 9, 1939; Carl V. Reynolds to M. V. Ziegler, April 17, 1940, SPH.

24. M. J. Rosenau to R. B. House, November 18, 1940, SPH.

25. Ruth W. Hay to M. J. Rosenau, September 11, 1940, SPH.

26. Harriet H. Barr and Helen Hanken, comps., *Health Education: Selected Papers of Lucy Morgan* (Chapel Hill: School of Public Health, 1986), ix–xii.

27. Lucy S. Morgan, interview with author, Asheville, N. C., December 19, 1988; Lucy S. Morgan, "Health Education in Extra-Cantonment Zones," in *Health Education*, Barr and Hanken, 10–13.

28. H. W. Brown to R. B. House, August 25, 1942, SPH.

29. Eunice N. Tyler and Lucy S. Morgan, eds., *Health Educators at Work*, Special Issue (May 1966): 41.

30. Morgan interview.

31. H. W. Brown to R. B. House, August 31, 1942, SPH.

32. Harold B. Gotaas, "Cooperative Health and Sanitation in the Americas," School of Public Health *News* 1 (Summer 1946): 3.

CHAPTER 3

1. M. J. Rosenau to W. K. Sharp, September 7, 1945, SPH.
2. Shepard is quoted in Ida Jenkins Gadsden, "The Historical Development and Social Implications of the Public Health Education Program at North Carolina College at Durham" (Ph.D. diss., University of North Carolina at Chapel Hill, 1968), 66. The most complete history of the program is Gadsden's. See also B. T. McMillon, "North Carolina College Makes Health Training Functional," *The High School Journal* 32 (1949): 217–219; Tyler and Morgan, *Health Educators at Work*, Special Issue, 59–62.
3. Morgan interview; Larsh interview.
4. Dorothy M. Talbot, "A History of the Public Health Nursing Program in the School of Public Health, University of North Carolina at Chapel Hill," (typescript in author's possession), 18–20.
5. Memorandum by E. W. McHenry, March 8, 1946, General Education Board records, Series 1, Subseries 3, Box 539, Folder 5769, Rockefeller Archive Center.
6. Edward H. Beardsley, *A History of Neglect: Health Care for Blacks and Mill Workers in the Twentieth-Century South* (Knoxville: The University of Tennessee Press, 1987), 273–309.
7. Larsh interview.
8. Morgan interview. See Gadsden, "The Public Health Education Program at North Carolina College at Durham," 12.
9. Rosemary M. Kent, "The Moment Between the Past and the Future," (typescript in author's possession), 25–6.
10. James S. Simmons to Frank P. Graham, January 24, 1946, SPH.
11. M. J. Rosenau to A. R. Mann, November 8, 1945, House Series.
12. "A. H. Bryan Heads New Department of Nutrition," School of Public Health *News* 2 (Winter 1946): 1.
13. H. G. Baity to R. B. House, May 15, 1946, SPH.
14. H. G. Baity to E. G. McGavran, March 1, 1947, Personnel File, Dean's Office, School of Public Health, University of North Carolina at Chapel Hill (hereafter cited as Personnel File).
15. Harriet H. Barr and Frances H. Barrie, *Edward G. McGavran: Guardian of the Body Politic* (Chapel Hill: The School of Public Health, 1979), 7–16.
16. E. G. McGavran, *Report to the Faculty* (Chapel Hill: School of Public Health, 1963), n.p.
17. "Proposed Field Training Program of the School of Public Health," n.d.; M. R. Kinde to E. G. McGavran, May 21, 1948, SPH.
18. "W. P. Richardson Heads New Department," School of Public Health *News* 3 (Summer 1948): 1.
19. Harold J. Magnuson to E. G. McGavran, February 7, 1950, SPH; "Syphilis Experimental Laboratory," School of Public Health *News* 4 (Summer 1949): 1–2.

20. Edward G. McGavran to R. B. House, July 30, 1948, SPH.

21. Barr and Barrie, *Guardian of the Body Politic*, 26–7.

22. Paul F. Whitaker and Frederick C. Hubbard, "The History of the North Carolina Medical Care Commission," in *Essays in the History of Medical Science and Medical Service, 1524–1960*, vol. I, ed. Dorothy Long (Raleigh, N. C.: The North Carolina Medical Society, 1972), 330–49. For a discussion of this process on a national and international level see Daniel M. Fox, *Health Policies, Health Politics: The British and American Experience, 1911–1965* (Princeton, New Jersey: Princeton University Press, 1986), 115–131, 149–168.

23. For McGavran's views on the Division of Health Affairs at the time of his retirement, see E. G. McGavran to William Aycock, June 4, 1963, Office of the Chancellor: W. B. Aycock Series, University of North Carolina Archives, University of North Carolina, Chapel Hill.

24. For a discussion of national postwar health policy see Starr, *American Medicine*, 347–363.

25. Fox, *Health Policies*, 153–8.

26. Edward G. McGavran to R. B. House, July 30, 1948, SPH.

27. H. E. Handley, Visit to the University of North Carolina School of Public Health, December 1–2, 1949, n.d., Commonwealth Fund records, Rockefeller Archive Center, p. 2.

28. Cecil Sheps, interview with author, Chapel Hill, N. C., November 4, 1988.

29. John J. Wright to Lowell J. Reed, December 19, 1945, SPH.

30. Report of Activities of the Department of Maternal and Child Health in the School of Public Health of the University of North Carolina, Under a Joint Project with the North Carolina State Board of Health and Sponsored by the Children's Bureau, n.d., SPH.

31. "Department of Mental Health," in *School of Public Health Annual Report, 1951–52* (Chapel Hill: School of Public Health, 1952), 1–3.

32. Rebecca Broach Bryan, interview with author, Chapel Hill, N. C., March 18, 1989.

33. Frances Gust, interview with author, North Myrtle Beach, S. C., June 21, 1989.

34. Geraldine Gourley, interview with author, Chapel Hill, N. C., August 31, 1989.

35. Gourley interview.

36. "Toward New Horizons," *The High School Journal* 30 (May 1947): 113.

37. Harcourt Morgan's philosophy is best expressed in Ellis F. Hartford, *Our Common Mooring* (Athens: The University of Georgia Press, 1941).

38. *School of Public Health Annual Report, 1951–1952* (Chapel Hill: School of Public Health, 1952), 11, 14.

39. Edward G. McGavran, "What Is Public Health?", *Canadian Journal of Public Health* 44 (December, 1953): 441–451.

40. Ibid., 445–7.

41. Memorandum by Dean McGavran to Faculty, December 9, 1952, SPH.

CHAPTER 4

1. Starr, *American Medicine* 347.
2. Daniel Okun, interview with author, Chapel Hill, N. C., September 23, 1988.
3. Department of Sanitary Engineering, *Sanitary Engineering in Peru* (Chapel Hill: School of Public Health, n.d.), 19; "UNC School of Public Health in Peru," *The Body Politic* 3 (May 1957): 1.
4. Department of Sanitary Engineering, *Sanitary Engineering in Peru*, 20.
5. Lucy S. Morgan and Hiawatha B. Walker, "A University's Focus on Indian Health," *Health Educators at Work* 11 (June 1960): 1–11.
6. Joe Fred Sills and Gilbert Trujillo, "Zuni—Center of the World—Reaches Out," *Health Educators at Work* 11 (June 1960): 25–32.
7. Starr, *American Medicine*, 343.
8. Goulson interview; Bryan interview.
9. Department of Biostatistics, "Report for the Year, July 1, 1951-June 30, 1952," in *Annual Report, 1951–1952*, 4.
10. Ibid.
11. Tyler and Morgan, *Health Educators at Work*, Special Issue, 30; McGavran, *Report to the Faculty*, n.p.
12. Gourley interview.
13. Department of Epidemiology, "Annual Report, 1953–54," in *School of Public Health Annual Report, 1953–1954* (Chapel Hill: School of Public Health, 1954), 3.
14. John Cassel to E. G. McGavran, October 1, 1958, Personnel File.
15. *School of Public Health Annual Report, 1958–1959* (Chapel Hill, School of Public Health, 1959), n.p.
16. E. G. McGavran to Sidney L. Kark, June 29, 1960, Personnel File.
17. Michel Ibrahim, interview with author, Chapel Hill, N. C., June 6, 1989.
18. Roger W. Howell to Edward G. McGavran, September 20, 1956, Personnel File.
19. The Ruth W. Hay Portrait Committee to E. G. McGavran, August 9, 1954, Personnel File.
20. Margaret B. Dolan, Curriculum Vitae, Personnel File.
21. Bryan interview.
22. Hilton Goulson, interview with author, Chapel Hill, N. C., July 12, 1989; Larsh interview.
23. Goulson interview; Larsh interview.
24. Larsh interview.
25. Larsh interview.
26. Okun interview.
27. McGavran, *Report to the Faculty*, n.p.; Okun interview.
28. "Construction to Start on New P. H. Building," *The Body Politic* 5 (May 1959): 5.
29. The letter included an editorial in support of the bond vote from *The Chapel Hill Weekly*, October 5, 1959, detailing the school's inadequate facilities.

30. *School of Public Health Annual Report, 1959–1960* (Chapel Hill, School of Public Health, 1960), 5.
31. E. G. McGavran, "Testimony Before the Committee on Interstate and Foreign Commerce Relative to the Proposed Bill H.R. 4998 (S. 1071) for Community Health Facilities and Services," May 4, 1961, SPH.
32. Rosemary Kent, *This Moment Between the Past and the Future* (Chapel Hill: School of Public Health, n.d.), n.p.
33. School of Public Health, "Self-Study Report," January 15, 1963, SPH, v–6.
34. Ibid., x–2.
35. McGavran, *Report to the Faculty*, n.p.
36. Goulson interview.
37. *Past, Present, and Future of Schools of Public Health* (Chapel Hill: School of Public Health, 1963).

CHAPTER 5

1. Starr, *American Medicine*, 367.
2. John E. Larsh, Jr., to Henry T. Clark, May 22, 1963, Vice Chancellor for Health Affairs, University of North Carolina Archives, University of North Carolina, Chapel Hill.
3. W. Fred Mayes, Curriculum Vitae, Personnel File.
4. *School of Public Health Annual Report, 1961–1962* (Chapel Hill: School of Public Health, 1962), 4; *School of Public Health Annual Report, 1972–1973* (Chapel Hill: School of Public Health, 1973), 21.
5. Weiss, "Historical Outline," 4.
6. Daniel A. Okun, "The History of the Institute for Environmental Studies," mimeograph, June, 1977, SPH.
7. *ESE Notes* 3 (April 1966): 1; *ESE Notes* 4 (January 1967): 1; *ESE Notes* 6 (July 1969): 1.
8. "Department of Biostatistics, UNC," mimeograph, November, 1974, SPH.
9. "Department of Biostatistics," in *School of Public Health, Annual Report, 1966–1967* (Chapel Hill: School of Public Health, 1967), 6, 29.
10. *A Guide to the Carolina Population Center and its Affiliated Programs* (Chapel Hill: Carolina Population Center, University of North Carolina at Chapel Hill, 1975).
11. Bernard Greenberg, "Memorial Speech for Dr. John C. Cassel," October 31, 1976, SPH.
12. John C. Cassel, "Summary of Major Findings of the Evans County Cardiovascular Studies," *Archives of Internal Medicine* 128 (December 1971): 881–9.
13. Greenberg, "Memorial Speech for Dr. John C. Cassel."
14. Larsh interview; Goulson interview.
15. Okun interview.

16. Okun interview.

17. William Herzog, interview with author, Chapel Hill, N. C., July 13, 1989.

18. Starr, *American Medicine*, 370.

19. W. Fred Mayes, "Personal Introduction—A Statement of Intentions and Expectations," September 17, 1963, SPH.

20. In 1967, the school also established an administrative board to comply with university policy, and the next year adopted a written constitution and bylaws.

21. Robert B. Moorhead, "Formal Goal Formulation in a School of Public Health" (M.P.A. thesis, University of North Carolina at Chapel Hill, 1972), 86.

22. Morgan interview.

23. J. Carlyle Sitterson to W. Fred Mayes, June 7, 1966; W. Fred Mayes to J. Carlyle Sitterson, June 22, 1966, Office of the Chancellor: J. C. Sitterson Series, University of North Carolina Archives, University of North Carolina, Chapel Hill.

24. Elizabeth Lovell McMahan, "A Study of the Department of Public Health Education, School of Public Health, University of North Carolina" (Ph.D. diss., Duke University, 1968), 269–82.

25. Memorandum by William Fred Mayes, January 3, 1969, SPH; Guy W. Steuart to Dean Mayes, August 24, 1971; Hiawatha B. Walker to Guy W. Steuart, July 30, 1971, SPH.

26. Herzog interview; Sagar Jain, interview with author, Chapel Hill, N. C., September 8, 1989.

27. Department of Public Health Administration, "Annual Report, 1966–67," in *School of Public Health Annual Report, 1966–67* (Chapel Hill: School of Public Health, 1967), 1–2.

28. Goulson interview.

29. Talbot, "History of Public Health Nursing," 32–4.

30. Ibid., 37–41.

31. Margaret Dolan to Charles Harper, August 24, 1966, Personnel File; Talbot, "History of Public Health Nursing," 45–7.

32. Weiss, "Historical Outline," 7.

33. John C. Cassel to Fred Mayes, November 5, 1964, SPH.

34. Gourley interview.

35. William Fred Mayes, *The University of North Carolina School of Public Health Relates to the Needs of a Changing Society: A Selective and Interpretive Account with Emphasis on the Decade of the Sixties* (Chapel Hill: School of Public Health, 1975), 53–4.

36. The SPH could look proudly at its own record in the black community and with black students. W. Fred Mayes to J. Carlyle Sitterson, February 24, 1969, SPH.

37. Gourley interview.

38. Herzog interview.

39. "Report of Temporary Committee on Student Organization of School of Public Health," n.d., SPH.

40. Jane Mathews, "Convocation Message," September 16, 1970, SPH.

41. PUBH Students to W. Fred Mayes, February 9, 1970, SPH.

42. School of Public Health "Self-Study Summary Report," (Chapel Hill, School of Public Health, 1975, Mimeographed), 372.

43. Herzog interview.

44. Herzog interview.

45. University of North Carolina at Chapel Hill, "Report of Chancellor's Study Commission on the Role of the School of Public Health," (Chapel Hill: University of North Carolina, 1971, Mimeographed), 7–14.

46. Ibid., 4.

47. Ibid., 63.

CHAPTER 6

1. Starr, *American Medicine*, 380.

2. *School of Public Health Annual Report, 1969–1970* (Chapel Hill, School of Public Health, 1970), n.p.; *School of Public Health Annual Report, 1979–1980* (Chapel Hill, School of Public Health, 1980), 17,26,45.

3. "A Statement of Concerns Regarding the Relevance & Responsiveness of the School of Public Health to the Needs of Black Americans," [1971], SPH.

4. William T. Small, interview with author, Chapel Hill, N. C., August 24, 1989.

5. Small interview.

6. Small interview.

7. Small interview; Minority Student Group to B. G. Greenberg, November 6, 1972, SPH.

8. John E. Larsh to Dorothea C. Leighton, June 15, 1972; Joseph C. Edozien to Dorothea C. Leighton, September 29, 1972, SPH. For an overview of the faculty's response to the report see Cecil G. Sheps, "The University of North Carolina School of Public Health," in *Schools of Public Health: Present and Future*, eds., John Z. Bowers and Elizabeth F. Purcell (New York: Josiah Macy, Jr. Foundation, 1974), 72–8.

9. Roy R. Kuebler to Emil T. Chanlett, January 10, 1972, SPH.

10. School of Public Health, "Self-Study Summary Report," 358–63.

11. Harriet H. Barr, Curriculum Vitae, Personnel File.

12. "Alumni Association," *The Body Politic* 1 (January 1973): 19; "A First: SPH Alumni Day 1973," *The Body Politic* 1 (June 1973): 1; "Darity Heads Alumni Association," *The Body Politic* 2 (August 1974): 1.

13. Charles L. Harper, "An Outreach Approach to Service," *The Body Politic* 6 (June 1979): 5.

14. "Highlighting Continuing Education," *The Body Politic* 1 (June 1973): 5; John Hughes, Curriculum Vitae, Personnel File.

15. Janice Westaby directed the program from 1969 to 1973, Lydia Holley from 1973 to 1974, and Bill Herzog until 1982.

16. Gust interview; "Bachelors Program Initiated in Public Health," *The Body Politic* 4 (October 1976): 16.

17. Dr. Cecil Slome and Howard Barnhill coordinated the program initially. "Area Health Education Centers Established," *The Body Politic* 1 (June 1973): 11.

18. "Dean Discusses School's Future," *The Body Politic* 1 (June 1973): 1.

19. Okun interview.

20. Cecil G. Sheps, *Higher Education for Public Health: A Report of the Milbank Memorial Fund Commission* (New York: Prodist, 1976), 211.

21. Ibid., 153.

22. B. G. Greenberg, "The Crisis in the Schools of Public Health: The Response," *The Body Politic* 2 (August 1974): 11.

23. Jain interview.

24. Jain interview; "A Conversation with Sagar Jain," *The Body Politic* 6 (January 1979): 1.

25. "Morris Heads Maternal and Child Health," *The Body Politic* 3 (November 1975): 4; Naomi M. Morris, "Child Advocacy a Major Role for MCH," *The Body Politic* 4 (October 1976): 1.

26. C. Arden Miller, Curriculum Vitae, Personnel File.

27. Memorandum by Review Committee of the Chairman of the Department of Nutrition, April 9, 1976, SPH.

28. "Medical Evaluation of Federal Program Completed," *The Body Politic* 4 (October 1976): 4.

29. "Project Established to Improve Maternal Nutrition," *The Body Politic* 9 (February 1982): 1.

30. "Rural Environmental Education Project End," *The Body Politic* 7 (January, 1980), 10.

31. "Program Begun to Strengthen Health Education in Cameroon," *The Body Politic* 6 (September 1978): 8.

32. A 1975 survey of the deans of the schools of public health ranked the University of North Carolina second overall. Epidemiology, environmental sciences and engineering, biostatistics, and parasitology and laboratory practice, however, ranked as the best in the nation. "SPH Ranked Second," *The Body Politic* 3 (March 1975): 2; "New Contract Awarded Lipids Center," *The Body Politic* 7 (October 1979): 6.

33. Val Lauder, "Re: The Russians," *The Body Politic* 4 (Summer 1976): 4.

34. Russell F. Christman, "ESE Looks Ahead," *The Body Politic* 3 (June 1975): 1.

35. "School Participates in Rubber Industry Research," *The Body Politic* 1 (June 1973): 6. Dr. Robert Lee Harris, Jr., the former director of the Bureau of Abatement and Control, of the National Air Pollution Control Administration, took over as director of the Occupational Health Studies Group in 1975. The group continued its arrangements with the rubber industry until the early 1980s, when it began investigating similar problems in other industries. See *School of Public Health Annual Report, 1975–76* (Chapel Hill: School of Public Health, 1976), 21.

36. "Hypertension in Rural Communities Studied," *The Body Politic* 7 (October 1979): 7.
37. *Annual Report, 1975–76* (Chapel Hill: School of Public Health, 1976), 27.
38. Small interview; *Self-Study Report, 1981* (Chapel Hill: School of Public Health, 1981), 131; "American Indian Recruitment Officer Named," *The Body Politic* 7 (January 1980): 2.
39. Small interview.

EPILOGUE

1. Institute of Medicine, *The Future of Public Health* (Washington, D. C.: National Academy Press, 1988), 19.
2. *Annual Report, 1978-79* (Chapel Hill: School of Public Health, 1979), 21, 29, 47; *Annual Report, 1988-89* (Chapel Hill: School of Public Health, 1989), 2-17.
3. *The Body Politic* 8 (November 1980): 1.
4. Ibrahim interview.
5. Ibid.
6. Ibid.
7. *The Body Politic* 12 (June 1985): 4.
8. Memorandum by Strategic Planning Committee, January 18, 1989, SPH.

Dedication Program

Michel A. Ibrahim, MD
Dean, UNC School of Public Health
Presiding

Greetings .... Michel A. Ibrahim

Remarks .... Earl J. Phillips, Chair
University of North Carolina
Board of Trustees

Memorial Presentations

- Edward G. McGavran .... Frances E. Williamson
  Ohio Department of Health
- Bernard G. Greenberg .... Delton Atkinson
  NC Department of Environment,
  Health and Natural Resources
- Herman G. Baity .... Emil T. Chanlett
  University of North Carolina
  at Chapel Hill

Acknowledgments .... Michel A. Ibrahim

Dedication .... Paul Hardin, Chancellor
University of North Carolina
at Chapel Hill

A reception and open house in the new buildings
will follow the dedication program.

Edward G. McGavran

1902 - 1972

Edward G. McGavran was born in Pachmari, Central Provinces, India where his parents were serving as missionaries for the United Christian Church. In 1910 he returned to the United States with his parents.

McGavran received an undergraduate degree from Butler University and M.D. and M.P.H. degrees from Harvard University, where he was a fellow in the Department of Comparative Pathology and Parasitology and involved in medical research with the Rockefeller Foundation in Egypt and India. He studied epidemiology with Dr. Milton J. Rosenau, who later became the first dean of the University of North Carolina School of Public Health. It was Dr. Rosenau who encouraged Dr. McGavran to practice medicine in a rural area before returning to Harvard for a public health degree.

When Dr. McGavran came to UNC in August 1947 to become the second dean of the School of Public Health and professor of epidemiology, he brought with him broad and rich experience in medicine, public health administration, epidemiology, and teaching. He also brought an enthusiasm for public health practice that endured throughout his life.

During the 16 years of McGavran's deanship, the student body tripled, the number of faculty increased from 16 to 83, and three new departments were added. Research expanded from a few studies in two departments to a multitude of studies, publications and scientific papers representing all departments. Rosenau Hall is a monument to the untiring efforts of McGavran and his staff to obtain adequate physical facilities.

Dean McGavran led the way for faculty service activities by serving as a consultant and an active participant in many professional associations. He was appointed one of three delegates to represent the United States at the Fifth Assembly of the World Health Organization in Geneva. He later studied public health problems in eight European countries.

As the Schools of Medicine and Public Health expanded and the dental and nursing schools were established, the need increased for coordination of all health affairs units. Dr. McGavran favored organizing the health-related schools and services into a Division of Health Sciences. He was chair of the committee that determined the organizational pattern and the first acting administrator of the division.

After retirement as dean in 1963, McGavran served as Ford Foundation consultant to the Indian Government in health and family planning. Returning to Chapel Hill in 1969, McGavran served as consultant to the School's continuing education and field service program, travelling throughout North Carolina to teach front-line public health practitioners.

Dr. McGavran was a stimulating and provocative teacher who knew his students well and valued their contribution to the development of the School. He was an able administrator who with characteristic modesty called himself the "executive secretary" of the faculty.

Dr. McGavran taught and practiced public health as the "scientific diagnosis and treatment of the body politic." He believed that local public health programs should be developed by the team of public health professionals and the people of the community. He never wavered in his belief that public health is a distinct scientific discipline and campaigned for a clear, concise statement of the mission, purpose and priorities of public health--a battle still being waged by his students, friends and colleagues around the world.

Bernard G. Greenberg

1919 - 1985

Biostatistician, teacher, scholar, administrator, renowned researcher, dean, public health professional. These words describe the life and career of Bernard G. Greenberg, Kenan professor of biostatistics.

Born in New York City, Greenberg attended the City College of New York, completing the B.S. degree in mathematics at the age of 19. His first position in public health as an assistant statistician at the New York State Department of Health played an important role in his choice of careers.

Following service in the United States Army, he earned the Ph.D. degree in experimental statistics from North Carolina State College. As a part of the doctoral program, Greenberg enrolled in public health courses at the UNC School of Public Health where he was a student of Dean Edward G. McGavran.

In 1949 Greenberg was recruited to Chapel Hill to establish and chair the Department of Biostatistics. He brought to this position a background in public health and strong ties to the Department of Mathematical and Experimental Statistics in Raleigh. During the 23 years of his chairmanship, the Department of Biostatistics grew to become the largest, and in the eyes of many, the best university biostatistics department in the world.

Greenberg was recognized worldwide for his research in the measurement of health and disease. His techniques of survey and analysis became standard practice for the National Center for Health Statistics. He served as a member of seven study sections in the National Institutes of Health. As chair of the Committee for the Study of Poliomyelitis Vaccine, National Academy of Sciences, he influenced polio immunization policy.

In 1972 Dr. Greenberg became the fourth dean of the School of Public Health. He insisted that faculty members "practice what they teach" and put their knowledge to use in service. His own service ranged from work with local and state health departments and private physicians to the U.S. Children's Bureau, Veteran's Administration, World Health Organization, and Pan American Health Organization. He was chair of the Governor's Task Force on Waste Management, which developed a comprehensive plan for the management and disposal of hazardous wastes in North Carolina.

Other accomplishments during Greenberg's deanship included the organization of the School's Division of Community Health Service and the establishment of the Bachelor of Science in Public Health degree to train persons for beginning level positions in local health agencies.

During his career Greenberg held many honors, including the American Public Health Association's Bronfman Prize in 1966, for significant contribution to public health, and the UNC O. Max Gardner Award in 1981. He was elected to membership of the Institute of Medicine, National Academy of Sciences, and appointed to the National Council on Health Care Technology.

As a teacher, Dr. Greenberg inspired and challenged his students. As administrator, he was sensitive to the needs of students, faculty, and staff and a creative and dynamic leader. As consultant and scientist, he bridged the gap between disciplines and was ever mindful of the need to apply new knowledge to the health problems of the world. As friend and colleague, he was always willing to provide wise counsel. Dr. Greenberg's illustrious career not only enhanced the reputation for excellence of the School and University but also contributed to the health and well being of the human race.

Herman G. Baity

1895 - 1975

Distinguished sanitary engineer, academician, and administrator, Herman Glenn Baity was born in Davie County, North Carolina. He attended the University of North Carolina, receiving the A.B. and the B.S.C.E. degrees in 1917 and 1922.

Baity began his engineering career as assistant sanitary engineer in the North Carolina State Board of Health. He interrupted service in this position to become a Rockefeller Foundation research fellow at Harvard University, earning the Master of Science in Sanitary Engineering and later the Doctor of Science degree in sanitary engineering, the first engineer in the world to earn this degree.

For a time after completing his studies at Harvard, Baity served both the State Board of Health and the University. He joined the faculty as associate professor of sanitary and municipal engineering, rising to the rank of professor, head of the department, and dean of engineering before the University transferred the engineering program to North Carolina State College in Raleigh.

In 1936 when the Division of Public Health was being created in the UNC School of Medicine, Baity was named professor and head of the newly created Department of Sanitary Engineering, joining Milton J. Rosenau and other early public health faculty in the task of building a program of graduate public health education with a strong sanitary engineering component.

This task was periodically interrupted when Baity was called to serve as director of the federal public works administration in North Carolina, as chief engineer of the Health and Sanitation Field Party at the Institute of Inter-American Affairs in Brazil, and as summer consultant in Latin America and Europe.

In 1952 Baity was appointed chief engineer and director, Division of Environmental Sanitation, World Health Organization, the first person to occupy this post. During the 10 years of his tenure, the global community water supply program of the World Health Organization was established and substantial progress was made toward the eradication of malaria. Baity had the rare opportunity of working with a network of former students who had risen to responsible positions in the United States and around the world. After retirement from the World Health Organization, he returned to serve many short-term consultantships, including a year's assignment in Tehran.

Among the many honors Baity received were the Clemens Herschel Prize in Hydraulics at Harvard University, the Hemisphere Award of the U.S.A. Section of the Inter-American Association of Sanitary Engineering, the certificate of life membership of the American Society of Civil Engineers, and the Doctor of Law degree from the University of North Carolina.

Herman G. Baity's life was dedicated to the mission of improving the standard of living and meeting the needs of people for sanitary water and safe food. His talents were recognized and demanded around the world. Each mission, whether at home or abroad, was carried out with dedication to his profession, a powerful intellect, competent and creative leadership and the ability to make hard judgements with a view to long-term benefits.

Baity's contribution as a distinguished teacher continues through the lives and work of former students who have translated their education into tangible action on the environmental problems of the world.